HOLDING
HEALTH CARE
ACCOUNTABLE

HOLDING
HEALTH CARE
ACCOUNTABLE
Law and the New
Medical Marketplace

E. Haavi Morreim

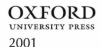

OXFORD
UNIVERSITY PRESS
2001

OXFORD
UNIVERSITY PRESS

Oxford   New York
Athens   Auckland   Bangkok   Bogotá   Buenos Aires   Calcutta
Cape Town   Chennai   Dar es Salaam   Delhi   Florence   Hong Kong   Istanbul
Karachi   Kuala Lumpur   Madrid   Melbourne   Mexico City   Mumbai
Nairobi   Paris   São Paulo   Shanghai   Singapore   Taipei   Tokyo   Toronto   Warsaw

and associated companies in
Berlin   Ibadan

Published by Oxford University Press, Inc.,
198 Madison Avenue, New York, New York, 10016
http://www.oup-usa.org

Library of Congress Cataloging-in-Publication Data
Morreim, E. Haavi.
Holding health care accountable : law and the new medical marketplace /
E. Haavi Morreim.
p. cm.   Includes bibliographical references and index.
ISBN 0–19–514132–6
1. Managed care plans (Medical care)—Law and legislation—United States.
2. Liability (Law)—United States.
3. Physicians—Malpractice—United States.
I. Title.
KF1183.M67 2001   344.73′0411—dc21   00–054846

9 8 7 6 5 4 3 2 1

Printed in the United States of America
on acid-free paper

in loving memory of Florence, my mother

with all my love to Paul, my father

with special love for Janet,
the newest member of our family

PREFACE

For the past twenty years I have watched, with a mixture of fascination, consternation, and bemusement, the enormous changes sweeping health care. A broad economic upheaval has precipitated a far-reaching reorganization of health care delivery that, in the process, is quite literally rewriting medicine. After nearly a half-century of lavish third-party payment for virtually anything a physician chose to order, businesses and governments finally began to enforce serious cost containment in the late 1980s and early 1990s. From well-funded norms of "if it might help and probably won't harm, do it" and "too much is better than too little," clinical medicine is now expected to embody "less is more" and "if you can't show it will help the patient, don't do it." The transition has been tumultuous for providers, patients, payers, and health plans alike. And it is hardly finished.

Another wrinkle confuses the picture even further. The tort and contract doctrines by which the law traditionally holds providers and health plans accountable for the quality and quantity of care they deliver have not kept pace with medicine's economic and clinical overhaul. Those legal obligations were shaped largely during an era of affluence, in which the providers who transformed scientific discoveries into clinical miracles rarely, if ever, needed to worry about the cost of providing them to patients. Accordingly, neither did courts worry. Courts have expected providers to deliver the same basic standard of care to everyone—a standard that has come to incorporate costly technologies—regardless of the patient's ability to pay.

In recent years, as those free-flowing reimbursements came to a screeching halt, the realities of what can be delivered no longer match the limitless demands. The new economic constraints have provoked a variety of coping mechanisms. Some of them have been salutary, as when physicians and health plans carefully reevaluate which kinds of care really help patients and which do not. Others are less benign, as when plans impose utilization review hurdles that delay or deny needed care, or when physicians refuse to care for patients who lack adequate insurance. Many patients, long invited to expect a medical miracle for every ailment, now face pervasive restrictions on providers and treatments, with procedural obstacles at every turn.

More to the point for this book, when legal expectations based on yesterday's flush economics clash with current financial finitude, some disturbing scenarios arise. Physicians stand to be held personally liable for limits on care that are imposed by third parties. And on the other side, courts often expect health plans to provide each patient with unstinting care, regardless of the implication that they must then do the same for an entire population within increasingly stringent fiscal constraints.

These tensions between legal traditions and economic realities have prompted some unhealthy responses. Increasingly, providers and plans feel forced to resort to subterfuge. Unwilling to risk saying aloud that "this intervention may have some value, but it isn't worth the money," health plans instead are more likely to declare the intervention "not medically necessary," as if the decision were dictated purely by science, and patients denied this care were not being deprived of anything important. Physicians, laboring under abrasive restrictions on their clinical autonomy and under fears about being forced to treat patients inadequately, increasingly resort to duplicity in order to deliver the care—and receive the payment—they think appropriate. So long as law demands a level of care that is no longer economically sustainable nor always medically desirable, the cycles of gamesmanship are likely to continue. And so long as that happens, we are impeded from determining, as openly and constructively as we should, what sorts of health care merit our investment as a society and as individuals.

I began writing nearly two decades ago about this tension between law's expectations and medicine's changing economics, building since then a fairly comprehensive body of thought through a variety of articles in law reviews and other publications. As society debates ever more intensely whether and in what ways plans and providers should be liable for the medical consequences of their cost-cutting, it seems propitious to collect some of the ideas in those works, scattered across time and venues, into a single volume. However, this book is not a collection of articles. Rather, it gathers, integrates, updates, enriches, and expands the ideas found in those works, knitting them together into a single, coherent whole that is, I believe, considerably greater than the sum of its parts.

Although a detailed preview is provided in Chapter 1, a brief overview might be useful here. Part I explains how medicine's economic upheaval has precipitated far-reaching changes in the ways health care is organized and clinical medicine is practiced. Part I then considers the conflicts that traditional legal doctrines create for physicians facing tort liability and for health plans facing both tort and contract liability.

Part II examines several proposals for bringing legal doctrines into harmony with changing medical economics and, finding them to be wanting, offers an alternative. A coherent, defensible approach to apportioning legal liability between physicians and health plans must begin not with the question of which party we want to hold liable for what sorts of adverse outcome, but rather with that of how best to achieve high-quality health care. Those who bear potential liability often feel impelled to exert control over the factors that can precipitate such liability, after all, and if we do not want a particular party, such as an HMO, to control a given aspect of health care, then we should not hold that HMO legally liable for adverse outcomes in that realm. As this book will propose, physicians are better suited to control some aspects of care, while plans are better suited to manage others. Under such a quality-oriented division of labor, each party should then face liability only for those aspects of care that it could and should have controlled.

Part II also proposes another distinction. High-quality health care often requires costly technologies, and a lack of funding often translates into a lack of care. Nevertheless, poor quality of care is not always the result of constraints on fiscal and physical resources. Good care also requires mental skills and personal diligence— knowledge, judgement, skill, and effort. Thus, it is important to distinguish between "resource" issues and matters of "expertise."

Within this distinction, physicians have obvious duties of expertise, but they also can have obligations regarding resources, particularly when they bear financial risk for the costs of the care they provide. Reciprocally, while health plans have obvious duties regarding resources, they can also have expertise duties, such as to exercise diligence and good judgment in their activities of business administration and quality surveillance. Part II proposes that resource duties, whether for plans or physicians, should be litigated through contract law, while duties of expertise should be examined in tort.

Finally, Part III shows that although familiar legal doctrines seem ill-equipped to address all of medicine's economic changes, and although this book's approach is novel in many respects, in fact the changes proposed here can be accommodated quite nicely within the most fundamental traditions underlying tort and contract law. As an added advantage, the expertise/resource distinction can improve the law in other areas, particularly by clarifying and enhancing courts' management of difficult issues currently litigated under the Employee Retirement Income Security Act (ERISA).

In sum, health law is currently lagging a bit behind the extraordinary economic changes reshaping health care. Though daunting, the situation presents important opportunities. Although the legal system must stand as a guardian to ensure accountability through this difficult transition, it need not cause obstruction and confusion. Rather, if undergirded by a thoughtful reconception of what society should rightly expect from its providers and its health plans, the law of tort and contract should actually be able to clarify, and even ease, that transition. This book aims to point the way.

Memphis, Tennessee   E. H. M.

ACKNOWLEDGMENTS

Excerpts and adaptations from the following articles are used in this book with permission from the respective publishers:

*Morreim EH. Playing doctor: corporate medical practice and medical malpractice. Michigan Journal of Law Reform 1999; 32(4): 939–1040.

*Morreim EH. Medicine meets resource limits: restructuring the legal standard of care. University of Pittsburgh Law Review 1997; 59(1): 1–95.

*Morreim EH. Cost containment and the standard of medical care. California Law Review 1987; 75(5): 1719–63.

(© 1987, by permission of California Law Review)

*Morreim EH. Moral justice and legal justice in managed care: the ascent of contributive justice. Journal of Law, Medicine and Ethics 1995; 23(3): 247–65 (© 1995, by permission of the American Society of Law, Medicine & Ethics. May not be reproduced without express written consent).

Other pertinent works by the author are noted throughout the text. The author acknowledges with deep gratitude the very helpful comments provided on various drafts of these papers by Peter Jacobson, JD, MPH; William Sage, MD, JD; Philip G. Peters, Jr., JD; Philip G. Peters, Jr., JD; Robert Jerry II, JD; Charles Key, JD; Susan Wolf, JD; Clark Havighurst, JD; Barry Furrow, JD; David Hyman, JD; Lance Stell, PhD; Nancy King, JD, Max Mehlman, JD; Larry Churchill, PhD.

CONTENTS

PART III   ASSESSING THE PROPOSED APPROACH:
PROSPECTS FOR JUDICIAL ACCEPTANCE

HOLDING
HEALTH CARE
ACCOUNTABLE

1

INTRODUCTION

In the past thirty years, health care in the United States has been rocked by two developments that seemed to threaten its very foundations. Tort law provided the first. Malpractice crises erupted in the early 1970s, then again in the mid-1980s, as the number of claims against physicians skyrocketed and the economic severity of awards from juries and from out-of-court settlements rose commensurately.[1] As malpractice suits became much more common, they also became distressingly unpredictable from physicians' perspective, because tort claims correlate poorly with actual episodes of negligent care: the great majority of negligence never leads to claims, while reciprocally the majority of claims filed do not appear to be tied to truly negligent care.[2] During these crises, the cost of insurance rose while its availability declined, driving the costs of care up and some physicians out of practice. Into the 1990s and beyond, liability coverage has been available, albeit costly, yet physicians continue to look back over their shoulders in virtually every aspect of patient care. Further, the discussion has broadened as we debate the extent to which insurers and managed care organizations should bear tort liability for their increasingly active role in determining the care that individual patients receive.

The second major development has been the economic upheaval that continues to transform our entire health care system. The rising cost of care was recognized in the 1970s and 1980s, but various efforts launched to address the problem were largely ineffective.[3] The most powerful forces—the ones that crafted managed care and rewrote many of the fundamental economic and even clinical assumptions underlying health care—did not reach full stride until the early 1990s.[4] As employers

3

began to demand lower costs and greater value for this very expensive fringe bene-fit, health plans realised that they could compete for employers' business only by cutting premiums, and with them, the provider fees and utilization levels that gener-ated the costs. The ensuing turbulence has left patients paying higher out-of-pocket costs in exchange for reduced levels of care and fewer choices among providers, while physicians watch their clinical autonomy and their incomes erode. Mean-while, more than forty million citizens still lack health care coverage.[5]

Both these phenomena are familiar enough to readers who follow the health care scene with a modicum of interest. What is only now becoming evident is how little we understand the interaction between these two factors that, individually, have had such profound influence.

This gap between legal challenges and economic changes is partly rooted in the fact that, as contemporary tort law regarding medical malpractice was developing from the 1950s through the 1980s, economics was not a major concern.[6] Most peo-ple enjoyed a generous medical insurance that emerged in the private sector during World War II and blossomed further in 1965 with the passage of Medicare for the elderly and Medicaid for the poor. Those government programs did not just broaden access to health care for millions of Americans, they also endorsed hefty payment arrangements that quickly became standard for private health plans. Physicians and hospitals could largely set their own fees and provide care as they saw fit, as payors reimbursed providers' "usual, customary, and reasonable" charges with little objec-tion.[7] Under this system it was fairly easy for physicians to provide, for virtually any patient, whatever kind and level of care represented prevailing practice. Even the uninsured could enjoy this affluent standard once they managed to get into the health care system, because providers routinely padded their charges to paying pa-tients to cover the uninsured.

The "Artesian Well of Money"[8] that flowed during those years also shaped the basic values underlying medical practice, fostering an unstinting standard of care. If money is truly no object, a host of inferences seems to follow: if an intervention might help, and it won't hurt, then surely it must be provided, regardless of cost; it is unethical for physicians to consider costs, because that would mean short-changing the patient to whom they owe their fidelity; every patient is entitled to the same quality of care, regardless of ability to pay; it is better to do too much than too little.[9]

So long as money flowed freely, it was reasonably easy for physicians to satisfy tort law's duty of care to provide the same basic quality of care to every patient whom they accepted for care, regardless of finances. That standard was largely identified according to physicians' prevailing practices, and with such generous third-party coverage, it became rather lavish. Malpractice suits were ordinarily an accusation of not knowing enough, not being skillful enough, or not being diligent enough. Litigation rarely reflected deficiencies of resources because there simply was not much need to conserve resources.

In like manner, little reason existed to worry about tortious misconduct by health plans. Their main role was to pay the bills, and they usually did so without hesita-tion. Insurers might, of course, balk if a particular type of service was clearly not covered, as with an explicit contractual exclusion of acupuncture or podiatry,[10] or if doubt arose that some physician actually had provided the service for which he billed. But since payors rarely refused to pay, they were of little interest to the tort system.

The economic upheaval of recent years has completely upended this cozy scene. Although physicians', hospitals', and other providers' legal duties of care were largely shaped during that era of generous third-party coverage, today's economic realities no longer support such liberal levels of care. Decades of relentlessly rising costs have fostered urgent efforts by employers to curb this major cost of doing business, while governments have been impelled to restrain the tax increases that would be required to support the endless increases in health care expenditures. Many health plans have sharply limited payments to providers so that physicians and hospitals can no longer afford to play Robin Hood[11] as they once did, charging more to paying patients in order to help the indigent.

To this fiscal shrinkage is added a wide variation in kinds and levels of coverage. Plans now differ markedly in their benefits, exclusions, and procedures, and many have adopted their own, usually proprietary and undisclosed, practice parameters to guide coverage decisions. As each health plan becomes more emphatic yet less predictable about what it will and will not cover, physicians' practices have become attuned less to what other physicians are doing and more to what each health plan expects. The relative uniformity of medical standards seen in the past is rapidly evaporating.

For all these reasons, the traditional legal standard of care, based on prevailing physician practices and requiring a fairly uniform level of care for everyone, has become economically and even medically anachronistic. That change, in turn, has precipitated a major jurisprudential challenge, in which physicians stand to be trapped between old legal demands and new economic realities—potentially held legally liable for economic constraints they did not create and cannot control.

The situation has become even more complex regarding health plans' liability. Whereas health plans once were little more than financial conduits, they are now active participants in decisions about care, because most insurers and managed care organizations (MCOs) must now cover a population of patients within a budget constrained by employers' and governments' (un)willingness to pay. And so the question arises whether, since health plans are now more active in monitoring and guiding patients' care, they should bear liability when they do a poor job of it.

To be sure, health plans have not been exempt from tort pressures. Beginning in the 1960s and accelerating in the 1970s and 1980s, courts began to identify duties for institutions such as hospitals, duties that were later extended to health plans. Indirect, or vicarious, liability addressed the failings of their employees while, under corporate negligence, a hospital or MCO could be directly liable for a failure to use due care in credentialing and supervising physician staff. More recently, a further question has arisen concerning whether MCOs and other institutions literally practice medicine, for instance when they undertake intensive utilization management that, by denying financial coverage for care, effectively denies the care itself. If health plans literally practice medicine, then perhaps they should be subject to liability for medical malpractice of the very same sort to which physicians have long been held.

With respect to health plans' potential liabilities, it is easy to be of two minds. On one hand, economic sobriety forces us to recognize the reality of resource limits. Health plans must now use finite resources to maximize the welfare of groups of people over time, and they cannot accomplish this if they provide every conceivable benefit to every patient. Courts need to appreciate that even the best policies, chosen on the basis of careful research and a thoughtful balancing of competing priorities, can sometimes produce a poor outcome for a given individual. That poor outcome should not automatically undermine the legitimacy of the policy.[12]

On the other hand, the tort system needs to maintain its traditional concern for the needs and rights of individuals who are entitled, among other things, to receive all the care they were promised by their health plans and to redress the very real injustices that sometimes befall them. This emphasis on individuals may sometimes go to excess in our current system, but it is important that individuals not be too conveniently subordinated to the greater good.

Federal law has greatly complicated these questions about health plans' liability. ERISA, the Employee Retirement Security Income Act of 1974,[13] governs benefit plans for most employees across the country. In exchange for various requirements that ensure that employers keep their promises to fund pensions and other benefits, Congress placed employee benefits under a single set of federal laws. Administration of benefit plans thus became far simpler under just one set of rules, instead of fifty sets for fifty states, so employers found it easier and more affordable to provide benefit plans.

However, this federal preemption of state laws also has had the effect of insulating MCOs and other health plans from tort litigation. This is because claims for malpractice, wrongful death, emotional distress, and the host of other claims patients might want to bring against health plans when a denial of care causes harm, lie within states' common law. No federal law equivalent exists. Aggrieved patients can, of course, sue under federal law, but remedies are limited to the financial value of the treatments that were owed, and sometimes attorneys' fees and certain other equitable relief. Patients cannot collect noneconomic damages, no matter what kind of suffering, disability, or death they have endured. Needless to say, the ERISA preemption has become a topic of hot debate, as patients injured by denials of care have sometimes been left completely without remedy.[14]

In sum, the separation between law and economics posed few challenges until the need to cut costs translated first into cuts in the care that physicians could provide and second into an intensive involvement by health plans in the specifics of the care delivered. In the face of these profound changes, the legal system can no longer pretend that money is irrelevant. The ways in which health care is financed and delivered have changed profoundly, and the legal system needs to acknowledge these changes as it determines what providers and health plans owe patients and how to hold them accountable for what they do. The old precepts of law must now be reconciled to the new economics of medicine. This book aims to address this gap.

Part I, consisting of Chapters 2, 3, and 4, discusses the problems that have emerged from the law–economics gap. Chapter 2 focuses on physicians. They, along with health plans, are a special focus of this book because physicians, unlike other providers in the health care system, have a unique sort of control. Their prescriptions and medical orders are a necessary, even if no longer sufficient, condition for patients to receive most health care interventions. Evolving scope-of-practice laws do now permit some allied health professionals, such as nurse practitioners, to exercise limited independent authority.[15] Even so, physicians still direct seventy percent to eighty percent of health care expenditures.[16] Accordingly, Chapter 2 discusses the traditional standard of care that tort law requires of physicians, why it once was reasonable, and why, in light of changing economics, it has now become untenable. Chapter 2 also discusses available tort theories that might, in principle, alleviate the problem—theories such as the locality rule and the practice variations permitted by the rule of reputable minorities—and explains why these are inadequate to the enormous task of reconciling old tort requirements with the new economic realities.

The rest of Part I focuses on health plans. Chapter 3 looks at plans' tort exposure, while Chapter 4 turns to health plans and contract law. Chapter 3 begins with the historical note that, until recently, health plans have had little vulnerability to tort litigation, partly because they were mainly financiers who rarely said "no" and partly because federal ERISA preemption has significantly limited otherwise available tort remedies. New avenues for liability are rapidly emerging, however. In the mid-1990s a significant chink appeared in health plans' ERISA armor to permitting a fairly large number of claims to proceed to state courts. Beyond this, two causes of action initially applied to hospitals have now been extended to health plans: direct corporate negligence and vicarious liability. Yet another inroad may be emerging via an updated version of the old corporate practice doctrines. Here, a court might find that when an MCO engages, for instance, in intensive utilization management (that is, making decisions about which services are "necessary" for a particular patient), the MCO is literally practicing medicine and should be held directly liable for medical malpractice, just as would a physician. This chapter introduces the questions surrounding corporate practice, while a resolution will be left for Chapter 8.

Finally, Chapter 3 identifies some of the problems and challenges associated with ascribing tort liability to health plans. First, such liability is not always assigned on the basis of well-conceived rationales. In this rapidly emerging area, judges must sometimes "make it up as they go along," thereby creating an unpredictability that makes it difficult for health plans to plan appropriately for legal risks. Second, because tort litigation traditionally focuses on injured individuals, it is difficult for courts to encompass health plans' needs to enforce policies geared toward the best interests of the broader enrollee population, policies that, even if excellent on the whole, inevitably will sometimes disadvantage particular individuals.

Chapter 4 turns to contract law. In discussions about physicians' liabilities, contract law has been only marginally relevant because, although technically the physician–patient relationship begins in contract, thereafter the physician's conduct has largely been judged in tort. However, contract plays a major role in health plans' accountability to subscribers. Patient–plan relationships do not just begin in contract, they are systematically governed by it. Prima facie, the health plan owes the patient whatever it promised to deliver in the contract, no more, no less. However, when health care resources are involved, several problems arise.

To begin with, some of the most basic conditions for effective contracting are often poorly met in the health care context. These contracts are usually quite vague, so it is often difficult for courts to determine whether a patient was entitled to receive a disputed service. Because such contractual vagueness is traditionally construed against the drafter, health plans increasingly find themselves covering services they had not intended to fund, thereby exacerbating their difficulties in planning care for a large population within a fixed budget. A primary culprit creating much of this vagueness is the fuzzy notion of "medical necessity" that serves as the contractual cornerstone of most health plan contracts. In addition, enforceable contracting usually requires that the parties have made free, relatively informed choices—often not the case when it comes to health care.

The challenges do not end with contract language, however. Even in cases in which the health plan quite clearly does not owe the patient a particular intervention, courts sometimes hesitate to enforce contractual limits on care when it appears that the denial of a particular service may lead to a medical disaster for the patient. Thus, some courts have freely awarded coverage for exotic care to desperate patients, contract language notwithstanding.

The deeper problem is society's profound ambivalence about living with the real, individualized consequences of resource limits. Although most of us agree, in principle, that even an affluent society cannot afford every conceivable medical benefit for every needy person, we are terribly uneasy when we see the personal consequences of a policy that, from a distance, we may have endorsed. The result is an exacerbation of the already formidable difficulty in creating an efficient, effective health care system.

Part I having identified these tort and contract challenges for physicians and health plans, Part II seeks answers. Chapter 5 proposes that we must begin with the right question: instead of focusing on how we want to hold physicians and health plans accountable for their conduct toward patients, we must instead begin with a question that is conceptually—and medically—prior. We must ask whom we want to be controlling what in the delivery of health care. This question should be answered first because our ultimate goal is good care. Restitution for injuries and inadequacies is obviously important, but it is arguably more important to foster the kind of health care delivery that can provide good care and prevent such misadventures in the first place.

Chapter 5 explores problems associated with asking first where liability should fall. One problem is that, once it is determined that a particular party bears liability in a given area, then that party ordinarily tries to exercise control to limit its liability risk. Unfortunately, when clinical control is exercised not on the basis of who can best deliver care, but rather on the basis of liability fears, the medical implications can be unfortunate, if not disastrous. Suppose, for instance, that we say health plans must bear complete liability for all unfortunate outcomes, including those caused by physicians' errors ("enterprise liability"). Although such an approach might simplify tort litigation and open greater resources to compensate injured patients, it is also quite possible that more patients might be injured in the first place. This is because if plans manage heightened legal risk by imposing greater control over physicians, they may intrude on clinical decision making and on the physician–patient relationship in ways that ultimately impede good care. Indeed, this is the very sort of intrusion we see when health plans micromanage medicine to manage economic risk. Adding to their legal risk might encourage even deeper and more clinically dubious intrusions.

If misplaced liability can thus breed misplaced control over health care, it becomes clear that the first question must be to ask who should control what in health care. Chapter 5 outlines how various responsibilities for patient care might reasonably be divided between physicians and health plans. Physicians' primary domains are familiar, as they build trusting relationships with patients, individualize care as needed, and help health plans refine their systems for delivering care. Health plans, for their part, should tend to four domains: business and administration; identifying and promoting patterns of good care; monitoring providers for poor care and taking appropriate remedial actions; and, in certain instances, literally practicing medicine. Under such a division of responsibility, liability should be assigned only for those aspects of care that the physician or health plan could and should have controlled.

Chapter 6 then introduces a crucial distinction. Once it is clear which party should be controlling which aspects of care, it can be inferred which party ought to shoulder any corresponding legal liability. However, a further question concerns just what sort of liability it should be—tort or contract. This, in turn, cannot be determined until it is clear just what sort of error was made. And this requires an important distinction: expertise versus resources.

Errors of expertise arise from a lack of knowledge, skill, or judgment or from a failure to apply such knowledge and skill with diligence and care. Errors regarding resources, in contrast, represent a deprivation of some particular service or product to which the patient was entitled, usually by contract. Errors of expertise are more commonly associated with physicians and medical malpractice, as when a surgeon reads a radiograph backwards and removes the wrong kidney. But as Chapter 6 will show, health plans are also capable of expertise errors, as, for instance, when they bungle their administrative responsibilities. Reciprocally, resource errors are more commonly associated with health plans, as, for instance, when the plan denies inpatient psychiatric care to which the patient was contractually entitled. However, under financial risk-sharing arrangements, physicians can have considerable resource control and thereby can be responsible for wrongful denials of resources. Once this distinction is outlined, Chapter 6 proposes that errors of expertise should be addressed as torts, while errors regarding resources should generally be handled under contract law.

Chapters 7, 8, and 9 explore the ways in which tort and contract liability should play out, once it is determined which party actually exercised control in a given situation and what sort of error (expertise versus resources) occurred.

Chapter 7 discusses liability for physicians. Errors of expertise—the classic scenarios of medical malpractice—should be handled as torts and governed by familiar tort standards. The amount and kind of knowledge, skill, and effort a physician owes a patient should be determined by examining the knowledge, skill, and effort prevailing elsewhere in the professional community. Standard caveats, such as for differing schools of thought and for reputable minorities, likewise can provide familiar sources of flexibility for medical knowledge to evolve over time.

Resource issues for physicians must be addressed very differently. The first question concerns what level of control the physician actually exercised over the resources the patient allegedly was denied. Under some kinds of financial arrangements between physicians and payors, that level can be considerable. In a capitated system in which the physician is paid a monthly fee for all of a patient's outpatient care, the physician may control most or all of the resources reserved for primary care, for instance; in full-risk arrangements, physician groups may control literally all the resources for patients' care, right down to hospital care, medical devices, and home nursing services. For such resource issues the appropriate standard for determining what the patient should have received is not the level of resources other physicians would have used in that particular situation. Rather, the standard should be the level of resources the patient (or the employer or government program) actually purchased in this particular plan. This is normally a question of contract, not tort.

Chapters 8 and 9 concern health plans' liability. Chapter 8 focuses on plans' tort liability for their deficiencies of expertise, while Chapter 9 considers plans' contract-based accountability for resource decisions.

Chapter 8 initially surveys the kinds of duties that health plans owe enrollees as obligations of expertise within their four domains of control, as outlined in Chapter 5. These begin with the business administration activities that are health plans' most familiar task. Expertise duties also include obligations to use care in selecting the medical guidelines by which they make benefit decisions and promote good care and by which they evaluate their physicians' performance. Health plans additionally have a duty to use appropriate knowledge, judgment, care, and skill when they engage in the practice of medicine.

To claim that plans literally practice medicine is controversial, and Chapter 8 addresses this question squarely. Many physicians insist that MCOs do practice medicine, because their utilization management decisions have such an enormous impact on the care patients actually receive. Conversely, health plans usually insist that they do not practice medicine at all but rather simply decide which benefits they owe the patient under the terms of the plan. A careful analysis of the concept of what it is to practice medicine reveals, in Chapter 8, that health plans do and sometimes must practice medicine. When they do, they should potentially be liable in tort for classic malpractice, of the same sort to which physicians are held. At the same time, this chapter argues that health plans currently practice medicine much too often. Because most contracts are founded on the notion of "medical necessity," health plans often must make medical decisions in order to make their benefit determinations. For a host of reasons, plans need to discard the notion of medical necessity entirely in favor of a far more specific iteration of what subscribers will and will not receive from a given plan. Once this is accomplished, plans will practice medicine sparingly rather than frequently, as they currently do.

Finally, Chapter 8 explores the ways in which tort litigation should proceed when health plans breach their duties of expertise. As in all tort litigation, once plaintiffs establish a duty and its breach, they must additionally prove proximate causation of an injury.

Chapter 9 turns to health plans' contract liability for resource decisions. As noted in Chapter 4, the conditions for effective, enforceable contracting often are not satisfied in the current health care market. Major corrections are required.

First, as argued in Chapter 8, vague promises to provide "medically necessary" care should give way to guidelines-based contracting. That is, instead of promising patients "we'll give you whatever we decide is necessary," plans should publish the guidelines on which nearly all benefit decisions are already, in fact, made and should offer their coverage on an open, specified basis: "If you buy this plan, here is what you will receive." Such guidelines-based contracting could provide vastly clearer information about each plan, on the basis of which a prospective subscriber could make far more informed choices than is possible at present.

Second, effective contracting requires options from which to choose, and information about those options. Enrollees need choices among health plans and ideally a range of choices within plans. Only when people have real options and reasonable information by which to make decisions will contracts that limit health care resources be more fully enforceable. And only when contractual limits on care can be enforced will it be possible not only for health plans to keep their premiums more controllable and predictable, but for citizens to decide how much of their resources they want to allot to health care and how much they want to reserve for other priorities.

Part III assesses the legal and theoretical acceptability of this book's proposed solutions to the gap between old legal expectations and new economic realities. Briefly, those proposals are: to distinguish between expertise and resource duties; to recognize that physicians and health plans can each bear and breach either type of duty; to address breaches of expertise as torts and breaches of resource duties as contract violations; to enhance enforceable contracting by promoting informed choices among real alternatives within and among plans; and to recognize that at least some measure of variability in contractual entitlements is legitimate in health care, just as it is for other important goods and services in a society that treasures free exchange.

Chapter 10 tests these recommendations against prevailing legal doctrines and existing case law and finds a surprisingly good fit. First, although it is ostensibly somewhat novel, the proposal to distinguish between expertise and resources, addressing the former through tort and the latter through contract, actually fits remarkably well with current legal traditions and case law. Second, although contract remedies are not as generous as are tort damages to compensate injured patients for wrongful denials of resources, they are, in fact, considerably more adequate to the need than one might initially suspect. Third, serious challenges nevertheless remain.

In particular, if guidelines-based contracting is theoretically attractive, some sobering practical obstacles must be overcome if such an approach is to be acceptably implemented.

Chapter 11 focuses on ERISA, the federal law governing employee benefit plans. The discussion begins by examining recent major trends that interpret the federal preemption clause. An emerging body of case law is beginning, albeit implicitly, to distinguish between expertise issues and resource issues in a way that appears fundamentally consistent with the letter and the spirit of the ERISA statute. However, courts have not quite articulated the distinction correctly, as analysis of a number of cases will show. If ERISA courts amend their thinking as proposed in this book, their preemption decisions will be considerably clearer and more rational. Although this book does not purport to resolve the question of whether ERISA's statutory preemption should itself be changed as it applies to health plans, a few thoughts will be offered on the matter.

Finally, Chapter 12 wraps up with a moment of reflection on the extraordinary transition time in which we find ourselves.

I

JURISPRUDENTIAL PROBLEMS

2

PHYSICIANS AND TORT LIABILITY

Although medical malpractice is a somewhat specialized area of tort law, it nevertheless embodies the basic elements of tort. Tort law emerges from the fundamental precept that citizens should comport themselves with a modicum of care in order to avoid unreasonably injuring one another. When someone breaches that duty, and when that breach has caused an injury, the costs should be borne by the one who has carelessly caused the problem, not by the blameless one who was harmed. The injured person may thereby have a cause of action for which he or she can collect damages.[1] Reciprocally, where an unfortunate event has not been caused by a breach of due care, the damages should lie where they fall.

Medical malpractice law does differ somewhat from standard tort law.[2] The duty of care physicians owe their patients is established not according to the reasonable person at large, but rather is set by the profession itself.[3] In practice it is generally an empirical appeal to what physicians do, that is, to the customary practices prevailing among reasonable and prudent physicians.[4] Exceptions have emerged over the years, such as for alternate schools of thought, for the views and practices of reputable minorities, for differences among various specialties, and for variations among localities. But these, like the prevailing practice approach, still empower the profession to establish its own duty of care and to resolve questions by appealing to what physicians actually do.

Two other features have come to figure prominently in malpractice law. First, as medicine has become highly technological, the standard of care has likewise come to incorporate this vast and rapidly growing array of costly technology, because

15

physicians often cannot care effectively for a patient without sophisticated diagnostic and therapeutic modalities. Antibiotics, not wisdom, cure bacterial pneumonia; chemotherapy, radiation, and surgery treat cancer; and computerized tomography or magnetic resonance imaging may be needed to diagnose a stroke or tumor. Thus, courts have held physicians liable for failure to order x-rays, laboratory tests, biopsies, intravenous pyelograms, pathologic examinations of tissue, and other diagnostic and therapeutic interventions.[5] As noted by Siliciano, "[t]he unitary standard [of care] . . . is relentlessly contemporary; past practice, no matter how efficacious, is rendered legally inadequate as soon as it is supplemented with or superseded by newer approaches."[6] Older, cheaper technologies become substandard simply by falling out of favor.

The other feature of keen interest here is that the same duty is owed to everyone, regardless of costs or patients' abilities to pay. This feature begins with the fact that tort law, in general, expects citizens to render the same duty of care to all fellow citizens. The motorist must look out for all vehicles and pedestrians, not just some of them. In medicine this means that physicians are expected to provide the same basic quality of care to every patient they accept for care.[7] The physician may refuse to accept a patient for any reason, including the patient's indigence.[8] But once the patient is accepted, "whether the patient be a pauper or a millionaire, whether he be treated gratuitously or for reward, the physician owes him precisely the same measure of duty, and the same degree of skill and care."[9] The duty of care "imports no discrimination based on economic status."[10] Thus, the physician may not perform an inadequate diagnostic work-up out of cost considerations,[11] nor may he abandon the patient at a critical juncture because the patient cannot pay his fees.[12] If a hospital lacks a computed tomography (CT) scanner, the physician may be obligated to send patients to a facility that can provide it, even if the hospital must pay with its own scarce dollars.[13]

This is not to say that physicians and hospitals must provide literally every therapeutic intervention that promises benefit. The law has never required physicians to deliver the highest possible standard of care,[14] nor has it required the physician to purchase the patient's prescription medications out of his own pocket. Indeed, it is not entirely clear just how far the physician must go to ensure that poorer patients receive the same basic quality of care as well-insured patients. Nevertheless, in principle, malpractice law requires that each patient receive at least "ordinary and reasonable" care, regardless of whether he can pay for it. "To date, medical malpractice law has refused to recognize formally the economic status of the patient as a factor legitimately influencing the kind or degree of care the patient receives. Instead, malpractice claims are assessed against a unitary, wealth-blind standard of care."[15]

These three crucial features of the medical standard of care—that it is set by what physicians actually do, that it can encompass costly technologies, and that it must be honored regardless of finances—have meant, in effect, that tort law expects physicians to commandeer other people's money and property in order to deliver the required standard. After all, physicians usually do not own the technical resources they use for their patients, ranging from hospital beds to operating rooms to CT scanners. And so they may be obliged simply to order whatever they feel the patient needs, letting the financial chips fall where they may.

This judicial indifference to costs is illustrated by the recent case of *Muse v. Charter Hospital, Inc.*[16] Although an adolescent patient's physician believed the boy should remain in a psychiatric hospital, the hospital discharged him after insurance and parental payments ended. Finding that a hospital has a duty not to interfere with a physician's medical judgment and citing with approval a case holding that "a hospital has a duty to the patient to obey the instructions of a doctor,"[17] a North Carolina appellate court held that Charter Hospital had a duty not to willfully interfere with a doctor's medical judgment by discharging a patient who could no longer pay for services. Clearly, the implication of this holding is that when a physician writes medical orders, others must simply provide the resources commanded, regardless of cost or payment.[18]

Similarly, a California appellate court noted that, although "[t]hird party payors of health care services can be held legally accountable when medically inappropriate decisions result from defects in the design or implementation of cost containment mechanisms . . . the physician who complies without protest with the limitations imposed by a third party payor, when his medical judgment dictates otherwise, cannot avoid his ultimate responsibility for his patient's care. He cannot point to the health care payor as the liability scapegoat when the consequences of his own determinative medical decisions go sour."[19] Other courts have echoed this view.[20]

A. ECONOMIC UPHEAVAL

For many years, these elements in the malpractice standard of care presented little difficulty. Before World War II physicians had relatively few interventions, costly or otherwise, to offer patients. As expensive technologies emerged, virtually unlimited third-party reimbursement encouraged physicians to provide patients with all services that promised potential benefit. Uninsured patients were covered by an informal cost-shifting system in which providers raised their charges to paying patients to cover those who could not pay. Though not all citizens had access to the health care system, those who did could usually receive its full range of its benefits.[21] Hence, so long as costs posed no obstacle, physicians could easily provide a uniformly high quality of increasingly technological care to any patient, regardless of ability to pay. Courts and providers alike could safely ignore the costs of care.

In recent years, however, a serious problem has emerged. Health care costs, predictably, skyrocketed. Between 1980 and 1993,

> private health insurance costs increased by 218 percent in inflation-adjusted dollars, while the inflation-adjusted gross domestic product per capita rose by just 17 percent. The increased costs were simply passed along by insurance plans to employers . . . In one year alone, 1988–1989, employers' health insurance costs rose by 18 percent. Between 1980 and 1993, spending by employers on health care as a percentage of total compensation to workers increased from 3.7 percent to 6.6 percent."[22]

Businesses and governments, deeply troubled by health care costs rising out of control, have resorted to increasingly stringent cost containment measures. As these payors ratcheted down the inflated fees that formerly included enough surplus to cover the uninsured, the initial result in the 1980s was a "stratified scarcity" in which physicians could not always provide uninsured patients with the same level of care they provided everyone else.[23] The discrepancy came to be particularly pressing at large, inner-city, public hospitals that cared for growing numbers of uninsured patients under stagnant, if not shrinking, budgets. As the medical director at one such hospital lamented, "We're a ship at sea, running out of coal, and starting to burn the furniture."[24] This economic shift precipitated a serious jurisprudential challenge, as physicians caring for the medically indigent stood to be caught between affluent legal expectations for society at large and the stringent realities of inner-city economics.[25]

Since then the economic picture has become considerably more complex.[26] After years of uncontrolled inflation in health care, employers now insist that health plans compete for their business. Although professing an interest in quality of care and value for their dollars, most employers look mainly, if not exclusively, to premium price.[27] But health plans cannot price their plans competitively without strictly limiting their expenses, which means limiting both their payments to providers and the kinds and intensity of services they provide to subscribers. In the process, plans have devised a staggering variety of ways to constrain and redefine the care they cover. In response, other players have purveyed their own, sometimes incompatible, expectations of physicians and the health care system. As a result, physicians' actual practices are now shaped by at least five very different factors.

1. Traditional Fee-for-Service ("Artesian") Standards

As noted in Chapter 1, the era of affluent insurance essentially provided a bottomless "artesian well of money" that promoted certain values: too much care is better than too little; any intervention that might help and is unlikely to harm should be used, regardless of cost; when a new drug or device is shown to be safe and effective, it should immediately be deemed "necessary" and approved for payment; if a new procedure is promising (even though unproven) for patients who urgently need help and who have no superior alternatives, it should be adopted; no one should be denied potentially beneficial care on account of inability to pay; high-tech is better than low-tech is better than no-tech.[28]

This technologically lavish standard is alive and remarkably well. Even if relatively few people retain the first-dollar coverage that many once enjoyed, indemnity insurance still occupies a significant sector of the market. Although insurers are scrutinizing their expenditures much more closely, denials of authorization for care are still relatively uncommon.[29] Moreover, many physicians regard artesian "cost is no object" values as part of their moral commitment to patients.[30] This belief is reinforced by the collective habits formed in medical training[31] and by courts' "judge-made insurance" rulings that look not at the actual contract language, so much as at patients' expectations. In some instances, courts have required plans to cover even very high-cost, relatively unproven technologies to patients who otherwise lack much hope for survival.[32] Hence, a rich standard of care still flourishes in many sectors of medicine.

2. Specialty Societies

Medical specialty societies are among the most prominent, respected creators of practice guidelines that purport to capsulize the best ways for physicians to treat a host of common conditions.[33] The American College of Physicians and many other organizations have undertaken extensive efforts to produce guidelines constructed by academic leaders who review medical literature and other factors such as costs.[34] A number of these guidelines have clearly enhanced the quality of care. For example, anesthesia standards have significantly reduced intraoperative hypoxic injuries.[35] However, although specialist guidelines may often be motivated by a concern for patients, they are sometimes accused of being vehicles for preserving turf in an increasingly competitive marketplace and for ensuring high utilization of profitable procedures.[36] Further, when guidelines are created by physicians in academic environments, they may reflect economically insulated artesian values more than the leaner realities of the marketplace.[37]

3. Managed Standards

Undoubtedly the greatest diversity among clinical practice guidelines comes from the many health plans providing "managed care," broadly defined here to include any health plan that attempts serious cost containment by directly or indirectly limiting the kinds and amounts of care provided for subscribers.[38] Nearly all health plans these days are "managed" in some sense because virtually none permit physicians and patients to consume whatever plan resources they want. A wide array of tactics is employed.[39] In this sense the term *health plan* has become essentially interchangeable with the term *managed care organization,* or MCO.

Managed plans vary widely,[40] but they do share certain values that starkly contrast with artesian precepts: more is not necessarily better; watch-and-wait is often preferable to quick intervention; and scientific evidence, rather than medical customs or anecdotal experience or local department chairmen, should determine which interventions are medically warranted.

Some managed care guidelines are commercial products, developed by commercial firms and sold to a large number of MCOs across the country.[41] Some other MCOs develop their own guidelines, sometimes strictly through their own efforts but more commonly by adapting guidelines found elsewhere in the marketplace. Smaller entities, such as physician group practices, likewise may develop or adapt guidelines for in-house use.[42] In a more recent development, some corporations now contract directly with health care providers rather than purchasing conventional health plans for their employees. Many of these corporations are instituting their own parameters to guide and monitor providers' care.[43] The federal government has also made a few forays into the realm of guidelines creation.[44]

Among these managed care guidelines, an extraordinary diversity reigns. Indeed, the full extent of the variety cannot be known because many of them are proprietary, kept confidential partly to ensure commercial salability and partly to limit physicians' ability to "game the system" for extra benefits.[45] Widely differing methods are used to construct the guidelines. As will be discussed in greater detail in Chapter 5, although some are based on carefully controlled scientific studies, many others are founded on less reliable data sources, and still others have no link with science whatsoever.[46] With such research deficits, guideline creators often must rely on consultants to fill in the gaps. Any such consensus-guidelines, of course, will be flavored by whatever process was used to choose the creators.[47] Finally, although many guidelines permit a modicum of flexibility, others afford rather little.

Even when several health plans ostensibly use the same guidelines, actual decisions about which patients should receive which interventions can fluctuate. For instance, although the federal Medicare program has a single set of rules regarding what interventions should be covered under what conditions, the numerous individual carriers who actually implement those standards make widely differing decisions.[48] Some managed care entities use no explicit guidelines at all. One study concluded that among physician groups who manage their own care, thirty percent of the groups did not refer to guidelines of any sort in their in-house utilization review.[49]

In such a setting practice patterns can change drastically through collective panic as physicians confront major, sudden changes in their payment arrangements. Cardiologists who shift from fee-for-service to a capitated form of payment,[50] for instance, may rapidly downplay costly nuclear treadmill tests in favor of cheaper stress echocardiograms and may decide to perform fewer ordinary treadmill tests.[51] Capitated obstetricians may perform fewer cesarean deliveries,[52] while gastroenterologists may decide that biopsies are needed less often during colonoscopy.[53] Reciprocally, capitated primary care physicians may perform fewer procedures themselves, once specialists likewise are capitated, because referrals no longer represent an extra expense to the health plan.[54]

Such practice changes may sometimes reflect mercenary interests. More often, however, physicians are reevaluating long-held practice patterns that probably should have been reconsidered long before. In either case, economic changes are sparking a staggering variety of practice changes under the rubric of "managing" care.

4. Malpractice Insurers

Guidelines promulgated by malpractice insurers aim not to save medical costs or protect professional domains, but to minimize the risk of lawsuit or, in the event of suit, to minimize damage awards. Here, guidelines tend to focus on such high-risk areas as breast cancer diagnosis, anesthesia monitoring, heart attacks, head trauma, antibiotics, and pulmonary embolism. Some insurers offer discounts to those who agree to abide by their guidelines, while at least one company has threatened to drop noncompliant physicians from its rolls.[55]

These standards aim to reduce litigation partly by ensuring that necessary interventions are undertaken and partly by improving chart documentation. Sometimes, however, they may require a level of care that is economically or practically unsupportable in some settings. For instance, a rural area may not have the malpractice insurer's ideal level of facilities and personnel.[56] In other cases, the level of care expected by the malpractice insurer may exceed that permitted by a particular health plan. Thus, the interests of managing legal risk may require extra time in a hospital or a more thorough diagnostic evaluation, while the patient's plan may discourage or outright deny these as "medically unnecessary."

5. Patients' Expectations

Because patients are the principal source of malpractice suits, their expectations pose a powerful influence on medical practices. Yet the direction of this influence is not always clear. To begin with, patients have widely varying expectations and preferences, including very personal goals for their lives and health care and a broad spectrum of willingness to accept risk. In some cases patients' understandings of their illnesses and of proposed interventions may be largely a product of cultural beliefs or idiosyncratic interpretations of the information their physicians provide. These can powerfully shape patients' demands, sometimes in unpredictable ways.[57]

Moreover, patients' attitudes toward economic factors can introduce another unpredictable influence. On the one hand, many patients, economically insulated from the costs of care, bring to the medical encounter an entitlement mentality demanding the best of care, spare no expense.[58] In the same manner, physicians' penchant toward defensive medicine may impel them to deliver every intervention the patient explicitly demands or presumably wants.

On the other hand, patients do not necessarily sue out of displeasure with the technical quality or quantity of their care. As noted in Chapter 1, the great majority of negligent medical injuries do not precipitate any kind of tort claim, while reciprocally many malpractice suits have little connection with negligence or even injury.[59] Thus, little correlation appears to exist between physicians' technical quality of care and their likelihood of being sued.[60] Often, the strongest predictor of whether a physician will be sued is the extent to which patients feel they are being treated with honesty, respect, and personal interest.[61] Even these more modest expectations, however, pose a formidable challenge. Patients who want their physician to take plenty of time, explain everything carefully, and invite lots of questions may be disappointed if the physician's heavy caseload—the "productivity" expectation from the MCO or group practice—does not permit such leisurely conversation.[62]

6. Net Result

In sum, physicians' actual clinical practices are pressured by a plethora of factors—formal and informal guidelines and constraints that vary even more than the widely disparate physician practices that such guidelines were created to supplant.[63] At the same time, tort law continues to expect physicians to provide a high, fairly uniform standard of care to all patients whom they accept for care.

Still, there may be an escape hatch. Tort law has always permitted a measure of variation and flexibility in the standard of care to accommodate reasonable differences of opinion and to permit the evolution of the profession over time. Relevant provisions include the locality rule, informed consent doctrine, empirical reliance on prevailing practices as the basis for the standard, and a deference to respectable minorities. One might hope these could provide relief. Unfortunately, as will soon be evident, none is entirely adequate to respond to the tremendous tension between legal traditions and economic realities.

B. INADEQUACIES OF CURRENT MALPRACTICE TORT LAW

1. Locality Rule

Perhaps the oldest legal leeway for resource variations comes from the locality rule. Since the late nineteenth century the locality rule has held that it is unfair to apply "urban" standards of care to physicians who, practicing in outlying rural areas, do not have access to the greater opportunities for learning and practice available to their colleagues in larger cities.[64] Over the past few decades the locality rule has largely disappeared as a basis on which to evaluate physicians' personal skills and knowledge. Standardized education and certification and improved communication have largely erased the regional differences of competence within various medical specialties, and so the locality standard has largely given way to national standards of knowledge and skill both for specialists and for general practitioners.[65]

Still, the locality rule does partly survive through some courts' recognition that physical and fiscal resources vary from place to place. For example, in *Hall v. Hilbun*,[66] the Supreme Court of Mississippi offered a "resources-based caveat" to the national standard of care when it held that a physician's duty of care should be discerned not only according to the nationwide level of knowledge and skill for physicians within his field, but also according to the particular level of facilities, services, and equipment actually available to that physician. If a remote village has neither a CT scanner nor access to one within a reasonable distance, then the physician would not be at fault for failing to order such a test, even if it is common practice to do so elsewhere. Under this approach, then, a court can take into account the resources of the local community when it applies a general professional standard.[67]

Unfortunately, this caveat does not help the physician caught between traditional tort demands and evolving economic realities, because in these cases the economic limits of an entire region are not the primary concern. Rather, the problem lies in the variation of financial resources within a given locality. The physician forgoes an intervention, not because it is literally unavailable, but because at some level a priority decision has been made that, for some subgroup of the population, this particular intervention is not cost–worthy relative to alternative uses of those funds within the same constrained budget. Thus, when an un- or underderinsured patient is denied an otherwise desirable intervention because of its cost, the locality rule would have to be stretched to apply, not to the patient's geographic location, but to his socioeconomic station. The locality rule was never intended to immunize cost-conscious decisions to refrain from using locally available resources.

2. Informed Consent

The principle of informed consent aims to enhance patients' control over their health care and reduce the imbalance of knowledge and power in the physician–patient relationship, by maximizing their knowledge.[68] Accordingly, some commentators have suggested that physicians ought to inform their patients about all medically reasonable options, even those that are not covered by their health plans.[69] The patient then has the option to pay for the additional health care out of his own pocket or to petition those who hold the purse strings. In principle, at least, the physician can thereby both enhance patient autonomy and honor his fiduciary promise to pursue his patient's interests above others', even in the face of economic constraints.

An updated version of this approach proposes that patients need only one opportunity for informed consent regarding economic constraints. When initially enrolling in a health plan, the subscriber would provide a "bundled consent" to the plan's particular set of rules, procedures, and incentives. Patients choosing that plan would thereby have consented to all the further decisions that emanate from the plan's rationing system, so that further disclosures about individual cost–benefit trade-offs need not be made at the bedside. Courts would regard enrollees as having implicitly consented to whatever rationing decisions are made.[70]

Under either approach, we can agree that enhancing patients' knowledge of and choices among health plans would be desirable for many reasons and that physicians have important disclosure obligations regarding the economic as well as the medical aspects of the care they propose.[71] However, disclosure will not suffice as a vehicle for directly immunizing physicians' reductions in the standard of care.

To begin with, since many citizens have little or no choice between health plans,[72] it is difficult to speak of "consent" to a plan's rationing policies. Moreover, as discussed in Chapter 4, courts have been quick to emphasize patients' vulnerability in contracts with health plans. As noted by one court, "[t]here is, of course, no public policy against allowing patients of [public] clinics to agree to fewer amenities, longer waits, or greater inconvenience in exchange for lower prices than they would pay elsewhere. . . . [t]here cannot, however, be any justification for a policy which sanctions an agreement which negates the minimal standards of professional care which have been carefully forged by State regulations and imposed by law."[73] Accordingly, courts are unlikely to accept as binding a patient's consent to let physicians deny care for economic reasons, particularly in a case where the denial is not one that the patient could reasonably have foreseen on the basis of a vague, generic disclosure at the time of enrollment in a plan he did not choose.[74]

A different sort of problem with the informed consent approach concerns trust. An economic informed consent could require the physician—often a pivotal agent of clinical allocation decisions—to inform the patient that she is withholding some intervention because of cost, or utilization rules, or other patients' greater need. When the patient lacks the money or political influence to secure the preferred care, it will hardly enhance his autonomy or trust simply to tell him that his care is inferior.[75] And yet if the physician makes an exception every time a patient then pleads for better care, cost containment will effectively be negated. Further, if the scarcity that prompted the cost-containment pressure is genuine, then each physician who refuses to abide by resource constraints will place unfair burdens on other physicians and their patients. Her unwillingness to say "no" to her own patients will mean that they must say "no" to their patients more often.[76]

These prospective consequences do not entail that physicians should therefore keep mum about economic issues. Indeed, appropriate disclosures are arguably required, even if delicate.[77] Still, the problems do provide reason to doubt that disclosures could be the primary answer to the tort–economics clash.

3. Medical Custom

As noted, the medical standard of care is based on the actual practices of the profession's members.[78] In the face of the economic changes described above, it is tempting to suppose that medical custom could be reshaped to take new economic constraints into account. Judicial reliance on prevailing practices has never been absolute, after all. Courts permit deviations from custom when evidence shows new medical techniques to be superior to old, and they permit noncustomary routes to the same medical goals by accepting the practices of respectable minorities, differing schools of thought, and the like.[79] Furthermore, tort law has explicitly made room for economic considerations in the standard of care. In the classic case of *United States v. Carroll Towing,*[80] for instance, Judge Learned Hand proposed that the duties placed on citizens to avoid harms should take into account the probability that the harm will occur, the gravity of the injury that may result, and the burdens of taking precautions.[81]

Accordingly, Furrow has argued that because the tort system has always been willing to accommodate a wide variety of acceptable approaches, a collective contraction of standards would be relatively low-risk. Moreover, maintaining tort pressures on physicians, and especially on institutions, can help these providers ensure that they make the best uses of available resources, weeding out error, inefficiency, and their associated costs whenever possible. Similarly, Hall argues that tort law "can amply accommodate massive cutbacks in care within the tremendous variations in practice patterns that the established custom encompasses. . . . [S]ignificant savings are entirely possible *without any departure whatsoever* from existing practice patterns; all that is needed is a relative shift in numbers toward the more conservative end of the vast array of established practice patterns, a shift that, in theory, should create no malpractice conflict."[82]

These arguments have considerable merit. Customary medical care is inflated by needless and marginal interventions. Defensive medicine, wherein physicians perform extra tests and procedures to ward off malpractice risks, both real and imagined, is said to cost billions every year.[83] More fundamentally, the clinical routines on which physicians often rely to guide their management of ordinary cases are not always based on careful thought and scientific reasoning. For decades, generous third-party payment policies encouraged physicians to undertake every intervention that promised even an "infinitesimal benefit"[84] for their patients.[85] Medical practices came to vary widely, not so much because of patients' varying needs, but because of facilities availability,[86] local customs and habits,[87] and similarly idiosyncratic, non-medical factors.[88] Moreover, costs have always played at least some role in shaping medical standards of care.[89] Physicians do not order a CT or magnetic resonance imaging (MRI) scan for every headache, even though the tests pose little or no medical danger.[90] Per Judge Hand, cost-motivated shrinkage of routines thus need not clash with tradition.

Accordingly, a goal of many clinical guidelines has been to trim excessive practices without reducing the quality of care. Such trimming offers at least a partial exit from the tort-versus-economics dilemma, because a broad-based deflation can change the customs themselves. Furthermore, streamlined clinical routines need not offend society's egalitarian values. More cost-conscious customs could guide all patients' care, not just poor patients' care. In fact, significant shifts in practice already have occurred. Lengthy hospitalizations once common for conditions such as myocardial infarction (heart attack) and osteomyelitis (bone infection) are largely a thing of the past, replaced by shorter inpatient stays combined with various strategies for follow-up care, such as home intravenous infusion services.

Unfortunately, this promising and somewhat useful avenue cannot entirely solve the challenge. Problems can arise whether customs shift informally through collective clinical changes or more formally by means of written consensus guidelines.

a. Informal Shift in Custom

The limited value of malpractice law's traditional flexibility becomes evident as we distinguish between means and ends, that is, clinical inputs versus patients' outcomes. Courts have permitted physicians to eliminate useless or harmful practices and to innovate and diverge from one another quite freely, but only so long as these changes generally lead to the same ultimate goal—comparable health outcomes for patients.[91] Hence, although there is little problem in reducing superfluous care, courts are much less likely to endorse practices that lead to documentably poorer outcomes in order to achieve financial savings that benefit not the patient, but outside economic interests.[92] Although less care is not necessarily worse care, at some point less really is less. And that is where courts are likely to draw the line.

For example, when a diagnostic or therapeutic intervention is eliminated because it helps too few patients to justify its cost, the patients who would actually have been helped by that intervention might cite the "loss of a chance" doctrine[93] to argue that they have been treated negligently. The elimination may not harm most patients and may even benefit some by avoiding iatrogenic injuries or diagnostic false positives. Nevertheless, the injured patients can argue that, had the more costly tradition been followed, their own illness would have been better diagnosed and treated.[94] Indeed, in many cases patients have successfully made that argument not only with

respect to customary interventions that have been deleted, but even regarding innovative care that has not been fully proven scientifically.[95]

If courts begin to see a significant backsliding of health care outcomes, it would
not be surprising to see a flurry of new rulings in the mode of *Helling v. Carey.*[96] In
that case the Washington Supreme Court court simply rejected a widely followed
professional custom in which physicians generally did not perform a tonometry test
for glaucoma in patients under age forty because the disease is so rare in this age
group. Noting that the test is inexpensive and the disease is serious, the court found
that the entire profession had made an unreasonable assessment and declared physicians' custom invalid as a matter of law.[97]

Few courts have followed this approach, but that could change. Recent analyses
suggest that deference to custom is declining overall in favor of a "reasonable physician" standard that is less interested in what physicians actually do than in what
they ought to do.[98] Moreover, even when courts do not order physicians to adopt or
return to costlier practices, legislatures can and have. In response to a general tight-
ening of hospital lengths of stay, for instance, many states and even the federal
government have mandated minimum hospital coverage for such conditions as
childbirth and mastectomy and have mandated coverage for specific treatments such
as autologous bone marrow transplant for breast cancer.[99] Interestingly, evidence is
highly equivocal regarding the question of whether twenty-four-hour hospitalization
for normal childbirth actually does lead to worse outcomes.[100] And recent evidence
shows that, despite its widespread use, autologous bone marrow transplant for breast
cancer is no more effective than standard chemotherapy.[101]

Chapters 9 and 10 will show that courts are increasingly willing to accept resource restrictions if they are clearly stated in contract. But for present purposes, the
upshot is that significant diminution of resource use is unlikely to come about
through tort law's traditional deference to professional practice. The lone physician
who dares to defy custom in the name of costs could incur significant legal risk,
particularly when a patient is worse off under the diminished practice than he would
have been under the more generous discarded practice.[102]

The problem is exacerbated for physicians who attend the uninsured. Even a
successful general deflation of custom could leave these physicians legally vulnerable. Because those who treat indigents sometimes have substantially fewer resources than most physicians for their patients' care, their services sometimes will
be literally sub-standard—that is, below the level available to the majority of the
population. So long as the law identifies the standard of care according to prevailing
custom, with little tolerance for care that produces predictably poorer outcomes,
then whenever these physicians are economically forced to provide a level of care
that is likely to lead to poorer outcomes, they will be at risk for malpractice liability.

b. Explicit Consensus Guidelines

If gradual shift in custom is not the answer, perhaps customs could be streamlined
through explicit consensus guidelines. When the profession, whether as a whole or
in prestigious specialty groups, declares that particular interventions, though hitherto
standard, are really of little or no value,[103] the individual physician can feel more

confident in trimming his own practices. As noted just above, medical societies are actively crafting such guidelines. Where they have, perhaps the individual physician can point to the professional consensus in the event his conduct is challenged in court.[104]

Although such a scenario may offer some hope, significant problems remain. When guidelines are designed mainly by leaders of the profession who practice at well-funded tertiary care centers, their cost-conscious new standards may still be too rich for private physicians practicing in economically leaner circumstances.[105] After all, it is difficult enough for a physician to measure up to the "anybody's guess" medical standards that emerge from competing expert witnesses in a courtroom. It could be nearly impossible to defend even an economically unavoidable deviation from a set of written standards established by colleagues for better-funded patients.[106] From a practical standpoint it should also be noted that in the face of the extraordinary diversity now emerging among the guidelines produced by various specialty societies, malpractice insurers, MCOs with their widely differing views on what is "necessary" care, and the plethora of other sources now telling physicians what to do, the very idea of achieving broad consensus across the spectrum of medical care seems quixotic.[107]

If deference to even a flexible version of "custom" is thus not entirely equipped to accept economically motivated reductions in care, perhaps some other familiar tort doctrines can, such as the "respectable minority," "accepted practice," and "reasonable physician" doctrines. These three concepts share a common heritage and a common defect and therefore will be considered together.

4. "Respectable Minority," "Accepted Practice," "Reasonable Physician"

As noted above, malpractice law has permitted substantial escape hatches for physicians whose practices deviate from the majority. Recognizing that medicine is an inexact science and that flexibility is essential to good care and medical progress, tort principles accept the practices of differing schools of thought and of reputable minorities of physicians. In the case of the "respectable" or "reputable" minority, some jurisdictions require the practice to be embraced by a considerable number of physicians; other courts expect only that the physicians in question be regarded as reputable by other physicians; and still other courts require both—that is, acceptance of the practice by a considerable number of physicians who, themselves, are respected within the profession.[108] By whatever formula, the principle holds that when an alternative approach is accepted by a reputable minority of physicians, then, even though it deviates from custom, its use is not substandard nor malpractice.[109] For example, an acceptable surgical treatment of early-stage breast cancer can be mastectomy or lumpectomy, each with varying options for adjuvant radiation or chemotherapy.

Several commentators have suggested that this concept may offer a suitable avenue for incorporating economic considerations into the standard of care.[110] If a physician can demonstrate that a respectable minority of colleagues provides a lean brand of care, perhaps he can avoid civil liability for his own cost-conscious practices.

A commendable modification, according to J.H. King and others, is to look not at what physicians actually do (whether as the majority or as a reputable minority), but at what the profession approves as good practice.[111] This "accepted practice" approach would seek from an expert witness his considered judgment concerning the profession's reasonable expectations for its members, rather than his guesstimate of a practice's popularity.[112] Because this approach is so much less dependent on preserving the status quo, it is said to be better suited than an empirically derived "prevailing custom" for incorporating considerations of cost-effectiveness while maintaining high standards of quality.[113] Essentially similar is the "reasonable physician" approach that many courts are now embracing.[114]

Unfortunately, these proposals will not resolve the problem. In order to address the most difficult cases, the "respectable minority," "accepted practice," and "reasonable physician" rules would have to go beyond merely stating that it is acceptable for physicians to eliminate useless or highly marginal interventions on economic grounds. That sort of change is already permitted. Rather, these rules would have to embrace the further idea that it is acceptable actually to reduce the quality of health care outcomes—to accept, for example, a somewhat greater possibility of failing to diagnose or cure, and in the process leave some patients worse off than they would otherwise have been—in order to conserve resources.

However, existing malpractice law effectively precludes this very step.[115] As noted above, each method of establishing the standard of care, whether custom or its variants, is sanctioned only insofar as it implements the same underlying principle, namely, that by whatever medical route, all patients' care should be aimed toward the same basic quality of outcomes. And yet that is one of the very issues at stake. Medicine has grown so lavish, and its cost has displaced so many other would-be spending priorities, that at a certain point we as individuals and as a society may want to spend less for health care, even if it means receiving less. Yet this is the very step that runs afoul of current tort doctrines.

The problem runs deeper. In the current economic mêlée, applications of the reputable minority doctrine are virtually guaranteed to offend the rules of logic by begging the central question. On the one hand, physicians who embrace old-style artesian values will regard many of the cost-conscious practices of managed care physicians to be disreputable compromises of patient welfare. Conversely, physicians who embrace a managed care approach will consider many artesian routines to be equally disreputable on the ground that they risk excessive iatrogenic (physician-caused) injury, waste money, and, in some cases, foresake the good of the larger population of patients in order to pursue a rather small or remote benefit for a few individuals. As a result, in litigating such disputes, one cannot determine whether a particular medical practice is "reputable" without antecedently determining which expert witnesses are sufficiently "reputable." And the answer to that question will depend on whether one favors artesian or managed approaches to care—the very question at issue. This is not a clash regarding esoteric scientific matters. It is a clash of basic values in which one side considers it irresponsible to ignore economics while the other side abhors letting costs influence clinical decisions.[116]

Consequently, it has become question-begging to appeal to what is "reputable," "reasonable," or "accepted" to determine which of the many diverging approaches to medical care are acceptable. Medicine is no longer characterized by a mainstream practice surrounded by a limited number of alternatives. It has become a plethora of minorities, each of which looks askance at the others. In any attempt to determine which minorities are respectable, we must first decide whose opinions to seek, thereby diving into circular reasoning.

5. Net Result

In sum, it appears that current malpractice law is inadequately equipped to resolve the rather novel situation that physicians now face. It is embroiled in a pervasive conflict between the legal necessity to provide the same basic level of care for everyone, regardless of ability to pay, and the economic necessity to attune each patient's kind and amount of care to payors' widely varying demands and restrictions. None of the methods by which the courts identify the standard of care is quite prepared to accommodate such nonmedical, third-party financial considerations.[117]

C. RECASTING PHYSICIANS' DUTY OF CARE

The foregoing considerations suggest that traditional appeals to physicians' prevailing practice have become untenable, if not outright incoherent, and should be abandoned in favor of a more rational, realistic approach to physicians' civil liability in health care. Several further arguments support this conclusion.

1. Diversity Has Supplanted Consensus

The essentially unlimited funding of the past made possible a strong consensus on the goals and values of medicine,[118] thereby permitting a remarkable level of similarity among physicians' practices. Physicians needed to answer only one basic question before a new drug, device, or procedure could be widely adopted: whether and under what conditions it was likely to be a medical benefit. Cost was essentially irrelevant. Naturally, opinions would differ in cases of significant medical uncertainty, such as an unusual illness or a radically new treatment, until time and experience could resolve the questions. But as long as the basic goals of care were shared, the practices of medicine could be fairly uniform.

Perhaps the most profound change spawned by the current economic upheaval is the introduction of competing goals into health care. Cost is now highly relevant, and patients' benefit is no longer the sole objective. Each expenditure raises questions about what other use, medical or nonmedical, might have been made of that money and how important these alternatives are relative to the proposed use. The answers will vary as greatly as the people who are asked. Hence, artesian fee-for-service differs profoundly from managed care medicine, and managed care itself speaks with many different voices. And as noted above, malpractice insurers, subspecialty societies, and patients introduce even greater diversity.

If any conclusion is obvious, it is that throughout much of medicine no particular practices "prevail."[119] There is no such thing as "the" standard of care. The variation reaches far beyond costly new technologies, down to the most ordinary details of care, such as which antibiotic to use for a given infection, how long to hospitalize someone with a particular illness, and what sort of outpatient care should follow hospital discharge.[120] Prevailing practice has been replaced by near chaos, and what is "customary" or even "medically indicated" depends upon who is asked. This diversity reflects deep division in the perspectives and objectives of the numerous, sometimes antagonistic players in the health care system.

The case of *Fox v. HealthNet*[121] illustrates this. Nellene Fox, a thirty-eight-year-old woman with advanced breast cancer, asked her HMO, HealthNet, to pay for high-dose chemotherapy with autologous bone marrow transplant (HDC/ABMT). It was supposedly the most advanced treatment for her condition and was recommended as her only, albeit slim, hope for survival. HealthNet denied coverage on the ground that it was experimental, while Fox claimed that it was widely practiced and therefore an accepted mode of care.

In fact, both sides were correct. Fox was right that the treatment had become widely practiced for breast cancer. This is partly because many physicians, acting on the artesian value that any potential benefit must be provided regardless of cost, have been willing to provide this treatment that seemed to offer a glimmer of hope to patients who otherwise had none. Court injunctions mandating insurance coverage, together with government mandates for coverage and insurance companies' acquiescence to threats of litigation, quickly provided widespread financial support for its medical proliferation.[122]

The health plan was also correct. Medicine purports to be based on science, not merely anecdotes and testimonials, and health plans have explained their refusals to cover this treatment by citing a lack of controlled scientific studies documenting that it is safe and effective. In fact, some early analyses had already indicated that HDC/ABMT for breast cancer provides no benefit over standard chemotherapy and actually diminishes patients' prognosis in certain categories.[123] In addition, although the National Institutes of Health (NIH) had a major study underway at the time, results were slow in coming. Because so many women had access to the treatment through their insurers, it became difficult to recruit enough women willing to enter controlled trials in which only half the subjects would receive HDC/ABMT.[124] When the NIH studies finally concluded, results indicated that HDC/ABMT had no advantage over standard chemotherapy.[125]

Thus, conflict rages over how to define the standard of care physicians owe their patients.[126] Given the diversity of the goals and guidelines among insurers, MCOs, employers, malpractice insurers, patients, and other major players in the health care industry, it is increasingly difficult to find physician practices that genuinely count as "prevailing."

2. Practices Do Not Always Reflect Professional Judgment

Admittedly, several arguments could still support the traditional appeal to physicians' prevailing practice for determining physicians' duty of care. In this realm of highly esoteric knowledge, laymen are not equipped to second-guess physicians, and so the best evidence of the profession's collective judgment may be what they actually do. Though the latest scientific research is, of course, important, physicians should only be held to developments that stand the test of time and experience. At the same time, the appeal to actual practices permits flexibility for medicine to evolve over time and for professional norms to be adjusted to the specific circumstances of each patient. Therefore, a certain plausibility inheres in the idea of looking to what physicians collectively do in order to determine what they ought to do.[127]

Nevertheless, critics point out that prevailing practice often does not reflect physicians' best judgment, either individually or collectively.[128] New technologies are sometimes adopted not because they are deemed medically best, but because they are new and exciting, and physicians hesitate to be out of step; because conformity to popular procedure is too often promoted for its own sake, regardless of whether the particular practice advances the desired medical outcomes or serves other values, such as fiscal efficiency;[129] and because physicians fear malpractice liability if they do not use the latest innovations. In other cases, inappropriate practices may disappear too slowly, while salutary changes may gain acceptance too slowly.[130]

Further, artesian financing has meant that economic considerations have been largely absent from collective customs. The fact that physicians adopt a particular clinical approach when costs pose no obstacle does not mean that their best judgment would be the same under more constrained conditions.[131] Physicians who are subjected to stringent utilization management or whose reimbursement suddenly shifts from fee-for-service to capitation, sometimes change their practices in ways that are based far more on urgency to cut costs than on careful reflection over time.[132]

3. Physicians No Longer Exercise Unilateral Resource Control

As noted above, by requiring an essentially equal and often high-technology, high-cost level of care, traditional malpractice law expects physicians to commandeer other people's money and property.[133] This mandate posed little problem so long as insurers provided a financial pass-through system that paid for virtually anything physicians chose to do. But those days are gone. An economic version of the "Golden Rule" now dominates the health care market: He who has the gold makes the rules. After years of facing costs rising out of control, payors that absorb the economic consequences of providers' medical decisions have two basic choices: controls or incentives. That is, they can limit their financial risk by directly dictating the decisions that generate the costs, or they can shift the economic risk, and with it a measure of resource control, to providers.

The control option includes explicit contract clauses excluding certain kinds of services, together with detailed guidelines and intense utilization management governing which interventions will be covered under what circumstances.[134] After all, every medical decision is also a spending decision, and a judgment about whether an intervention is "medically necessary" usually carries with it a decision about whether it warrants coverage.[135] Physicians and patients who agree to be bound by these plans' cost containment provisions have made a contractual commitment that cannot be dismissed merely because of *post hoc* regrets or inconvenience. Courts are increasingly willing to enforce contractually explicit limits.[136]

The risk-shifting approach includes incentive arrangements such as financial bonuses, penalties, fee withholds, and capitation.[137] Here, physicians can exercise considerably greater clinical autonomy than they can under tight utilization controls, but at a significant price. Physicians will personally lose money or professional standing and even risk "deselection" (being fired) if their clinical habits are too costly.

Either way, physicians no longer control medical resources with the freedom they enjoyed only a few years ago. The situation poses serious challenges. Courts continue to expect physicians to deliver a roughly uniform level of care to all their patients, regardless of the patients' ability to pay.[138] But because those who actually own or control those resources now restrict physicians' access to them, physicians stand to be held legally liable for resource limits that may be almost completely beyond their control.[139]

The problem is exacerbated when the patient's health plan is an employment benefit covered by federal ERISA law.[140] ERISA's preemption provision shields employee benefit plans from state-based tort and contract claims.[141] Hence, in many cases, because suits against the health plan for the harms caused by resource denials are preempted by ERISA, the patient's only remedy may be against the physician. Courts have recognized this point but have not seemed particularly disturbed by it, indeed in some cases expressing relief that the patient still has someone to sue.[142] ERISA will be examined in considerably more detail in Chapter 11.

4. Physicians Have No A Priori Entitlement to Determine the Values Underlying Health Care Resources

One more important reason not to base physicians' duty of care on professional custom is normative. Historic arrangements have given physicians enormous power to determine how much money other people must spend on health care services and products. Through its deference to custom, tort law has permitted, and even required, physicians unilaterally to determine what level of care all patients should have, regardless of who must pay how much. Concomitantly, so long as health plans defer to "accepted medical practices" in determining for which services and products the plan will pay—as many still purport to do[143]—they, too, permit physicians to dictate the economic underpinnings of health care.[144]

It is not clear what qualifies physicians to make such far-reaching social judgments for other people and their money. Resource questions go well beyond science and involve important trade-offs between benefits, costs, and other values.[145] As Bovbjerg noted more than two decades ago, many medical decisions concern risk reduction.[146] For instance, a physician might choose a more potent antibiotic not because it is the only one that can work, but because it marginally increases the likelihood of cure even though it is far costlier.[147] Similarly, tissue plasminogen activator and streptokinase are both effective in breaking up blood clots that cause heart attacks. The former may (or may not)[148] save one percent more lives, but at vastly higher cost than the latter. Likewise, radiologists can choose between traditional contrast dyes to highlight anatomic features for radiographic tests versus a newer but vastly more expensive low-osmolar version. The new dyes can reduce mortality in people who are at special risk for allergic reaction to the older agent, and they improve comfort for nearly everyone.[149] But as David Eddy points out, a decision to use the costly dyes for everyone, instead of just for those at special risk, carries significant opportunity costs. In one particular HMO, other uses of the same money could save thirty-five lives if used to increase mammograms to detect breast cancer, 100 lives if used for pap smears to detect cervical cancer, or 13 lives if diverted to improved cardiac care.[150]

Clearly, major value choices are often embedded in ostensibly "medical" decisions. As will be discussed in greater detail in Chapter 8, an intervention is not so much "necessary" or "unnecessary" per se, as it is useful to one degree or another toward some particular goal. Those goals are mostly matters of value, as are decisions about how much money is appropriate to spend and how much risk is acceptable in reaching for that goal.[151] As Justice David Souter pointed out in *Pegram v. Herdrich,* a cost-conscious health plan is more likely to witness ruptured appendixes from too few appendectomy surgeries, while a generous fee-for-service approach is more likely to produce unnecessary appendectomies.[152] Choosing which is "better" is a matter of values, not science. Health plans must constantly weigh the benefits that an expenditure will bring to a few individuals against the need to serve all their other enrollees. Those decisions in turn are limited by available premium dollars and by the uncertainties of future needs.

The implications of such trade-offs are hardly confined to health care. People have many priorities for their limited incomes, from housing and clothing to education and recreation. Just as the money spent on one kind of health care is not available for other kinds of health care, so, too, is it unavailable for other important goods and services.[153] There is no particular reason to grant physicians the unilateral power to make these value choices on behalf of everyone else. Although physicians' scientific knowledge and professional values surely warrant giving them a voice in the ways they will provide their services—and thereby some real influence over the ways health care resources are used—the greater voice surely should belong to those who purchase and receive the care and who forego other things of value every time their money is spent on health care.[154] Because different people can evaluate risk very differently and set their health care goals very differently, surely it is appropriate to permit individuals greater power than they now have to determine the direction of their own care.

D. CONCLUSION: THE TRADITIONAL CUSTOM-BASED APPROACH TO SETTING THE MEDICAL STANDARD OF CARE SHOULD BE ABANDONED, AND A NEW APPROACH TO PHYSICIANS' MALPRACTICE LIABILITY SHOULD BE IDENTIFIED

Little justification exists for retaining the traditional, uniform, physician-set, practice-based standard of care. As resource availability degenerates into ever wider variations, no particular practice routines "prevail." We cannot presume that actual medical practices reflect considered professional judgment. We cannot reasonably single out which among the plethora of minority practices are reputable or disreputable, because doing so presupposes highly disputable values. We cannot fairly insist that physicians owe to patients a panoply of resources they neither own nor control. And surely we should not penalize physicians because those who do own and control resources have refused to provide them. Finally, we should neither expect nor permit the medical profession unilaterally to choose the values that will set the amounts and purposes for which other people must spend their money.[155]

In sum, we must fundamentally reconceive physicians' legal duty of care toward their patients. After examining comparable challenges in tort and contract for health plans in the next two chapters, we will try to answer these challenges in Part II.

3

HEALTH PLANS AND TORT LIABILITY

This chapter begins with an historical focus, discussing why tort liability has not posed a major challenge for health plans until relatively recently. A principal factor is plans' tradition of merely paying for, rather than attempting to shape, the care that patients receive. Additionally, federal ERISA law has provided a powerful shield.

Thereafter the recent growth of tort liability for health plans is explored. A significant chink in ERISA's protective armor has now opened up, permitting tort causes of action even against employment-based plans. Beyond this, two tort causes of action previously applied to hospitals have now been extended to health plans: indirect liability for the actions of plans' employees and agents and direct liability for plans' own duties to their subscribers. Additionally, a somewhat new avenue for liability focuses on the question of whether a corporation such as a health plan can, in the most literal sense, practice medicine and thus be accountable for medical malpractice in the classic sense levied against physicians.

Finally, this chapter discusses some of the problems spawned by health plans' emerging tort vulnerability. First, such liability is not always ascribed on the basis of well-conceived rationales. Because judges must sometimes "make it up as they go along," it is difficult for MCOs to plan appropriately for legal risks. Second, because tort litigation traditionally focuses on injured individuals, it is difficult for courts to attend adequately to health plans' need to enforce policies that serve the best interests of their broader population of enrollees—policies that, even if excellent on the whole, will sometimes disadvantage particular individuals.

A. HISTORICAL OVERVIEW

Until the last few years, health plans were not often accused of causing harm by denying coverage for care, for the simple reason that they rarely denied coverage. Third-party payors were mainly cost-plus, pass-through financiers who rarely challenged how much or for what services they were asked to pay. Indeed, payors actually benefitted from the rising cost of health care, reaping higher profits as long as employers simply absorbed their annual premium increases.[1] In addition, because reimbursements were retrospective, patients had already received care by the time any denial of payment was made. As a result, disputes concerned monetary issues to be settled in contract, not denials of care that might have precipitated tort claims.

The other major source of tort insulation for health plans has been federal ERISA law. A brief description will suffice here, because Chapter 11 explores in depth the issues surrounding this law. ERISA, the Employee Retirement Income Security Act of 1974,[2] was enacted during an era of economic "stagflation"[3] in which many businesses appeared unable to meet their commitments to fund employees' retirement. "In fact, it was becoming increasingly apparent that many long time employers might be unable to meet benefit obligations owed to aging work forces. . . . At the same time, Congress was concerned that the Social Security system, itself strained by the increasing demands made on it by retired workers, could not be relied upon to provide adequate retirement benefits for the vast majority of covered workers."[4]

Against this background, Congress passed ERISA to ensure that employee benefit plans are established on financially sound principles and, as part of that goal, to ease the burdens that arise for employers operating in more than one state as they tried to fit their benefit plans to fifty different sets of laws. The statute established a quid pro quo: In exchange for requiring that pension plans be funded and administered under federal specifications, all benefit plans (not just pensions, but also welfare benefits such as health plans) were placed under a uniform set of federal rules that would ease their administration, minimize unanticipated expenses, and thereby make it easier for firms to offer and maintain such benefits. State-based claims against benefit plans were thereby preempted in favor of purely federal causes and remedies.[5]

Through this preemption ERISA has largely shielded insurers and MCOs from such familiar causes of action as malpractice, wrongful death, fraud, breach of contract, and the like because these claims all reside in state law rather than in federal law. Equally important is the fact that, even though ERISA plan beneficiaries can sue their health plans in federal courts, available remedies are very limited. Unlike states' allowances for punitive damages, noneconomic damages, and the like, ERISA generally limits recovery to the actual economic value of whatever benefits were wrongly denied, plus limited additional remedies such as attorneys' fees.[6] As a result, plaintiffs are sometimes left with no remedy at all for an injury that might under state laws have been a tort permitting substantial damages.[7] In other cases the plaintiff collects only the relatively small sum an MCO should have spent on health care, and no further compensation when a denial of care has caused death or lifelong disability. Over the years ERISA has thus posed a formidable obstacle to those hoping to make health plans pay for the consequences of allegedly wrongful denials of coverage.

B. GROWTH OF LIABILITY FOR HEALTH PLANS

These historic shields are rapidly eroding. ERISA's tort protection for health plans, hardly anticipated during the 1970s, has been controversial. In response, Texas state legislation has explictly broadened health plans' tort liability when they make treatment decisions negligently,[8] a move upheld in federal court.[9] Several other states have enacted similar legislation.[10]

Further, recent case law has opened a significant chink in the ERISA armor. Courts have begun to distinguish between the question whether benefits were improperly denied, versus whether the benefits that were provided were of adequate quality. In this emerging line of cases, disputes about the quantity of benefits continue to be restricted to federal courts and remedies. But when the plaintiff disputes the quality of the benefits he received, courts are increasingly willing to remand these cases to state courts for exposure to the full panoply of state-based causes and remedies.[11] Chapter 11 will discuss this shift in detail.

Outside the ERISA context, liability for health plans has grown, largely on liability models established earlier for hospitals.[12] For many years it was thought that hospitals could not be held liable for the conduct of physicians practicing within their walls. After all, physicians are independent contractors applying highly esoteric knowledge, skill, and judgment, and hospitals should not try to direct their professional actions. Indeed, any attempt to exert that sort of control might have been regarded as an illicit attempt on the part of the hospital to engage in the corporate practice of medicine.[13] Absent such control, no room existed for traditional vicarious liability, which is applied to employers regarding employees whose conduct, by definition, the employer controls.

With *Bing v. Thunig,*[14] however, that began to change. Although charitable hospitals had long been immune from liablility for medical (as opposed to administrative) errors committed by doctors and nurses within their walls, in 1957 New York state's highest court challenged this tradition. It is both good morality and good law, the court declared, "that individuals and organizations should be just before they are generous, and there is no reason why that should not apply to charitable hospitals."[15]

Darling v. Charleston Memorial Community Hospital[16] opened the door wide to hospitals' vicarious liability for physician conduct. The Illinois Supreme Court held in 1965 that hospitals have a duty to use care in selecting and supervising their physician staffs. *Johnson v. Misericordia Community Hospital*[17] extended these principles as the Wisconsin Supreme Court held that a hospital could be held negligent for carelessness in selecting physicians, allowing a physician to perform procedures for which the hospital knew (or should have known) him to be unqualified, and failing to investigate when the hospital had (or should have had) reason to believe a physician was unqualified to practice. The court required, among other things, "that a hospital should, at a minimum, require completion of the application and verify the accuracy of the applicant's statements, especially in regard to his medical education, training, and experience."[18]

From these and other landmark cases, two types of liability have emerged, first concerning hospitals, then applied to health plans: direct and indirect.[19]

1. Direct Corporate Liability

Under direct corporate negligence, hospitals and health plans owe certain duties directly to patients. A widely followed 1991 Pennsylvania case, *Thompson v. Nason Hospital*[20] found that hospitals have direct duties to (1) maintain "safe and adequate facilities and equipment"; (2) "select and retain only competent physicians"; (3) "oversee all persons who practice medicine within its walls as to patient care"; and (4) "formulate, adopt and enforce adequate rules and policies to ensure quality care for patients."[21] In 1998, *Shannon v. McNulty* explicitly extended these duties to health plans.[22]

For health plans the first of these duties, regarding facilities and equipment, applies mainly to MCOs that own their own hospitals, clinics, and other facilities, though in principle it could extend to MCO duties to ensure that any independent facilities with which MCOs contract are likewise safe and adequate. The remaining three duties require, among other things, that health plans review staff physicians' credentials and, if evidence suggests problems in qualifications or competence, take appropriate remedial actions, restrict their practice, or remove them from the medical staff. For health plans the fourth duty, regarding rules and policies, has been additionally interpreted to encompass defective design or implementation of utilization review mechanisms.[23] Other courts have echoed this overall approach, so that direct negligence has become a standard liability concern for health plans whenever ERISA does not preempt such suits.[24]

2. Indirect Liability

Indirect, or vicarious, liability comes in two forms.[25] The more traditional form is vicarious liability for the misdeeds of employees. This can include not just nurses and technicians, but also physician-employees.[26] As with direct corporate negligence, hospital law was the progenitor of the doctrines now applied to health plans.[27] In these cases, a central question often is whether the physician or other provider in question is actually an employee, subject to the direction and control of the hospital or plan, because employment or another relationship of control is prerequisite for a finding of standard vicarious liability.[28]

An updated version of this traditional *respondeat superior*, dubbed *implied authority*, particularly applies to MCOs. Even when a physician is an independent contractor, an MCO may bear vicarious liability for that physician's medical malpractice if it has "exerted sufficient control over the alleged agent so as to negate that person's status as an independent contractor, at least with respect to third parties. . . . The cardinal consideration for determining the existence of implied authority is whether the alleged agent retains the right to control the manner of doing the work. . . . Where a person's status as an independent contractor is negated, liability may result under the doctrine of *respondeat superior*."[29] In other words, implied authority applies when the independent contractors (here, the HMO's physicians) are effectively, even if not contractually, employees.

The other form of vicarious liability, called *ostensible agency* or *apparent authority*, again begins with the fact that ordinarily a hospital or health plan cannot be held liable for the actions of independent contractors because they do not employ these individuals or control their actions. However, when the plaintiff has been induced to believe that the physician is an employee or agent of the hospital or plan, the hospital or plan may be liable as though it were an employer.[30] In today's vigorous marketplace such beliefs may be invited, for instance, by hospitals' and plans' energetic advertising. Overall, "to establish a hospital's liability for an independent contractor's medical malpractice based on ostensible agency, a plaintiff must show that (1) he or she had a reasonable belief that the physician was the agent or employee of the hospital, (2) such belief was generated by the hospital affirmatively holding out the physician as its agent or employee or knowingly permitting the physician to hold herself out as the hospital's agent or employee, and (3) he or she justifiably relied on the representation of authority."[31] Accordingly, health plans are now sometimes held liable even for the actions of physicians over whom they have little or no control on the ground that the patient looked to the health plan rather than to the physician for help, such that the physician thereby was ostensibly the agent of the plan.[32]

Other causes of action against health plans have also been lodged, of course, including breach of contract, bad faith breach of contract, breach of warranty, fraud, tortious interference with business relations, and the like.[33] These are of less interest in the context of this discussion, which focuses on liability for personal injuries caused by negligent or insufficient health care.

Notably, neither direct nor indirect liability claims propose that the health plan itself actually practiced medicine and is liable for medical malpractice in the classic sense alleged against physicians. Although suits have often listed "medical malpractice" as one of the causes of action against a plan, in fact most of the actual charges have been either for direct negligence or vicarious liability.[34] The plan is potentially liable not for practicing medicine on its own, but for the malpractice committed by its physicians.

3. Corporate (Mal)Practice of Medicine

This situation is changing, however. An entirely different avenue for health plan liability is now emerging, alleging corporate (mal)practice of medicine. These allegations are a marked deviation from historical concepts about corporate practice of medicine. As the doctrine emerged, largely through case law in the 1930s, courts held that corporations were forbidden to hire professionals such as physicians, attorneys, dentists, and optometrists.[35] Among various reasons, the most powerful arguments were that such ownership threatened to place laymen in control of delicate professional decisions and to place professionals in untenable divisions of loyalty.[36]

Indeed, a primary reason why early courts were so concerned about firms that employ physicians is that, by definition, employment relationships are those in which a master controls the nature and manner of a servant's work.[37]

The original, employment-focused doctrine is now largely (though not entirely[38]) defunct, either through judicial neglect or through a variety of explicit legislative exemptions granted to hospitals, academic medical centers, HMOs, professional practice groups, and the like.[39] Nevertheless, the doctrine's underlying concerns about lay control of medicine and the division of professionals' loyalty are as lively today as ever. New allegations are arising that, amidst the turbulent economic changes in contemporary health care, corporations themselves are beginning to practice medicine and should accordingly be held liable. Some of the relatively few courts that have considered the question directly have held that a corporation cannot literally commit medical malpractice because corporations are incapable of practicing medicine and because corporate practice of medicine is prohibited.[40] In other cases courts have avoided deciding the issue, holding that the cases were preempted by ERISA, therefore to be addressed in federal courts.[41] Still, the debate is heating up.

On the one hand, physicians and other commentators have pointed out that MCOs' economic judgments have an enormous impact on the care patients receive. When an MCO undertakes close utilization management (UM), it tells the physician or patient precisely which interventions it will and will not cover as "medically necessary." On this view, such detailed second-guessing of clinical decisions is clearly a form of medical practice, and, when MCOs thereby change or significantly influence the patient's course of care, these commentators conclude that the health plan is practicing medicine.[42]

On the other hand, MCOs generally insist that they do not practice medicine because, even with very detailed UM, they are simply interpreting contracts and making coverage decisions.[43] Providers remain free to treat patients as they wish, even when the plan declines to finance their care.[44] Moreover, states' licensing laws typically define the practice of medicine in terms of actions to "diagnose, treat, operate or prescribe for any human disease, pain, injury, deformity or physical condition."[45] Clearly, an MCO cannot physically examine, treat, prescribe for, or operate on a patient in the literal sense portrayed in these statutes.

The question cannot be resolved without more thoroughly discussing the concept of medical practice. That task is reserved for Chapter 8, which will show that health plans do, and sometimes must, practice medicine. When they do, they may face the same kind of malpractice liability physicians face, in addition to the more familiar causes of action for direct corporate negligence and vicarious liability.

C. CHALLENGES IN ASCRIBING TORT LIABILITY TO HEALTH PLANS

Clearly, health plans are as capable as any other corporate entity of making errors that can wrongfully harm the clientele they aim to serve. And equally clearly, they should bear appropriate accountability toward those whom they injure, just as do other human and corporate persons in society. However, recent expansions of health plans' tort liability raise challenges that must be considered carefully.

Courts need to develop a coherent, defensible account of health plans' duties to their enrollees and apply it with reasonable consistency from case to case. This is the essence of sound common law, but, unfortunately, in the current scene such sound reasoning is sometimes hard to find. As the economics and organizational systems of health care change at breathtaking speed, courts have produced remarkably diverging opinions. When plaintiffs have sought cutting-edge technologies such as bone marrow transplant, for instance, courts have been unpredictable. Some have gone to great lengths to identify contractual ambiguities that permit plaintiffs to prevail, while other courts have cited the "plain language" of a contract to find that the technology is clearly not covered.[46]

Similarly, as noted above, courts have varied widely on questions such as whether health plans, including ERISA plans, can be liable under theories of ostensible agency.[47] Some of this confusion, of course, comes from health plans themselves when they fail to state clearly just what they will cover and what procedures they will use to decide the borderline cases (more on this in Chapters 4 and 9). But in many cases courts seem truly perplexed by a flurry of first-impression issues created by a host of very new mechanisms for financing, providing, and controlling health care. As a result of this confusion and unpredictability, it can be difficult for MCOs to plan appropriately for legal risks.

An even more profound challenge is for tort law to appreciate health plans' obligation to meet the needs not just of the individual who happens to be the plantiff in a given case, but of a whole population of subscribers. This recognition is sometimes lacking, as illustrated by two cases cited in Chapter 2.

In *Fox v. HealthNet*,[48] it will be recalled, an HMO denied autologous bone marrow transplant for a woman whose breast cancer had spread to her bone marrow, citing the lack of scientific evidence for the procedure's safety and efficacy.[49] Nevertheless, the jury awarded $89 million, including $77 million in punitive damages.[50] When courts look only at the desperate plaintiff, it seems reasonable to insist that health plans offer any treatment that might offer even the faintest glimmer of hope. Unfortunately, such glimmers can cost other patients dearly. When health plans fund every faint hope, they ultimately spend large sums on dubious interventions, leaving less money to meet obligations to all their other subscribers. By the time it was learned bone marrow transplant was ineffective for breast cancer, some 30,000 women had received the treatment at a cost estimated around $3 billion.[51]

Similarly, in *Muse v. Charter Hospital, Inc.*[52] an appeals court held that a psychiatric hospital had a duty not to "willfully interfere" with a physician's medical judgment by discharging a patient who could no longer pay for services. Without commenting on whether this particular hospital could or should have made greater effort to continue this patient's care,[53] it should be immediately apparent that if a hospital routinely provides uncompensated care simply because a physician wants his patient to have it, that hospital will not long remain open to serve anyone. Hospitals and other health care institutions must serve not just a lone individual, but large populations with diverse, competing, and often costly needs.

Leahy's discussion of screening protocols highlights the tension between individuals and populations powerfully.[54] Screening protocols recommend how often a particular test should be used to detect the presence of illness in otherwise asymptomatic individuals. They include mammography to screen for breast cancer; the occult fecal blood test to detect colon cancer; the prostate-specific antigen (PSA) test to look for prostate cancer; the Pap smear to identify cervical cancer; and a host of others. As Leahy notes, screening protocols are based on the certainty that a particular disease will occur, albeit with uncertainty regarding to whom. The objective is to minimize morbidity and mortality in cases in which treatment can cure or ameliorate the disease, but with trade-offs in cost and inconvenience. In the following extended excerpt he notes that

> at some point society must make a policy decision regarding how much expense and inconvenience it is willing to bear to address a given risk of disease. Once that policy choice is made, regardless of where the line is drawn, there will *always* remain a certain incidence of disease. . . . There will always be false positive results (causing needless further investigation), false negative results (causing failure to diagnose), and cases for which the chosen testing interval is too long (causing failure to diagnose in time to avert morbidity or mortality).
>
> The inconsistency arises when these predictable cases are realized, and the unfortunate patient—now plaintiff—develops disease despite conscientious application of the screening protocol. From the medical or epidemiological point of view, the case is straightforward: this is one of the cases that was predicted to occur, given the interval of testing and the limitations of the test chosen. The event is simply an instantiation of the prior known risk.
>
> In the courtroom, however, this statistical certainty that has been accepted at the policy level and integrated into a screening program may translate into personal liability for physicians implementing that policy. Juries focus retrospectively on the individual plaintiff before them who allegedly has been 'injured.' Retrospectively, the relevant legal question is reformulated to focus on the individual—could anything have been done to prevent this unfortunate individual from being injured? Could the screening test have been performed more frequently? Could another test have been done that might have led to a more timely diagnosis in this case?
>
> The answers to these questions will often be yes. But juries are not required to consider these questions from the prospective point of view in which injured individuals cannot be identified ex ante. . . . Nor does the jury consider the societal burdens of cost, convenience, and test-related morbidity of alternative testing protocols; it need not consider that other testing parameters suggested by plaintiff would have to have been implemented on a massive scale to have prevented plaintiff's injury. Instead, the jury focuses on the injured *individual,* and no currently enforced legal principle precludes its finding that the failure to use a different screening protocol or test 'proximately caused' the plaintiff's injury, and that compensation is therefore due.
>
> The problem with this process is that juries are performing a function which they are neither called upon nor qualified to perform. Under the auspices of addressing individual complaints, juries are reassessing and reformulating on an ad hoc basis all of the policies and medical evidence underlying the development of screening programs. The same logic applies to established diagnostic or treatment guidelines—carefully considered policies designed to serve society's best interests, and

based on the best available data, will be directly undermined if juries are permitted to overrule or ignore these guidelines in individual cases. From the defendant's point of view this is simply unfair, and from a societal point of view, it is simply bad policy.[55]

As Leahy notes so eloquently, tort law seems inadequately equipped to look beyond the needs and circumstances of individual litigants. No matter how well a resource policy maximizes good care overall, some people will be better off in this or that instance if a different policy had been adopted. Given that the outcome of focusing predominantly on individuals may thus be to thwart reasonable resource policies, it has become imperative to reconsider the ways in which tort law identifies health plans' duties to their members, both individually and collectively.[56]

Although subsequent chapters will attempt to resolve this challenge, a few reflections may be useful here. In principle, at least, tort law already contains a key element for a resolution. Tort law has never demanded perfection, only reasonableness—a notion that stems from broader concepts of fairness. On one hand, we believe it is unfair for an innocent victim to bear the costs of someone else's intentionally or carelessly harmful conduct. At the same time, we also believe that we should not ordinarily require someone to pay for others' misfortunes when his conduct was careful and prudent—hence, the usual tort interest in ascribing fault.[57] To determine whether someone is at fault, we generally ask whether his conduct was reasonable because we do not expect citizens to avoid all risks of harm, only unreasonable or unnecessary risks.[58] In that evaluation we appeal to the concept of the "reasonable person," or, in the case of medicine, to the reasonable and prudent physician.[59] In 1947 Judge Learned Hand brought economic concerns within the ambit of reasonableness by asking courts to weigh the seriousness and the likelihood of the harm we wish to avoid against the burdens incurred in avoiding that harm.[60]

Accordingly, malpractice law as applied to physicians has long accepted the fact that not every poor outcome, not every avoidable poor outcome, and not even every error amounts to negligence.[61] Rather, the important issue is whether an injury was caused by a breach of the physician's duty of care. If the physician acted with adequate prudence—a procedure- rather than outcome-oriented standard—then he is not at fault for negligence.

Health plans should be accorded the same leeway. The question should not be whether an enrollee fared poorly, or whether she might have done better if the health plan had made a different coverage decision. Rather, the question should concern procedures, in particular whether the plan undertook to answer the coverage question with adequate care and with fidelity to its contractual and other obligations. Within this sort of analysis, reasonableness balances the well-being of particular individuals against the specific obligations the plan agreed to undertake, and, indeed, against the well-being of all the other subscribers in that plan. Arguably, those others are owed a duty of "contributive justice,"[62] in which fairness requires attention to the needs and expectations of all those whose contributions make the plan possible and who rely on the plan for their care, just as does the plaintiff.

The challenge for courts in this setting is to ascertain where the balance of fairness and reasonableness lies. They must assess more clearly what health plans' duties to their enrollees are and what constitutes a breach of such a duty. They must define what constitutes culpable negligence on the part of a health plan and distinguish this from unfortunate but predictable outcomes of a reasonable resource policy. Some concrete proposals regarding this mission will be offered in Chapters 6 and 8.

4

HEALTH PLANS AND CONTRACT LIABILITY

Contract law has played a much larger role for health plans than it has for physicians because, although technically the physician–patient relationship begins in contract,[1] thereafter it is generally addressed in tort—a "contorts" approach, so to speak.[2] In contrast, the relationship between health plans and their enrollees is permeated by contract issues. Whether via indemnity reimbursement for incurred health care expenses or via a prepaid HMO that delivers a particular set of services, health plans perform insurance functions.[3] They spread the risks and costs of health care across a population, and in exchange for a premium payment they promise to reimburse or directly to provide a specified array of goods and services. Hence, when a health plan declines to cover an intervention desired by a subscriber, breach of contract, breach of warranty, or other contract-oriented claims are likely to figure prominently. Until fairly recently such claims were relatively uncommon, because health plans usually paid what was asked of them. A bit of history explains why.

The first Blue Cross plan was created in 1929 at Baylor University in Dallas, Texas, primarily to ensure that people could afford to pay for hospital care. Blue Shield plans were added soon thereafter to cover physicians' services.[4] Health care rapidly became a standard workplace benefit during and immediately following World War II, and when the federal government added Medicare and Medicaid in 1965, the great majority of citizens were covered by a system that was essentially a cost-plus, pass-through arrangement that paid providers virtually whatever they asked, to perform virtually whatever services they wanted to do.[5] Such a system was highly inflationary, of course,[6] but health plans continued to defer to physicians' judgments about what care a patient ought to have and how much their services were worth. Medical care, after all, is complex and esoteric; surely such decisions are best left in the hands of professionals.

By the 1960s, however, rising costs prompted insurers more frequently to question obviously pointless or noncovered kinds of treatments. And as costs began to rise more dramatically, they also tried to restrict payment to only "medically necessary" care. When enrollees challenged denials of coverage, however, courts commonly construed *medically necessary* in favor of subscribers and awarded benefits. In response, insurers began to specify that they, not providers, were entitled to determine which interventions were medically necessary. They also wrote increasingly explicit exclusions to deny experimental and investigational treatment,[7] ultimately incorporating specific, detailed lists of services and products they would not cover.[8]

The judicial system's reinforcement of generous, largely unquestioning reimbursement has been dubbed *judge-made insurance.* The term refers to many judges' tendency to interpret insurance contracts according to what the beneficiary might reasonably have expected or should have been entitled to expect, rather than according to a literal reading of contract or according to this particular beneficiary's actual expectations.[9] As noted in one study, it was almost irrelevant how narrowly or broadly a health plan wrote its exclusions: "This is because courts so frequently fault insurers for not making their coverage exclusions more explicit. When insurers attempt to correct this defect, however, they are criticized for making the exclusion too narrow or technical."[10] As Chapter 10 will explain, such judicial favoritism toward beneficiaries began to abate significantly in the mid-1990s[11] as courts showed increased deference to contractual language. Still, health plans can face significant judicial hurdles when they attempt to deny coverage.

Contract claims against health plans can figure in three basic litigation scenarios. The first scenario is prospective: the patient wants treatment that the plan has thus far denied and it is still medically reasonable to pursue the treatment. These cases typically arise as requests for injunctive relief. If the plan is an HMO, the request is for actual treatment, while if the plan is an indemnity insurer, the focus is usually on advance assurance of payment.[12] As one court noted, "due to the high cost of major medical treatment, individuals who obtain such treatment typically depend upon insurance of some kind to cover much if not most of the bill. In the current healthcare market, absent pre-claim verification of insurance coverage, patients may be forced to leave a hospital without receiving needed treatment."[13]

The other two scenarios are retrospective, meaning that they take place after treatment decisions have been made and carried out. In the second scenario, a plaintiff who has already been fully and timely treated, or in some cases the providers who provided that treatment, may sue to recover reimbursement in a purely financial action.[14] The third scenario arises after treatment has been either denied altogether or has been received but significantly delayed. Here, the plaintiff seeks damages under breach of contract and in most cases will also pursue tort action if the delay or denial has caused injury.

A. OBSTACLES TO EFFECTIVE CONTRACTING

Contract issues can figure prominently in all three of these scenarios, even if tort takes the spotlight in the third.[15] In the case of health care, however, contracts tend to differ from more typical business contracts, such as those for building homes or purchasing supplies. One difference, unfortunately, is that health plan contracts fail to satisfy some of the usual requirements for effective, enforceable contracting. In particular, they tend to feature ambiguity, adhesion, and arbitrariness.

A long-standing principle of contract adjudication is that ambiguity in the terms of a contract should resolved against the drafter. This traditional doctrine, called *contra proferentem,*[16] is based on the fairness principle that, since the party writing the agreement had the opportunity to make the wording clear, its failure to do so should not harm the party who lacked that opportunity.[17] Hence, in the presence of genuine ambiguity, judges have little alternative but to favor the patient.

Ambiguities pepper health care contracts, primarily from two sources. First, health plans generally define covered benefits not by enumerating precisely which particular products and services an enrollee is entitled to receive under what conditions, but rather via vague terms such as *medical necessity.*[18] That is, plans essentially promise to cover medically necessary care within whatever coverage categories the contract includes,[19] subject to whatever exclusions the plan lists. So long as a service is within an accepted category and is deemed necessary (i.e., is not excluded as unnecessary), ostensibly it is covered. As Chapter 8 will explain in detail, the vagueness of *medical necessity* creates a host of problems.

The second source of ambiguity stems from plans' tradition of operationally defining medical necessity by deferring to "accepted professional practice."[20] Until recently, this approach was relatively unproblematic, justified largely by the fact that clinical medicine is too complex to permit specifying every detail of care for every ailment.[21] Moreover, so long as funding was generous, physicians' practices were relatively consistent because they were predicated on the medical question of whether an intervention was safe and effective, uncomplicated by other dimensions such as cost-effectiveness.

As noted in Chapter 2, however, plans are no longer willing to defer so readily to physicians' customs. Increasingly, plans seek to limit what they cover. Many have substituted their own proprietary, undisclosed clinical guidelines to assess ordinary care and have adopted specific procedures to assess new technologies and innovative procedures.[22] At this point health plans exhibit endlessly varying interpretations of their medical necessity language. They have also been writing more exclusions into their coverage, yet even these are often worded rather vaguely.[23] Accordingly, through all this vagueness and variety, judges must often favor plaintiffs, and plans have a difficult time enforcing contractual limits.[24]

At least some measure of vagueness is unavoidable in health care contracts. To specify exhaustively which interventions are covered, an insurer would have to describe all of medicine—what diagnostic and therapeutic interventions are indicated under exactly what conditions and nuances of conditions. Clearly this is impossible.

Still, the situation is not hopeless. Chapter 9 will explore ways to ameliorate the problem significantly.

Conditions of adhesion pose a related but distinct obstacle to enforceable contracting. In a contract of adhesion, "the parties to the contract [are] of unequal bargaining strength; the contract is expressed in standardized language prepared by the stronger party to meet his needs; and the contract is offered by the stronger party to the weaker party on a 'take it or leave it' basis."[25] Thus, a contract might be very clearly written, avoiding problems of ambiguity. But if the drafter has an advantage because of the other party's vulnerability, courts will still scrutinize the arrangement with a skeptical eye.

Adhesion can figure prominently in health care. Individual subscribers ordinarily have no opportunity to negotiate the terms of their plans, and even corporate employers often have limited leeway to specify what they, as distinct from other firms, want in their health plans. When individuals have so little control over the terms of a contract that secures such an important service, courts have tended to be very deferential to the vulnerable individual. Historically, for example, courts have invalidated so-called exculpatory clauses, in which the patient agrees to waive his right to sue for substandard care as a condition for receiving care.[26] In other cases, courts have discarded arbitration clauses when they were deemed adhesory.[27]

In health care an added source of adhesion arises from the fact that many patients cannot even choose their health plans, because most employers who provide health coverage offer only one or two options.[28] When this is the case, it is even more difficult to argue that the subscriber should be held to contractual terms and limits of someone else's choosing.[29]

Arbitrariness poses the third major obstacle to effective contracting in health care because it, too, requires judges to favor the subscriber over the plan. Whereas ambiguity concerns the written language of the agreement, arbitrariness focuses on the human process of implementing and interpreting whatever is written. Unfortunately, the inevitable vagueness in health plan contracts virtually guarantees some measure of arbitrariness as different administrators decide which medical interventions are necessary, unnecessary, or experimental. Even when several health plans ostensibly use the same guidelines, actual decisions about which patients should receive which interventions can fluctuate significantly.[30]

In a further entrée for actual or apparent arbitrariness, it was noted above that many health plans' definition of medical necessity is now shifting away from the traditional reliance on professional customs toward detailed guidelines that vary from one plan to the next. Because these guides are often proprietary and undisclosed, little opportunity exists to ascertain, in advance, just what kinds of care each plan is likely to consider necessary for which medical indications. So long as plans purport to cover all medically necessary care and then base necessity judgments on covert guidelines,[31] an appearance of arbitrariness is inevitable.

The same problems affect health plans governed by federal ERISA law.[32] Although courts generally must defer to benefit decisions made in good faith, particularly when made by administrators who are ERISA fiduciaries obligated to serve the best interests of beneficiaries,[33] judges can override decisions they deem arbitrary and capricious or an abuse of discretion.[34] Unfortunately, the widely differing ways in which plans' guidelines and utilization review procedures interpret contracts' already vague language has precipitated the appearance (and sometimes the reality) of arbitrariness. Courts have therefore overturned benefit denials in in a number of ERISA cases.[35]

B. CONSEQUENCES OF INEFFECTIVE CONTRACTING

The net result of these problems of ambiguity, adhesion, and arbitrariness is that when health plans try to enforce limits on the amounts and kinds of resources they provide, they can easily lose when challenged in court.[36] This creates serious problems. Perhaps on a superficial level it might seem desirable for individuals routinely to prevail over health plans when litigating contract disputes. After all, the individual is relatively defenseless against the large, well-funded health plan. Each of us is a health care patient at least some of the time, and so when we picture ourselves as that lone soul fighting the behemoth, it is tempting to cheer for the "little guy."[37]

However, ineffective contracting combined with poor judicial enforcement even of clear contract limits can ultimately work to virtually everyone's disadvantage. Two scenarios help to illustrate the problems.

In the first scenario, suppose the contract is genuinely unclear about whether the patient should receive a particular intervention. At the level of the individual dispute, obviously the plaintiff should prevail—*contra proferentem.* But on a broader level, the lack of clarity itself poses important problems. As noted previously, health plans now vary widely in what they cover for various conditions. Some of that variation is desirable (a point reserved for Chapters 9 and 10), but when real differences among plans are hidden, it becomes difficult for citizens to make intelligent, informed choices about which plan to buy, at what price, with what opportunity-cost to their other priorities. Vagueness is thus a failure to achieve the "meeting of the minds" that is ideally a hallmark of contracting and which, when achieved, permits citizens to make decisions that reflect their values.[38] At the same time, only if contracts are enforceable in court will citizens be free to make such choices in the first place.[39]

In a second scenario, suppose that a contract is reasonably clear and states that a particular resource is not covered. If the patient nevertheless prevails, another serious problem arises. Again, although on the immediate level it may seem appealing for someone to receive care beyond what his plan covers, the ultimate price is high. By implication of both fairness and rationality, anyone else with a similar, also-not-covered need should receive a similar measure of extracontractual benefits. After all, the essence of justice is to treat similar cases similarly.[40] The cumulative cost can be substantial, and the money available for patients elsewhere in the plan is diminished. Health plans, after all, must serve all the needs for an entire population from a finite financial pool.

The diminution of resources available to others in the plan may not be visible in obvious morbidity and mortality statistics. Rather, the price will more commonly be paid in quality of life: reduced physical therapy for those recovering from stroke or accident; reduced nursing staff and longer waits to receive pain medications; longer delays to see one's primary care physician.[41] The extra benefits that are given to a few thus represent a betrayal of faith toward those who have lived within the limits of their contract and who will be adversely affected by the reduction in funds available for their care. The imbalance thus offends contributive justice.[42] Further, to the extent that courts impose costs that health plans had not anticipated, future premiums must rise, which in turn may well mean that some individuals or some employers will no longer be able to afford health care coverage. Diminished affordability can thereby lead to diminished access—already a major problem in a nation in which over forty million citizens lack assured health care access. According to one estimate, every one percent increase in premium costs results in loss of insurance coverage for 400,000 Americans.[43]

Perhaps even more vexing, when health plans are effectively precluded from saying "no" openly and when they must still limit expenditures, they may feel impelled to resort to less up-front approaches. Plans may create cumbersome bureaucratic procedures, routinely modify those rules, deny payments to those who violate them, or delay payments even to those who punctiliously follow the rules.[44] This much-hated "hassle-factor" may sometimes be the only means health plans have for the necessary task of limiting expenditures. Physicians, in response, feel ever more free to lie and "game the system" if patients are to receive the care they need and if physicians are to be paid what they want for doing what they think they ought.[45]

Such wars serve no one very well.[46] They consume enormous amounts of time that should otherwise be spent on serving patients' needs; they extinguish much of the joy that many physicians once found in their profession; they make life hellish for patients caught in the middle; and, ultimately, they do not even serve health plans' need to disperse resources as they are obligated while limiting them as they must.

In sum, contract terms and contractual liability for health plans need a major overhaul. When standard conditions for effective contracting are satisfied, two parties have the freedom to come together in an agreement that expresses their values and priorities and can generally promote their best interests. But in health care, conditions for effective, enforceable contracting are not well satisfied. Contracts tend to be ambiguous; they are commonly concluded under power imbalance and a take-it-or-leave-it adhesion; and, largely because they are so poorly constructed, their administration tends too often to be arbitrary. As a result, courts often have been reluctant to enforce health plans' resource limits, particularly when a desperately ill patient seeks costly but possibly life-prolonging treatments.

Such contractual confusion poses problems for virtually everyone. Patients cannot be sure precisely what they buy when they sign on to a health plan, and sometimes they cannot find out without layers of appeal or even litigation. Neither can patients make informed choices among health plans when the content of those plans is unclear or when an employer chooses the plan for them. Providers likewise are ill-served if they must spend too much time wrangling over whether this or that intervention will be paid for. Plans, for their part, face increasing difficulty in enforcing resource limits. No health plan can do everything for everyone, and when plans are forced to deliver more than they had intended, the actuarial process of setting realistic premiums and of keeping the plan fiscally sound enough to serve all its members can become a major challenge.

II

ADDRESSING THE PROBLEMS: RESHAPING LEGAL STANDARDS

5

PINPOINTING THE ISSUES

Chapters 2, 3, and 4 of Part I suggest that legal accountability for physicians and for health plans, in both tort and contract, has reached a jurisprudential crossroads.

Chapter 2 showed that the familiar standard of care physicians owe their patients has become untenably simplistic. Traditionally, physicians' duties to patients emanated from prevailing practices that, under affluent third-party payment, took little note of economic concerns. As new technologies emerged they often became standard, still regardless of patients' ability to pay. Resource constraints have changed the picture dramatically, however, as physicians are now subject to a wide and often conflicting array of guidelines and expectations from MCOs, specialty societies, colleagues, malpractice insurers, and patients. It has become incoherent to speak of "the" standard of care. Physicians no longer can, and arguably no longer should, unilaterally determine what kinds and levels of care should be purchased for which patients. Accordingly, tort law's physician-made, one-size-fits-all duty of care no longer describes what physicians can provide, let alone what they should legally owe their patients. But if the usual standards are no longer defensible, it is unclear just what should replace them.

Chapter 3 observed that for health plans, tort liability is on a rapid upswing. Direct, corporate duties now require that health plans exercise reasonable prudence in selecting and retaining their physicians, in creating and administering their policies and procedures, and the like. *Respondeat superior* can hold health plans, like other employers, responsible for employees' errors. And under ostensible agency and related doctrines, plans can even be liable for the actions of independent physicians whom they do not control. A new avenue of liability may also be emerging via a modified version of the old corporate practice doctrine. The high cost of health care has meant that MCOs' decisions about which care they will cover as being medically necessary can have an enormous impact on patients' care. If this constitutes practicing medicine, then, perhaps MCOs should be held liable for classic medical malpractice of the same kind as physicians.

These developments raise important questions. First, the rapid evolution and unpredictable fluctuation of liability make it difficult for MCOs to plan for and meet their legal responsibilities. Second, traditional tort law focuses mainly on injuries to identified individuals, with relatively little attention to the rationale behind whatever policies may have led to this individual's injury. Yet MCOs must meet the needs of a whole population, and sometimes even well-justified policies will adversely affect individuals. As tort law attempts to hold MCOs more accountable for how they treat enrollees, it becomes important first to identify what their duties are, to whom they are owed, and how duties to individual patients are to be reconciled with duties to the entire population.

Finally, Chapter 4 argued that conditions for effective, enforceable contracting are not well satisfied in the realm of health care. Health plans' contracts are vague in what they promise; patients have little or no power to negotiate the terms of their contracts or even to choose among plans; and daily decisions about who gets what within a plan can seem and sometimes be arbitrary. As a result, courts often have balked at enforcing MCOs' denials of coverage. To the extent that MCOs have difficulty enforcing limits on resource use, they sometimes must turn to other approaches to limit expenses and assure fiscal solvency. They may raise premiums or, when that is not feasible, may feel impelled to "game" providers and subscribers, creating a hassle-factor that effectively, even if not overtly, denies resources.

The upshot of these three chapters is a portrait of wide-ranging disarray in the law of tort and contract for health care. The implication: a new approach must be forged. The very essence of law, as an institution for regulating human conduct in society, requires that the demands of law be reasonable, or else they will not command the respect that is a precondition of obedience. And they must be fairly clear and predictable, or else citizens will not be able to plan their conduct in accordance with them.[1] These requirements, in turn, require a coherent rationale about what sort of conduct tort and contract law should expect from MCOs, employers, providers, and patients.

Chapter 5 begins by exploring two prospective answers to this challenge. The first would free health plans considerably from these emerging liabilities by demanding that they bow out of their intense involvement in medical decision making. They would not be liable for practicing medicine or denying care because they would no longer be interfering with medical judgments. The other proposal, from the opposite end of the spectrum, would have health plans bear all legal liability for mishaps in health care.

As the flaws in each approach are examined, this chapter will argue that an appropriate reconstruction of tort and contract law for health care cannot be framed until we begin with the right question. Instead of asking whom we want to hold liable for what, we should inquire what conditions are necessary for delivering high-quality health care. This focus, in turn, gives rise to the question of whom we want to control what in the delivery of health care. Only after we determine who should be controlling what can we then go on to establish what duties are owed to patients by health plans and what duties are owed by physicians. And only then can it finally be discerned who should be liable for what, via breaching those duties. Once this central issue of control has been identified, Chapter 5 then proposes a rough outline of how health plans' and physicians' respective realms of control and responsibility might plausibly be allocated.

A. TWO PROSPECTIVE ANSWERS TO THE JURISPRUDENTIAL DILEMMAS

1. Proscribe Interference with Physicians

The first proposal for addressing the legal challenges posed by medicine's changing economics is to fix the flaws in the old corporate practice ban. In a nutshell, health plans could hire physicians, as many now do, but would be expected to refrain from controlling physicians or interfering with medical care. They would not need to fear malpractice liability because they would stop practicing medicine.

The original corporate practice doctrine, which prohibits corporations from hiring physicians as employees, has largely become anachronistic as hospitals, staff-model HMOs, and a variety of other entities routinely hire physicians. This is part of a massive, ongoing reorganization of the economic structures by which health care is now delivered.[2] However, it has also been recognized that an employment relationship is hardly the only means by which MCOs exert control over physicians. Health care is often so costly that patients can ill afford to pay out of pocket, and providers straining under reduced fees and increasingly frequent reimbursement denials and delays are less able to provide care gratis. Hence, a denial of coverage or even a sluggish utilization review process can exert a powerful influence over which services are realistically available.

Notwithstanding such broadened opportunities for corporate control of medicine, it can also be argued that the flourishing diversity of economic arrangements for health care delivery has helped to spawn useful innovations and to contain costs that had previously been spiraling out of control. Indeed, the Federal Trade Commission (FTC) has long opposed the traditional corporate practice ban for just such reasons. In the 1940s the Supreme Court held that the American Medical Association (AMA) had illegally restrained trade when it tried to discourage its physician members from practicing in an HMO setting.[3] And beginning in 1975, the FTC ordered the AMA to remove its ethics-code restrictions on contract- and corporate-practice on the ground that these provisions stifled innovation and illegally restrained trade.[4]

Accordingly, one approach now advanced by a number of commentators would retain but significantly modify the corporate practice doctrine. The focus should shift away from whether corporations hire physicians to emphasize issues of control: corporations must not interfere with physicians' clinical decisions. They must abstain, that is, from practicing medicine. Thus, Mars argues that "[u]nless a corporation is truly interfering with its employed physicians' medical judgments, there seems to be no sound basis for the continued blanket and unconditional prohibition on contractual employment arrangements."[5] He suggests that "[t]he line of demarcation that courts have drawn, based on structure, should be reanalyzed in terms of whether the form of arrangement is truly interfering with a physician's freedom of action. . . ."[6]

Several states have moved in this direction. In 1996, for instance, Tennessee enacted legislation freeing hospitals from the corporate practice ban while mandating that they not interfere with physicians' medical judgment.[7] Similarly, a South Dakota statute, while continuing to ban corporate practice per se, stipulates that employing physicians does not constitute practicing medicine so long as the relationship does not "'[i]n any manner, directly or indirectly, supplant, diminish or regulate the physician's independent judgment concerning the practice of medicine or the diagnosis and treatment of any patient.'"[8]

Superficially the proposal seems attractive. After all, the real concern about corporate practice of medicine is not the employment status, but rather MCOs' control over physicians. And so instead of proscribing particular structural arrangements, the proposal is to require plans to stop intruding their own medical judgments into patient care decisions.[9]

Such intuitive appeal, however, fades quickly as the proposal's implications are traced out. "Interfering" in clinical decisions seems to be defined as any action that might cause a physician to alter or diminish her proposed course of care. This definition seems implicit, for instance, in the case of *Muse v. Charter Hosp. Winston-Salem Inc.,* discussed previously.[10] A sixteen-year-old boy, admitted to a psychiatric hospital for suicidal ideation, was discharged by the hospital when his insurance funding ran out. The North Carolina appellate court held that, by discharging the boy merely because funding had expired, the hospital had "interfered" with the physician's medical judgdment.[11] Such reasoning implies that a hospital—or, by extension, a health plan or any other entity that might employ or closely contract with physicians—must permit physicians to use whatever resources they want, lest the hospital or plan "interfere" with medical judgment and thereby practice medicine.[12]

The problem with this approach is that it fails to recognize that every medical decision is also a spending decision. If physicians have unfettered medical freedom, ipso facto they also have unfettered economic freedom to spend others' money and consume others' resources. By implication, MCOs would have little or no direct power to control costs. In an era when the cost of care has risen to nearly unbearable levels, effectively precluding access for millions of citizens, it is difficult to defend giving any single party so much control over shared financial resources.

Admittedly, if MCOs were forbidden to guide physicians' practices directly, they could still exert other forms of cost containment, such as by transferring financial risk to physicians.[13] Under these kinds of arrangements, physicians are freer to deliver care as they please because they personally bear the costs of their medical excesses. Such risk transfers create significant problems of their own, however, because they place physicians in systematic conflicts of interest, raising ethical and perhaps also legal problems.[14] Beyond that, so long as the MCO has the contract with the patient, the MCO must ensure that enrollees receive the quantity and quality of care for which they have paid. This responsibility can in turn require MCOs to monitor physicians very closely and sometimes to redirect patients' care.[15]

In the final analysis, once we agree that MCOs may—perhaps must—"interfere" at least sometimes with physicians' spending decisions in order to conserve resources[16] or, in a risk transfer setting, "interfere" sometimes to ensure that the appropriate quality and quantity of services are being provided, we are left with powerful questions about who should be controlling what in the delivery of health care. That issue will be addressed below, but not until after we see this very same question about control arising via another route.

2. Enterprise Liability

While the above approach would reduce MCOs' liability by insisting that they stop practicing medicine and stop controlling physicians, an alternative would have MCOs shoulder all legal liability, including malpractice, because they are viewed as the best locus of legal responsibility. This "enterprise liability" approach was originally proposed as a way to address broader flaws in the tort system.[17] By consolidating tort liability at the locus where most malpractice incidents happened—identified at that time as the hospital—and by focusing all litigation on just one party, it was hoped that faster, less costly resolution of tort claims might be achieved. Further, it was hoped that hospitals might use their influence to enhance the quality of care delivered within their walls and, reciprocally, that physicians no longer under litigation pressure could avoid the heavy costs of malpractice insurance and might feel less impelled to resort to costly defensive medicine.

Enterprise liability as a hospital-oriented proposal did not gain much foothold, partly because changing economic conditions soon meant that MCOs rather than hospitals became the more important locus of control over the financing, delivery, and accountability of care.[18] However, some commentators now support translating the essential concepts underlying enterprise liability into the world of MCOs. As Clark Havighurst, one of its leading advocates, proposes, MCOs "should bear exclusive legal responsibility for the negligence of physicians treating their subscribers."[19] In a more recent, somewhat revised version of this view, Havighurst recommends a default rule whereby "a health plan is vicariously, and exclusively, liable for medical malpractice and other torts committed by health care providers whom it procures to treat its enrollees."[20] Plans and providers would be contractually free to shift risk to downstream providers,[21] but plans would bear "ultimate responsibility . . . for the quality of the health services their enrollees receive."[22]

Several rationales support this approach. For one thing, when MCOs are the main agents of cost containment, they may need the threat of legal liability to keep their cost cutting from paring down quality.[23] At the same time, MCOs are better positioned than are individual physicians to serve as the centers for information technology, disease management, and other population-oriented health care improvements.[24]

Because these system-wide factors are often the root causes of adverse outcomes, MCOs should bear responsibility and, in the process, become prime movers for monitoring and improving quality of care. In addition, it might be hoped that "physicians—relieved of many concerns over individual liability—might participate more readily in cooperative decisionmaking and might be less resistant to clinical practice guidelines and other efforts by health plans to induce cost-effective practice on a system-wide basis."[25]

Finally, "the market-oriented health policy of the 1980s and 1990s could easily give way to heavy-handed government regulation of MCOs unless private-law remedies for torts and breach of contract are perceived to provide adequate deterrence of quality lapses."[26] Such regulatory intrusions could squelch a wide array of potentially useful cost-saving and quality-enhancing innovations in health care delivery. Accordingly, Havighurst concludes that enterprise liability, recast as vicarious liability through a default rule, is the "logical legal culmination of the shift to de facto corporate responsibility that is revolutionizing American health care."[27]

In sum, on this view, conferring legal accountability onto MCOs may be the only way to deflect undesirable regulation, legitimize managed care in the eyes of the public and its political representatives, ensure a reasonable level of quality, and secure a viable level of market freedom to assure continued innovation and improvement of care into the future.[28]

Up to a point, these are cogent arguments for expanding health plans' legal accountability. Plans need to be more careful about the quality implications of their cost cuts and, on the positive side, should take a greater role in improving overall quality of care. However, requiring MCOs to bear all of the liability—for all physicians' errors as well as for their own lapses—is a very different proposal, and it has major drawbacks.

The first challenge is empirical, questioning the assumption that holding plans liable for every aspect of physicians' care is actually likely to enhance the quality of care. To cite a potentially analogous situation, if health plans respond to this proposed rise in their legal risks the same way plans responded to recent years' rise in their economic risks, there is good reason to wonder. Arguably, health plans' cost controls have often been medically and sometimes even financially counterproductive.

Some of the tactics have been quite crude. Some MCOs, for instance, required physicians to seek approval for every intervention costing more than $200, sometimes forcing them to wait long periods, only to speak with a utilization clerk lacking the education or medical sophistication to understand the request.[29] Other MCOs have been said to "deselect" a physician merely for ordering an ambulance to transport an unconscious patient; or to limit specialist referrals to just one visit, thereby introducing considerable inefficiency and discontinuity of care; or to contract with hospitals far from members' homes, potentially exacerbating an illness or injury while a patient is en route to the distant site.[30]

Other tactics have been subtler but not necessarily wiser. Tightly constrained pharmaceutical formularies, for instance, may save short-term drug costs but can raise rates of hospitalization and emergency room use, as some patients experience greater side-effects and adherence problems with older, cheaper, or generic drugs that are not fully equivalent to their newer counterparts.[31] Standard utilization review and gatekeeping arrangements are costly and may be only marginally effective.[32] Failure to make timely specialist referrals can generate multiple visits, extensive testing, and treatment failures.[33]

If MCOs' increased economic risks have precipitated clinically counterproductive intrusions, increasing their legal risk could have a similar effect. After all, whoever bears risk, whether economic or legal, has an incentive to take whatever measures might limit that risk.[34] And those measures, particularly if undertaken by people who have legal or business expertise but no medical expertise, can potentially impede good patient care.[35]

Indeed, another instructive parallel may come from physicians' malpractice experience. Evidence suggests that there is, at most, a tangential connection between the existence of negligent injury and the filing of a tort claim. As noted previously, most negligent injuries do not lead to a claim, and reciprocally most claims are not associated with negligent injuries.[36] At least partly because of this unpredictability, many physicians respond to the tort threat not with systematic, quality-focused improvements in care, but with costly defensive medicine tactics that are often medically pointless even if they soothe physicians' nerves.[37]

Hence, the empirical challenge: we have seen that health plans have not always responded in prudent, clinically well-founded ways to their enormous economic pressures and that, elsewhere in the system, physicians do not always respond in prudent, clinically well-founded ways to their legal pressures. It is not clear why, then, we should expect that health plans would respond in prudent, clinically well-founded ways if suddenly they bear all legal liability for everyone's errors. Perhaps they would respond magnificently. But given the indications to the contrary, the burden of proof is on whoever would insist that massive expansion of plans' liability would help more than harm. Bona fide quality improvement is costly and extremely complex. And since the majority of suits arise not from poor quality of care, but from poor relationships,[38] it may be far more likely to see plans respond to increased legal pressures by improving their public image and by doing the kinds of things that make people feel loved and cared for, regardless of whether they are getting good care.

These empirical concerns are only part of the problem.[39] An even deeper problem concerns how courts should identify the standard of medical care to which health plans should be held when they are exclusively, vicariously liable for physicians' professional malpractice. That is, if plans shoulder all liability for the quality of physicians' care, how should we define the plans' duty of care? As noted in Chapter 2, current common law usually permits physicians to set their own standard of care, largely via prevailing practices—a flawed approach that, as is argued there, needs to be overhauled. In the context of enterprise liability, however, an unusual twist emerges. Because physicians would no longer shoulder liability for their own conduct, it is unclear whether courts would or should continue to let physicians determine, through prevailing practices or any other means, just what sort of care they should provide for their patients. If the whole idea of enterprise liability is to place health plans under pressures to improve quality, then courts would have little reason to permit physicians to continue to determine what "quality" is, even regarding their own professional services.

Three scenarios are possible. In one scenario courts might choose, purely on their own authority, what sorts of care health plans and physicians should have delivered to which patients, for which particular medical conditions. The untenability of this idea is readily obvious. Medicine is extraordinarily complex, and the judiciary and its lay jurors are in a poor position, except perhaps in unusual cases,[40] to determine what tests and treatments physicians and health plans ought to have provided, with what level of skill and expertise. Surely the bulk of the medical standard of care should be set by those who are well-versed in health care, even if, as argued in Chapter 2, physicians should not exercise unilateral authority.

Alternatively, courts might permit MCOs to establish physicians' standards of care. A major objective of enterprise liability, after all, is to promote greater MCO influence over day-to-day clinical practice.[41] Below it will be argued that plans should indeed have a role in developing and implementing the guidelines by which clinical care is delivered, but for now we must note that the merits of any guideline or episode of care must ultimately be appraised with at least the aid of medical science and professional judgment. Health plans can gather important statistical information about how well its enrollees fare overall under what sorts of protocols, but this cannot reliably tell us what sort of care—or what exceptions to those protocols—are warranted for particular individuals. Plans must serve populations, but they must still do so by caring for human beings, one by one. If health plans are permitted to determine, unilaterally and completely, what constitutes "adequate" quality of care, it is plausible to envision major deteriorations in quality as managers with a keen eye toward the bottom line and perhaps too little clinical knowledge decide what to call "good enough." As discussed below, the guidelines that many MCOs currently use are not always of the highest scientific calibre, and even well-founded guidelines do not apply to every patient.[42]

A third scenario remains. Even if all liability is shifted from physicians to health plans, physicians could still establish the standards for their own services via their prevailing practices, as is traditional. MCOs would then be liable when their physicians deviated from their peers' prevailing practices.

Yet even this option is fraught with hazards from two directions. From one side, it could defeat an important purpose of enterprise liability, namely, to encourage MCOs to influence physicians' standards in positive ways, as Havighurst suggests they can by creating centers for information technology, error reduction, disease management, and other population-oriented health care improvements. These improvements can be implemented only if MCOs modify, rather than uniformly defer to, physicians' customary behavior.

From the other side, MCOs bearing sole liability for adverse medical outcomes might require their physicians to adhere closely to MCO-chosen guidelines, that is, to insist that their physicians' prevailing practices be the ones the MCO has chosen for them. After all, if courts define medical malpractice in terms of physicians' actual conduct, as stipulated in this third scenario, plans could ensure that their

MCO guidelines *become* the prevailing standard simply by requiring rigid adherence from their physicians. Once that happens, then adherence will almost always be legally adequate to ward off adverse malpractice judgments, even if the guidelines were created ineptly and even if patients fare poorly under them. The more rigidly and uniformly the MCOs enforced their guidelines, the more security they would have that even a patient with an adverse outcome would fall within the standard of care—the empirical standard that they themselves created and enforced.

The problem of who sets the standards rums deeper. Quality in a realm so complex as health care is unlikely to be achieved by a strictly one-way flow in which information, guidelines, and instructions go from the MCO to the physicians, as the former "supervises" the latter to ensure that its standards are met. Optimal quality of care requires that physicians reciprocally "supervise" the MCO to advise when a guideline is not effective or when it does not serve a particular patient's needs. Checks and balances are essential. However, if MCOs bear all legal responsibility for adverse outcomes, and if, indeed, the very adoption of a particular guideline will tend to make that guideline the standard of care, then MCOs may not be warmly receptive to physicians' challenges. Important clinical input may never reach the MCO.

Reciprocally, physicians in such a system may be loath to challenge their MCOs. Under the current system, the prospect of a malpractice suit does, of course, haunt physicians. But physicians also know that the great majority of adverse outcomes do not lead to malpractice claims, even when the injury was the product of negligence.[43] Physicians can also take reasonable steps to ward off suits, partly by emphasizing rapport and good communication,[44] and partly by documenting carefully both their care and the reasoning behind it. Moreover, when tort claims are filed, the financial costs of litigation and adverse judgments are usually covered by malpractice insurers. Nothing can completely remove the unpleasant threat of malpractice suits, but for these reasons in most situations the issue can remain reasonably well in the background of daily clinical practice.

The scene would be strikingly different under enterprise liability. Here, the MCO, not the tort lawyer, poses the threat. And that threat is constant and up-front, not intermittent and residing in the background. The prospect of being fired by the MCO or of having one's privileges or income reduced may be much more likely and more immediate than the chance that a tort claim may be filed. After all, a vigilant MCO that is constantly monitoring its physicians' every move will be far more likely than the average patient to spot an error—defined as any deviation from what the MCO deems appropriate. Moreover, the financial damages of being disciplined by the MCO are borne, not by an insurer, but by the physician himself, and those costs could be substantial.

One answer is, of course, for the physician to ensure that his care is of high quality. But more realistically, the physician may feel impelled to ensure that his care is high-quality *as perceived* by the MCO. He will be rewarded for following the guidelines, not for challenging them. If the MCO's guidelines are poor, then let the MCO bear some well-deserved liability. Under such a scenario, where the physicians may be penalized for challenging the MCO but not penalized for failing to challenge, physicians may not be eager to help improve quality by pointing out MCOs' guidelines flaws.

As a further disincentive to being the "squeaky wheel," physicians would also be aware that MCOs typically evaluate them not just on their medical quality, but on their economic performance. Being a costly physician could trigger an unfavorable review, just as being a poor-quality physician could. Thus, although enterprise liability may theoretically give health plans an incentive to strive for quality, it may actually give physicians perverse incentives to cooperate with the quality quest in only superficial ways. Such a "don't-rock-the-boat" complicity could produce a mediocrity that no one would embrace.

In the end, such heightened MCO control over clinical practices raises the very spectres that prompted the original corporate practice bans so many years ago: lay supervision over intimate, medically sensitive decisions between physicians and their patients and a dividing of physicians' allegiances between patients and corporations. As noted by the Indiana Supreme Court: "The master is in a position where he may dictate to his servant the manner of conducting his business, the kind and nature of the goods to be sold and furnished to the patient, in order to procure the most favorable financial gain to the employer. And this may be done without regard to the public health. . . ."[45] And as the New York Court of Appeal observed in a case involving corporate practice of law:

> "The relation of attorney and client . . . involves the highest trust and confidence. It cannot . . . exist between an attorney employed by a corporation to practice law for it, and a client of the corporation, for he would be subject to the directions of the corporation, and not to the directions of the client. There would be neither contract nor privity between him and the client, and he would not owe even the duty of counsel to the actual litigant. The corporation would control the litigation, . . . and the attorney would be responsible to the corporation only. His master would not be the client but the corporation, conducted it may be wholly by laymen, organized simply to make money and not to aid in the administration of justice which is the highest function of an attorney and counselor at law."[46]

In sum, where corporations feel pressed to control every detail of the medical care for which they bear legal risk, even beyond the economic risks they now bear, the implications are troubling.

B. THE REAL DISPUTE: WHO SHOULD CONTROL WHAT

An important lesson has emerged from examining these two attempts to answer the jurisprudential challenges precipitated by medicine's rapidly changing economics. Statutes forbidding health plans from "interfering" with physicians' clinical judgment would avoid the problems of "nouveau-corporate practice" of medicine, but at the cost of handing virtually all clinical, and thereby all economic, control to physicians. Reciprocally, however, enterprise liability would give all legal responsibility, and de facto thereby virtually all clinical control, to the health plans. Their opportunities to practice medicine would burgeon, quite likely to patients' detriment at least some of the time. Between these unsavory alternatives—ceding all economic control to physicians versus ceding all clinical control to health plans—there must surely be a better answer.[47]

It begins with the suggestion that these two analyses start with the wrong questions. The first approach begins with the implicit question of how to preserve clinical control in physicians' hands, a view presupposing that all control should, indeed, be in the hands of physicians. In the second approach, proponents of enterprise liability begin with the question "whom do we want to bear liability in health care," a view presupposing that the most important question is who should bear the costs of adverse outcomes. As argued above, however, we should not assign liability to an MCO for anything we do not wish the MCO to control. If we do not want MCOs to create all the guidelines for medical care and force physicians into lockstep compliance, even when good clinical judgment would dictate otherwise, then we should not place upon MCOs the kind of liability that could inspire them to exert such control.

Accordingly, instead of asking "how do we preserve physician control" or "who should bear liability," the lead question should focus on how to achieve the kind of quality clinical care we want—whom do we want to control which aspects of health care. That is, if we want good health care and good health care systems, we must ask which party is best able to perform a given function in providing care. On the obverse of the same coin, if we do not want a particular party to exercise control over some aspect of health care, then we should not assign liability to that party. Instead, liability should be aimed toward those who, by antecedent analysis, could and should have exercised control.

The answer to the question of who should control what aspects of health care is neither simple nor self-evident. As the following analysis suggests, high-quality health care should best be achieved by a sharing of control and responsibility, appropriately distributed between physicians and health plans. It will be useful, first, to consider some of the reasons why neither health plans nor physicians should have exclusive, unilateral control over health care before outlining, after that, a rough sketch of how controls and responsibilities might be most fruitfully allocated.

1. Limits on Health Plans' Control

In any high-quality health care system, physicians must be able to exercise a considerable degree of independent clinical discretion in the care of individual patients.[48] The initial reasons are classic and familiar.

First, medicine requires complex judgments. The physician must bring scientific generalities and finely honed skills to the care of individual patients whose personal and biological idiosyncrasies may defy any standard routines of care. Unlike more mechanistic vocations such as plumbing or carpentry, the hallmark of any profession is the need to make judgments that combine an esoteric, expansive knowledge with a host of uncertainties and peculiarities inherent in individual situations, toward the objective of meeting deeply important human needs.[49] At some point, only a physician who has personally examined a patient can discern the specific character of that person's signs, symptoms, and statements and bring these together into a coherent picture of what is happening and what could or should be done. Although more distant observers can comment intelligently, a professional directly involved with the patient is almost always in the best position to determine whether those suggestions actually fit the realities of the case.

Second, in this era of high-technology medicine it has become impossible to provide even simple, mundane kinds of care without ready access to an array of resources. An orthopedist cannot diagnose a fracture without radiographs and cannot surgically reduce that fracture without a well-equipped operatory theatre; an oncologist needs sophisticated pharmaceuticals, radiation, and chemotherapy, even if optimal use of those agents should be subject to broader discussions; an infectious disease specialist needs quick access to laboratory tests and antibiotics to treat bacterial meningitis or pneumonia, again even if some of the specific therapeutic choices can legitimately be influenced by resource constraints; a primary care physician must be free to provide a variety of common tests and treatments. Admittedly, not all medical routines are well-conceived, and vexing questions surround new technologies. As argued below, health plans have a legitimate role in providing general guidance for both medical and economic efficiency in health care. But in daily clinical care, physicians should not be required to plead "mother may I" for literally every resource for every patient at every turn. Endless delays to secure innumerable approvals can be medically hazardous and demoralizing to physicians and patients alike.

Third, good health care is often impossible to provide without a personal relationship between patient and provider. The patient who does not trust her physician may be unwilling to disclose medical history that can be crucial to diagnostic accuracy, or she may be unwilling to adhere to treatment if she does not believe the provider is both knowledgeable and devoted to her best interests. Physicians can examine and prescribe endlessly, but if patients refuse to cooperate, it is to little avail. Reciprocally, the patient who asks for a particular intervention may be deeply suspicious if her physician, embedded in financial incentives or in an MCO-controls-all health plan, suggests that such an intervention is unnecessary. The result can be a gamesmanship that thwarts both clinical quality and economic prudence.

Such physician–patient trust requires that physicians have sufficient flexibility to be able to negotiate with patients to reach mutually acceptable courses of action. If the physician does not have the discretion to offer choices that will suit the patient's personal circumstances and values, then in an important sense, the physician and patient do not relate to each other. They relate instead to a third party who tells each of them what to do.[50] The more severely that MCOs limit physicians' capacity to fine-tune guidelines to patients' needs, the less is the opportunity for trust, and the poorer those patients' care may be.

Finally, even though physicians can, of course, err, and even though their clinical routines are not always based on the best of science and judgment, MCOs are not necessarily better suited to do the job. In particular, the tools by which MCOs currently second-guess physicians' judgments are often deeply flawed. Although practice guidelines have proliferated in health care,[51] many of those by which MCOs make benefit determinations and utilization management decisions, and which they expect physicians to follow, have a seriously inadequate scientific basis. The reasons are numerous.

Many important topics in medicine have not been studied scientifically.[52] Although new drugs and devices must be scientifically proven to be safe and effective before they can be approved for commercial marketing, much of clinical medicine does not fit this mold. Surgeries and other invasive procedures are under no such regulatory requirements, and they can be difficult to study under rules of classic science.[53] Thus, although coronary artery bypass surgery was first performed in 1964, its efficacy was not scientifically evaluated until 1977. Similarly, angioplasty to open clogged arteries in the heart was "performed in hundreds of thousands of patients prior to the first randomized clinical trial demonstrating efficacy in 1992."[54]

In like manner in 1988, a national conference on antithrombotic therapy (anticlotting treatments used to prevent stroke, pulmonary embolism, and the like) evaluated the scientific foundation for various recommendations on which physicians based treatment. The American College of Chest Physicians found that only twenty-four percent of those recommendations were based on appropriately scientific studies, while fifty-five percent were based on uncontrolled clinical observations. Ten years later, forty-four percent of the recommendations were science-based, although this was largely because of Food and Drug Administration requirements for testing new drugs.[55]

In a related area, a number of medical devices have never been subjected to systematic scientific evaluation because the government does not require this for devices already in use at the time device regulations were enacted. As a result, some devices, such as the pulmonary artery catheter, introduced in the 1970s for monitoring the cardiopulmonary function of critically ill patients, have not been thoroughly studied. Recent evidence seems to indicate that this device, although widely used, may actually do more harm than good, and some critics have called for a moratorium on its use until further evaluation can be undertaken.[56]

Once a drug or device is approved for a given indication, physicians can use it as they wish. For "off-label" uses, and indeed throughout ordinary clinical care, physicians often have little science on which to base their decisions, so that a large proportion of clinical practice is off-label. Until fairly recently, for example, much of the scientific testing required for new drugs did not include children or fertile women as research subjects.[57] The omission was intended to protect children and potential fetuses, and yet the result is that we have only limited knowledge about important differences in the ways drugs work in and are metabolized by children and fertile women.

One kind of research emerging to meet this deficit is called *outcomes studies*, intended to establish better correlations between what physicians do during clinical care and the results that patients actually experience, both long- and short-term. Unfortunately, outcomes studies in general suffer from a lack of standardized methodologies—what counts as an outcome, which costs should be tallied, etc.[58] Among legitimate methodologies, each has distinct advantages and disadvantages. For instance, administrative databases (hospital billing records) permit great breadth, quantity, and easy availability of data but are often littered with gaps and inaccuracies.[59] Furthermore, because many organizations undertake their outcomes studies independently, it is difficult for any single project to be large enough to achieve statistical significance.[60]

In other cases, studies may seem scientific yet lack any acceptable methodology at all, while still others may be corrupted by researchers' personal conflicts of interest.[61] One pharmaceutical company, for instance, compiled an extensive registry listing patients who had had a particular illness (e.g., heart attack) and what treatments they received with what outcomes. The registry paid physicians to provide considerable information about the use of drugs manufactured by the company, but not about patients who received alternate treatments. As a result, not only were there no controls, there was no comparative information. Though such a study has the look of science and is often cited by physicians, it is not seriously scientific.[62]

In the worst examples, some of these industry-sponsored outcomes studies are simply marketing devices with no scientific merit whatever. One such "study," for instance, was ostensibly intended to

> assess the efficacy and tolerability of [the company's drug] in controlling mild-to-moderate hypertension. The sponsor used its sales force to recruit 2500 office-based "investigators" who were frequent prescribers of drugs in the therapeutic class in question. Each investigator was to enroll 12 patients (for a total enrollment of 30,000) and was offered reimbursement of $85 per patient enrolled, or $1050 per physician. The "study" was not capable of achieving even the modest objectives stated. There was no control group, and the study was not blinded. There was thus no possibility that it would generate useful data on efficacy and little likelihood that it would produce data on safety other than the potential for detecting a rare adverse event.[63]

A significant portion of outcomes studies and pharmacoeconomic research is undertaken by drug and device manufacturers, insurers, managed care organizations, and employers, any of which can be affected by substantial conflicts of interest.[64] Such conflicts do not automatically taint the research with bias, but the hazards cannot be dismissed. At the other end, studies undertaken by government or academic groups may ignore considerations of economics and cost-effectiveness.[65]

As a result of such factors, when MCOs or other entities create the guidelines that are then used to shape clinical care or to make benefit decisions, those guidelines may not be based on adequate science. In such situations, guidelines creators may simply rely on the Merck manual, Medicare guidelines, "an administrator who 'asked friends who are doctors,' or an insurance company's employee-physician (usually not a specialist in the field in question) who reads textbooks and discusses the issue with other insurance company physicians."[66] As several commentators have observed, "materials such as the practice guidelines prepared by Milliman and Robertson, a well-known actuarial firm, often rely on insurers' own decisions rather than on well-designed scientific research."[67] Even when scientific studies are available, they are not always incorporated into guidelines because groups and organizations that construct guidelines may have agendas other than scientific purity, or they may simply fail to perform a sufficiently thorough search for available studies.[68]

Often, a dearth of good studies prompts guidelines creators to assemble panels of experts who provide their professional experiences and opinions. Here, further opportunities for bias arise if those who choose these experts have a financial interest in the conclusions these panels reach.[69] Even when panelists attempt to remain as free as possible from bias and conflict of interest, their personal values can shape their final recommendations powerfully, as, for example, when they assess the desirability of various outcomes.[70] Even if an MCO manages to produce an excellent set of guidelines based on the best available evidence and the most careful reasoning of a well-chosen panel, there is always the further challenge of keeping those guides up to date as new technologies emerge and as knowledge about them continues to evolve.

Yet the problems do not stop here. Even the best-designed, most scientifically well-founded guidelines will not apply well to every patient. The most pristine kind of science, the randomized, double-blind, controlled trial, can be particularly problematic. In order to test strictly for the effects of the specific drug or procedure under investigation, scientific study design must be restricted to patients who fit a narrow set of eligibility criteria. Typically, they must suffer exclusively from the particular disease whose treatment is being studied, with a minimum of other diseases and medications because other diseases and treatments can make it difficult for scientists to distinguish between the effects of the study treatment and other potentially confounding factors.[71] Once the study is complete, however, its results are applied in clinical practice to all those complex patients who would never have been eligible to be test subjects in the study.[72] For example, regarding coronary artery bypass surgery, Gellins and colleagues observed that "only 4 to 13 percent of the patients who now undergo this operation would meet the eligibility criteria for the randomized controlled trials that established its efficacy."[73]

Thus, the more highly controlled and perfectly scientific a study is, the less its enrolled subjects resemble the ordinary souls, with their multiple problems, for whom ordinary physicians care. No guidelines can be detailed enough to accommodate patients' vast variability; their biological idiosyncrasies, complex conditions, and atypical presentations do not always fit into preestablished categories.[74] Hence, to the extent that guidelines are plainly inapplicable in an individual case, physicians must have discretion if they are to do what that patient needs.

Equally important, guidelines do not always leave room for issues that are personally important to patients. Many studies collect data on only a limited array of outcomes, such as mortality or tumor shrinkage, and do not include factors such as a treatment's effects on quality of life.[75] Neither do they routinely allow for patients' personal preferences,[76] which can be crucial for long-term adherence to therapy—especially important in chronic illness.

In sum, MCOs cannot at present claim to provide anything resembling an immaculate conception of how health care should be delivered.

2. Limits on Physicians' Control

The story does not end here, however. Unlimited clinical discretion for physicians is not the best way to optimize health care, either, even aside from financial concerns. Contrary to common assumptions, physicians—even subspecialists—do not necessarily share a basic foundation of knowledge and skills. Actual clinical practice varies widely, often with no underlying basis in patients' illnesses.[77] And those practices often are not based on sound science. "[S]everal studies estimate that only 15 to 20 percent of medical practices can be justified on the basis of rigorous scientific data establishing their effectiveness."[78]

Part of the problem is that medicine is permeated with uncertainties. As noted above, many features of human physiology and function and of the medical tests and treatments applied to them have not been adequately studied. Moreover, no individual physician knows everything that the profession as a whole knows, nor will any one physician master every skill with proficiency. And patients sometimes present biological idiosyncrasies that defy the textbooks. As a result, most clinical scenarios permit a number of acceptable approaches. Choosing one approach over another is less a matter of science and medicine than a matter of values regarding the management of uncertainty.[79] It becomes difficult for physicians to insist that they, and they alone, should be entitled to make all these nonmedical judgment calls.[80]

Perhaps more important, physicians do not always adhere even to those practices that are widely agreed to be appropriate. Overuse, underuse, and misuse of medical interventions are common, presenting significant problems in the quality of health care throughout the United States.[81] As one analysis suggested, "there are large gaps between the care people should receive and the care they do receive. . . . [A]bout 50 percent of people received recommended [preventive] care. . . . An average of 70 percent of patients received recommended acute care, and 30 percent received contraindicated acute care. For chronic conditions, 60 percent received recommended care and 20 percent received contraindicated care."[82]

Specific examples of overuse—excessive care—are not hard to find. Antibiotics, for instance, have often been used with unnecessary frequency and potency, with the result that resistant organisms are increasingly a problem.[83] In the realm of heart disease, evidence suggests that coronary angiography and revascularization (by-pass surgery) is used significantly more in the United States than in Canada and Europe, with no apparent justification in terms of patients' degree of illness or infirmity.[84] Although the jury is still out, recent studies suggest that the aggressive, interventionist approaches common in the United States do not necessarily reduce the rate of heart attacks compared with drug-based approaches and that aggressively treated patients may have a higher rate of treatment-associated adverse events.[85] Even the use of some heart drugs appears excessive.[86]

In the same vein, intensive surveillance of women in preterm labor "had no effect on the primary outcomes . . ., but did lead to significantly more unscheduled visits and greater use of prophylactic tocolytic drugs."[87] Another study found that, according to one set of utilization guidelines, nearly eighty percent of tube insertions to treat children's middle ear infections would have been judged unwarranted.[88] A particularly disturbing study concluded that between 1991 and 1995 psychotropic medications prescribed for preschool children increased dramatically despite inadequate evidence of safety and effectiveness in this population of two-to-four-year-olds.[89] Doubts likewise can be raised about the use of growth hormone therapy in children who have no growth hormone deficiency or other recognized medical need for the treatment.[90]

In other cases, underuse is the problem. Heart disease again provides some leading examples. During a myocardial infaction (MI, or heart attack) thrombolytic (clot-busting) agents can dramatically improve survival rates, yet these drugs are seriously underused.[91] Similarly, for patients who have survived an MI, aspirin and beta-blocker (β-blocker) drugs can significantly reduce the likelihood of a second episode. Yet studies show that an average of only thirty-seven percent of physicians actually prescribe these drugs for their post-MI patients.[92] In another study, "less than 50% of cardiologists' patients were taking β-blockers."[93] Likewise, it is well known that patients with congestive heart failure (CHF) can benefit greatly from angiotensin-converting enzyme (ACE) inhibitor drugs, yet in one study of patients with CHF "only three quarters of eligible patients were taking an [ACE] inhibitor, and only 60% of those were at doses known to be efficacious."[94]

In like manner, it is well known that many surgery patients are at significantly increased risk for thromboembolism (blood clots). Although an array of safe and effective means can greatly reduce this risk, they often are not used. In a study of Medicare patients from twenty community hospitals in Oklahoma, appropriate preventive (prophylaxis) "measures were implemented for only 160 (38%) of 419 patients studied. . . . Only 97 (39%) of 250 patients . . . at very high risk received any form of prophylaxis and of these 97, only 64 patients (66%) received appropriate measures."[95]

In the same vein, many physicians, particularly primary care providers, fail to prescribe standard anti-asthma medications, such as inhaled corticosteroids.[96] Physicians also commonly fail to order standard diabetes care, such as frequent glucose monitoring, regular cholesterol checks, and annual retinal exams.[97] Physicians widely fail to prescribe diuretics for hypertension, despite evidence that they are safe and effective. Instead, prescriptions for hypertension and many other common conditions lean more toward high-cost, highly advertised newer drugs such as calcium-channel antagonists that may, in fact, have greater risks and lower efficacy.[98] More broadly, evidence indicates that physicians may sometimes unwittingly base treatment and drug selection decisions more on the basis of drug advertisements than on medical literature.[99] In still other examples, physicians often do not: recognize and treat depression in the outpatient setting; use anticoagulents for patients in chronic atrial fibrillation; use breast-conserving surgery for women with localized breast tumors;[100] wash their hands between patient visits.[101] In sum, a broad variety of simple, widely accepted, routine health interventions are often neglected.[102]

Misuse likewise presents significant problems. "Researchers studying elderly patients found that 38 percent of those who received antidepressants, 19 percent who received oral hypoglycemics, 18 percent who received sedatives, and 13 percent who received nonsteroidal anti-inflammatory drugs (NSAIDS) were given a poten-tially inappropriate drug."[103] Peptic ulcer disease is often mistreated. It is now known that this condition is often caused by a bacterium, for which antibiotics are the treatment of choice. Nevertheless, one study showed that "physicians continued to use traditional and ineffective [drugs] as their preferred approach for 72 percent of all patients."[104]

Another study concerned the new Cox-2 arthritis medications. The main virtue of these costly new drugs is to reduce the risk of causing gastrointestinal bleeding for patients, such as people with arthritis, who must use pain relievers continually. The new drugs offer no better pain relief than otherwise comparable pain relievers, so there is no reason to prescribe them for patients who need only short-term relief. Nevertheless, one large physician group found that within nine months after these drugs appeared on the market, physicians were routinely prescribing them for the wrong patients.[105]

A further example of misuse emerges when improvements highlight earlier errors. Salt Lake City's Latter Day Saints Hospital created computer algorithms to guide proper antibiotic use for patients in intensive care. Physicians were free to override the computer's suggestions, but those who followed them achieved a seventy-six percent reduction in patients receiving antibiotics to which they were allergic, a seventy-nine percent reduction in excessive drug dosage, and a ninety-four percent reduction in patients who received the wrong antibiotic. These patients also left the hospital 2.9 days earlier than those whose physicians overrode the computer's rec-ommendations.[106]

Diagnostic accuracy is not always better than therapeutic choices. In a ten-year retrospective review of autopsies at a major New Orleans medical center, re-searchers discerned that of the 250 tumors found at autopsy, 111 were undiagnosed or misdiagnosed. Of particular concern, in fifty-seven percent of these patients, the underlying cause of death was directly related to the undiagnosed or misdiagnosed malignancy.[107] In other diagnostic areas, studies suggest that "simple clinical predic-tion rules have proven superior to physician judgment in the diagnosis of acute abdominal pain . . . , acute myocardial infarction . . . , tonsillitis . . . , pneumonia . . . , intracellular vs. extracellular causes of jaundice . . . , presence of ankle fracture . . . , survival after diagnosis of Hodgkin's disease . . . , [and] coronary artery disease."[108]

Even standard techniques of physical examination may not always be mastered. A recent study evaluated the ability of trainees in internal medicine and family practice to recognize important sounds when listening to patients' hearts. Overall, the residents recognized only twenty percent.

> [A]ll residents we tested had great difficulty in identifying 12 commonly encoun-tered and important events. Residents were incorrect 4 of 5 times, improved little with year of training, and were not more accurate than a group of medical students. Indeed, trainees in both residencies were less accurate than students [for certain kinds of heart sounds]. . . . [W]e found minimal gains, if any, as a result of resi-dency training. Deficiencies of this type will probably persist even after residents

enter practice. Indeed, increasing evidence in the literature seems to suggest that errors in physical diagnosis are commonly encountered among generalists. These errors may even lead to greater utilization of resources and a higher cost of care.[109]

When significant clinical deficiencies such as those listed above are directly pointed out to physicians, they do not always change their clinical practices. Studies suggest that concerted, systematic attempts to encourage physicians to adopt improved approaches are often unsuccessful.[110] Some observers have suggested, perhaps somewhat cynically, that entrepreneurial concerns may sometimes be relevant in this preservation of old routines.[111]

Error rates of institutional providers such as hospitals have also been studied. A widely cited study of New York hospitals during the mid-1980s concluded that the rate of adverse events was 3.7%. Although an error per se does not entail substandard care, researchers found that the overall rate of negligent adverse events was 1%.[112] A more recent study found that over an eight-year period the rate of medication prescribing errors increased significantly.[113] More recently, an Institute of Medicine study concluded that errors in hospitals may cause as many as 98,000 deaths per year.[114]

These serious, rising rates of error, overuse, underuse, and misuse of medical interventions are not entirely surprising, and they should not prompt hasty condemnation of the medical profession. During the past several decades, "an explosion has occurred in the proliferation and supply of drugs, the availability of technological tests and bedside procedures, and the array of high-tech diagnostic methods and invasive therapeutic maneuvers. Each of these changes creates new opportunities for error."[115] As medical science becomes increasingly complex, and with it the health care systems through which it is provided, it has become unreasonable to expect physicians to continue their traditionally unilteral responsibility for care and for outcomes.

C. WHO SHOULD CONTROL WHAT: SEEKING A REASONABLE BALANCE

At this point several observations sit somewhat uneasily together. On one hand, forbidding health plans to "interfere" with physicians' judgment would effectively require them to give physicians unfettered clinical discretion—probably medically suboptimal as well as financially costly. On the other hand, the guidelines by which health plans exert clinical control often are based on inadequate science, and even scientifically based guidelines cannot supplant the need for professional judgment to fine-tune clinical care to individual patients' distinctive biological and personal needs.

If one conclusion seems evident, it is that neither physicians nor health plans should monopolize clinical control. A thoughtful division of labor based mainly on which party is better suited to do which tasks appears to make better sense. What follows should not be deemed some sort of hard-and-fast recommendation for distribution of control. At most it suggests one reasonable approach to allocating responsibilities between health plans and physicians. Neither does it propose a rigid separation. As health care delivery evolves, considerable fuzzing of these boundaries is likely. Nevertheless, some kinds of tasks seem more suitable for the organization level, while others seem more suited to the personal, clinical level. This discussion will focus primarily on health plans because their role is under such vigorous evolution.

1. Health Plans

Clearly, there are some things that only physicians or other individual practitioners can do.[116] Only a human clinician can physically examine a patient, ask about medical and social history, and discuss the delicate, private matters that can make a crucial difference to a particular patient's diagnosis and treatment. Only an individual surgeon can decide what should be done at the moment something goes wrong in the operating room. Health plans cannot hope to review every physical exam and history, cannot scrutinize the differential diagnosis[117] for every patient with vague complaints; can not second-guess every reading of every x-ray or ultrasound;[118] can not build a warm, deeply trusting relationship with each patient, and cannot determine, on their own, when their guidelines do not fit a particular patient. In short, health plans have no choice but to trust that, for the most part, their physicians know how to practice medicine in the care of individual patients.

Accordingly, rather than obsessively peering over shoulders and second-guessing individual clinical encounters, health plans should concentrate on global issues, filling four main functions. First, they must focus on the business aspects of running a health care system. Next, when plans undertake to provide or directly arrange for care, rather than merely reimbursing it, or when they limit subscribers' choices among providers or treatments, they should monitor what happens under their auspices. There are two aspects to this. On a positive note they should identify and encourage the delivery of good care—their second function. And on a more negative dimension they should identify and take reasonable steps to remedy defective care—the third function. In both these realms health plans must focus not so much on individual episodes as on overall patterns of care. Fourth, in certain circumstances health plans must also practice medicine. Each of these deserves further discussion.

a. Business Functions

Health plans' first and most obvious domain is the business dimension. The chief function of a health plan is, of course, to ensure that the right care (or payment) flows to the right people, for the right purposes, in a timely fashion, as promised in the contract. For an indemnity plan this will be financial payment, whether to reimburse patients for expenses incurred or to pay providers directly for goods and services rendered. In an HMO-type plan this will mean directly arranging for enough of the right kinds of providers and facilities to be available in enough of the right locations to ensure that the full spectrum of promised services will be readily available to enrollees. It also means forging workable, appropriate contractual and financial relationships with such providers. Transferring high levels of financial risk to physician groups who are too inexperienced to manage resources under capitation, for instance, might be a poor business move that, in turn, could have serious medical implications for subscribers.

Admittedly, such business matters cannot always be distinguished crisply and cleanly from medical issues. Any decision to cut business costs will almost certainly have medical implications, whether immediate or long-term. Still, some functions are obviously business related and clearly are the health plan's responsibility—from arranging for facilities and housekeeping, to purchasing and maintaining equipment, to reimbursing covered medical interventions, to paying the electric bills.[119]

b. Patterns of Good Care

Regarding the second function, identifying and encouraging patterns of good care, it should be noted that modern health plans virtually cannot operate without using some sort of clinical guidelines by which to decide which care is covered under the plan. It is a business necessity with obvious clinical implications.[120] Ideally, when functioning as a coherent, scientifically well-founded set of protocols that suggest routine ways to handle routine problems, guidelines have become an important tool for promoting consistency of care, for integrating new information into clinical practice, and for shaving off practices that are pointless or injurious.

Good guidelines are especially needed regarding serious illnesses and injuries. Here, at the cutting-edge of medicine, where life and death are the most uncertain, where excesses and inadequacies of care can have the most dire consequences, where the newest technologies may or may not deliver the wondrous results they promise, and where the greatest sums of money are spent,[121] it is particularly important for health plans to ensure that care is provided effectively and that resources are used wisely.[122] Systematic technology assessment should be the cornerstone of health plans' coverage decisions in this difficult realm.[123] The resultant guidelines can help health plans to make more rational, evidence-based decisions and to respond more fairly and consistently to treatment requests from members. Such fairness is particularly important with respect to dire illness and cutting-edge care.[124]

Guidelines need not dwell exclusively on determining what is and is not financially covered. HMOs especially are defined at least partly by the fact that they reach beyond being financial agents and directly arrange for enrollees' care. They can and should actively seek to ensure that high-quality care is delivered. This means assuring not only that their physicians refrain from delivering treatments that an enrollee does not need or did not purchase, but reciprocally that physicians do provide the care the plan has promised. As noted above, physicians do not always provide even the care that is of obvious, agreed-on benefit.[125] Accordingly, standards for such things as preventive care and the routine management of chronic illnesses such as diabetes, arthritis, and asthma will be important areas in which health plans can undertake affirmative leadership.

As a practical matter, health plans are ordinarily in a better position than the lone clinician to identify effective patterns of care. Few physicians have time for the kind of systematic literature review that can help them distinguish between solid research that warrants changing their clinical routines and more transient findings that do not warrant change. Health plans can and should make it their business to evaluate ongoing research and scientific consensus, especially regarding those aspects of medicine that are most amenable to general guidelines. Because all health plans must choose the levels of care they will cover, and because some directly furnish that care, they should do so on the basis of the best available evidence.[126] Fortunately, a number of efforts are underway to collect, evaluate, and promulgate evidence-based guidelines.[127]

The mandate to choose, scrutinize, and improve guidelines need not mean that each health plan should work in isolation from other plans. Indeed, collective investigation, if undertaken by consortia of health plans and other research entities, is more likely to produce credible results than if each plan reinvents its own peculiar wheel.[128] Neither does it mean lock-step, one-size-fits-all mandates. Since not even the best guidelines will fit every patient, and since various purchasers have different goals and different levels of resources to spend on health care, ranges of options with flexibility are important. This will be explored further in Chapter 9. Nevertheless, guidelines for routine care do help remind physicians that, in the absence of contraindications or other exceptional circumstances, certain things should generally be provided for people with particular conditions.

As health plans do the homework for continually improving routines of care, they can also institute mechanisms for helping physicians learn and implement these routines. The ordinary physician, busy each day with large numbers of patients, may know very well about inhaled steroids for asthma, anticoagulents for atrial fibrillation, and retinal exams for diabetics. But a hectic pace may make it difficult to remember everything that must be done during ever-briefer office or bedside visits.[129] MCOs can help physicians remember what each patient needs, and they can help reduce errors[130] by providing computer-based reminder systems and the like to help physicians implement improvements to care. A number of such initiatives have been very successful.[131] MCOs can also provide opportunities for continuing education by working with medical leaders in the community.[132] And they can undertake their own health-promotion initiatives, such as initiating support groups, education, and exercise classes for patient groups such as diabetics, asthmatics, and the elderly.[133]

c. Patterns of Poor Care

Just as health plans should work, in a positive sense, to establish the patterns of care that should be provided, so must they, on a more negative side, strive to identify and remedy poor-quality care. This is their third proposed area of major responsibility. As argued above, health plans neither can nor should try to second-guess every individual clinical encounter. To do so would require enormous resources—virtually an entire extra layer of physicians to check up on clinicians' every move, with perhaps yet another layer to monitor the monitors. More important, such intense supervision would be intrusive and, if the medical staff is chosen with reasonable care, generally unnecessary.[134] On the whole, plans should reserve intense scrutiny of individual cases for those situations in which it appears that an egregious error has been committed—one that could betoken a serious lack of skill or care, or physician impairment, or some other major problem—and for individual case studies that might be part of a random system of spot-checking for quality.[135]

Accordingly, health plans' primary focus should be on patterns of conduct in which a physician systematically fails to render an appropriate quality or quantity of care or in which patients' outcomes are consistently worse than what should have been expected.[136] The American College of Physicians' remarks on utilization review apply well to quality review: "Evidence suggests that the principal process of review, the case-by-case review, may not be cost-effective and may not be conducive to improving quality."[137] Instead, the College "recommends that routine case-by-case reviews be abandoned and replaced by profiling of patterns of care."[138] Such profiling can aim, on the positive side, to ensure that physicians are providing important forms of standard care, such as routine preventive care. On the negative side, it can monitor adverse incidents to ascertain whether a given physician has simply committed an individual error or whether isolated incidents have begun to constitute a pattern.

When deficiencies appear, plans can respond by providing education or supervision, imposing practice restrictions or, if necessary, removing personnel. In some instances it may be the plan's own guidelines, rather than physicians' behavior, that need to change. Throughout this process the health plan's question is not whether a physician erred in a given instance or whether that physician owes redress to a patient. Such personal debts from physicians to their patients are generally better addressed within classic malpractice tort law. Rather, the health plan's task is to determine whether a given physician should remain on its panel and, if so, what remedial actions should be taken to improve performance. Such evaluations might be undertaken directly by the MCO or may emerge from traditional kinds of physician-conducted peer review. Either way, the process should be geared not toward punishment but toward quality improvement.[139]

d. Practicing Medicine

In their fourth function health plans literally practice medicine. This subject will be explored in more detail in Chapter 8, which will provide a more precise definition of medical practice and its place in the context of health plans and tort. Suffice it here to note that even if health plans ordinarily provide only general guidance on the optimal management of chronic illnesses, even if they look mainly for patterns of inadequate care rather than trying to pinpoint every error or dubious judgment, and even if their business administration duties are not ordinarily "medical" in character, nevertheless, at certain points the health plan will affect a member's clinical care in a way that can only be described as practicing medicine because they will be making medical judgments that directly determine, or at least substantially influence, a patient's specific care and outcomes. Because of this, health plans could find themselves practicing medicine in any of their first three domains as identified above.

In the first domain lie the most obvious opportunities for practicing medicine. Most of this discussion is reserved for Chapter 8, but it can be noted here that almost all health plan contracts are based on the notion of medical necessity. As a result, even when plans are ostensibly doing nothing more than interpreting their contracts to determine who should receive which goods and services, the medical necessity standard requires them to make medical judgments before they can finalize their business decisions about coverage. Suppose, for instance, that a physician indicates one of his patients needs a more extensive diagnostic work-up for chest pain than is typically permitted under the plan's general guidelines for that particular problem. To determine whether that exceptional care is medically necessary, the plan must carefully consider the facts and use its own medical evaluation to discern whether this patient's case is truly atypical and whether the extra tests will be appropriate in this instance. In the process, the plan's medical judgments will quite likely have a significant impact on the patient's care and thereby, arguably, constitute the practice of medicine.[140]

In essence, any time an HMO must interpret its own contractual or clinical guideline ambiguities in order to determine which care it will cover for a specific enrollee, or any time it must consider exceptions to its usual limits on covered care for a patient who doesn't fit the guidelines, a fairly high probability exists that the plan will be practicing medicine. Note that these instances will mainly arise in situations in which the HMO exercises direct utilization management over which care is provided or covered. In cases in which the plan has transferred financial risk to physicians, as through capitation, physicians are usually free to provide as much care as they wish so long as they provide no less than that to which the patient is contractually entitled. In these cases, the physician, not the plan, typically makes the medical/financial judgments.

The business domain might also provide other, less obvious occasions for practicing medicine, because a host of business decisions can have medical implications. For instance, if surgeons on an HMO's staff request that a certain piece of equipment, such as a new type of laser, be purchased, for instance, the HMO may need to undertake an independent evaluation of the surgeons' claims that this new laser will produce better outcomes than do current procedures. If the HMO decides that these medical claims are not fully credible and thereby declines to purchase it on medical grounds (rather than on straightforward cost grounds), its decision will directly affect the health care of the enrollees who would otherwise have been treated with that laser. In such cases the health plan may have practiced medicine in the course of making business decisions. These cases will be debatable because the impact of the HMO's business decisions on individual patients' care and outcomes will be considerably more remote than other, more obvious instances. Nevertheless, it is possible at least to envision scenarios in which such business decisions could involve practicing medicine.

Additional opportunities for practicing medicine lie in the other two domains, namely, fostering good practice patterns and addressing poor performance patterns. Both these activities require the plan to choose specific clinical guidelines that are then applied to the care of real patients and also to the selection, supervision and sometimes deselection of medical staff. As noted in Section B-1 above, among the plethora of guidelines that plans have created, adopted, and adapted, some are medically credible and others assuredly are not. It takes medical knowledge and judgment for a health plan to discern which is which.[141] Because these standards can have such an enormous impact on patients' care, both directly and indirectly, and because they require sophisticated medical evaluations, it may be reasonable to argue that guideline selection can potentially be a form of practicing medicine. More on this in Chapter 8.

2. Physicians

If the foregoing are the kinds of things that health plans can and should control, physicians likewise have their distinctive domains. As noted, physicians must have the freedom to exercise considerable clinical discretion so that they can examine patients, form diagnostic hypotheses, explore those hypotheses, discuss medical options and their respective benefits and risks, and, in the process, build the personal trusting relationship with each patient that is so indispensible to good care. Physicians should not have to spend endless hours justifying ordinary decisions for over-the-shoulder, second-guessing MCOs, because the MCOs should be looking mainly at practice patterns, not moment-by-moment decisions.

Beyond these obvious patient care duties, physicians also have an important responsibility to identify instances in which patients do not fit the health plan's guidelines, because even the best clinical protocol will not fit every patient. The physician has the professional training and the responsibility to recognize such instances and to pursue acceptable alternatives on behalf of that individual.

More broadly, physicians also should be expected to help plans recognize when the guidelines themselves are not working and when they need to be improved or replaced.[142] It is a task that can only be fulfilled by those who live and work at the intersection between the general (the science and guidelines of care) and the particular (the patients).

3. The Balance

In sum, health plans and physicians each can claim a fairly distinctive role. The MCO's job is to find better ways to shape clinical patterns of practice and to find minimally intrusive ways to draw physicians in that direction. MCOs cannot escape practicing medicine at certain points. But those occasions should be limited to such instances as when guidelines are unclear and require interpretation or when a patient's atypical presentation or unusual situation requires special attention. MCOs should not be in the position of having to practice medicine virtually every time they make a benefits decision, as Chapter 8 will discuss further.

Although the foregoing is at best a rough sketch of the ways in which control might be distributed between physicians and health plans, it emphasizes that a focus on quality of care should guide decisions about who should control what in providing health care. Although admittedly sketchy, this structure lays sufficient groundwork to move into a discussion of liability issues. As noted, health plans and physicians should bear liability only for those aspects of care that they can and should control. As Chapter 6 will now show, a further important distinction must be drawn before we can properly determine what sorts of liability physicians and health plans should bear and for what kinds of errors.

6

A BASIC DISTINCTION

Chapter 5 suggested that between health plans and physicians any reasonable formulation of who ought to be liable for what should be based on a plausible account
of who ought to control what. If we do not want health plans dictating, day to day,
what a particular person's diagnosis is or which patients should have which routine
lab tests or x-rays, then we should not make health plans preeminently liable for
errors in such decisions. If we want a health care system in which quality medical
care is the primary goal, then the first question should be to determine which party
is better positioned to provide that quality, for which aspects of care. Those domains
of control then become each party's respective areas of primary medical responsibility—and legal liability.

As discussed in Part I, profound changes in the economic organization of health
care have precipitated equally profound jurisprudential challenges for the ways in
which errors in health care have traditionally been addressed, both in tort and in
contract. A major conceptual shift is required. As proposed here, that shift must be
based on a fundamental yet under-recognized distinction between matters of expertise
and matters of resources.[1] Whereas Chapter 5 proposed a general division of labor
between plans and providers, this chapter distinguishes two different kinds of obligation that plans and providers can owe within their respective domains of control.

The first kind of obligation, called a duty of expertise, concerns the obligation to
have and to use special kinds of knowledge, skill, and judgment, and to use these
with an acceptable level of diligence and care for the betterment of someone (usually a patient) who needs specialized service. These are obligations to use one's own

mental and physical faculties and energies, something over which each person exercises control simply by conducting himself in certain ways. A deficiency of expertise occurs when someone who is obligated to have such knowledge and skill does not possess it or does not exercise it. For instance, a surgeon might remove the wrong leg,[2] or a radiologist may fail to discern a breast mass on mammography.[3] An oncologist could prescribe vastly excessive doses of chemotherapy drugs,[4] or a physician's assistant might puncture a tympanic membrane while cleaning out impacted ear wax.[5] In another scenario, a physician might neglect to provide required information to an MCO, so that the patient's care will not be paid for. In each case the duty might have been fulfilled better if the person had known more, been more skillful, proceded more carefully, or taken more time.

Special duties of expertise are not placed on ordinary people in the course of their ordinary conduct; these people are expected only to behave like reasonable, prudent persons. Rather, duties of expertise are typically placed on those who hold themselves out as being able to perform some special service with a level of quality that permits people to entrust themselves to such a person for some important need. As discussed below, members of professions such as medicine explicitly hold themselves out in just this way. But other people can likewise have duties of expertise when they act in certain capacities. As we will also see below, those who administer health plans can also have duties of expertise.

Whereas expertise concerns faculties over which a person has direct, personal control, a very different genre of obligation concerns fiscal and physical resources. Here, the obligation cannot be fulfilled simply by engaging personal thoughts and energies. Something material, something outside oneself, must be delivered, transferred, utilized, or made available—resources such as a hospital bed, a diagnostic machine, the services of a home nursing organization, or cash to pay others for products or assistance.

Resource duties are usually established by promises: an insurer promises to make reimbursement payments under specified conditions, or a hospital promises to have equipment and facilities in good working order. Resource duties are often more complex than expertise duties because, especially in health care, a number of different parties often must cooperate in order to provide the resource in question. A hospital may purchase a new piece of diagnostic equipment, but that technology will not ordinarily be available to a patient without a physician's prescription, assurance of payment for its use, adequate personnel to operate and maintain it, and the like. Thus, unlike expertise duties, which require only the use of one's own faculties, the fulfillment of resource duties often requires certain structures for control, authorization, and cooperation.

The distinction can be illustrated by exploring the careful factual inquiry that would be required when an adverse outcome prompts an investigation into who breached what duty. A failure to diagnose cancer, for instance, might be mainly attributable to a physician's failure to undertake an adequate history and physical examination—a problem of expertise. Alternatively, it might result from the failure to order sophisticated tests such as computed tomography (CT) or magnetic resonance imaging (MRI). A failure to use resources like these would require closer analysis because it does not necessarily represent a denial of resources. If the physician simply did not know the test was needed, the basic problem would still concern expertise. However, if the physician knew the testing was indicated but did not order it because the patient's insurer refused to pay, the situation poses a resource issue. Even with this further information it would not yet be clear who, if anyone, breached a resource duty. If the physician provides services under a group contract that covers cancer screening tests, then the physician or his medical group may have been the ones who breached the resource duty. In contrast, if an insurer was obligated to cover the test and failed to do so, then the insurer breached a resource duty. However, if the patient's health plan simply does not cover this test, and if the patient declined to purchase it out of pocket, then quite likely no one breached any resource duty to the patient. Only a careful factual investigation can determine, in any given case, whether an expertise or a resource deficiency, or both, or neither, caused the patient's adverse outcome.

Though it may sometimes be difficult to sort out the facts in individual cases, the distinction is conceptually pivotal to an adequate reconstruction of the law by which medical mishaps are litigated. If a person is required to have special expertise, that duty can be fulfilled entirely, so to speak, "under one's own steam." A standard of knowledge and skill is identified, and the person either measures up to that standard or does not, according to his own abilities and efforts. In contrast, when resources are to be delivered, obligations arise from prior agreements and from networks of authorization and control.

Once these points are clear, it becomes obvious that a physician cannot owe the patient a resource that some other party owns and controls, nor can a health plan literally owe the patient a specific exertion of thought, judgment and energy from a physician. The plan might owe its own effort to credential and monitor that physician, but it cannot owe what is under someone else's control. Thus, physicians and even health plans can owe only what is theirs to give. One can only owe what is under his personal control or under his legitimate authority, whether that authority comes through contract, through legislation, through property rights, or through some other means.

The next section of this chapter specifies in a bit more detail the expertise duties and resource duties that can be owed, respectively, by health plans and by physicians. Although physicians have the most obvious expertise duties, health plans also can owe a certain level of expertise to their enrollees. Reciprocally, although resource duties are most obviously associated with health plans, physicians, too, can owe resources to their patients. The discussion here will be brief because details will be fleshed out more fully in Chapters 7, 8, and 9. The final section argues that breaches of expertise duties should be litigated under the law of tort, while resource duties should be addressed in contract.

A. EXPERTISE

Expertise, as noted above, concerns knowledge, skills, judgment, and effort—cognitive capacities and personal diligence under one's direct control. Regardless of resource availability, one still has one's fund of knowledge and ability and can exert effort as one sees fit. Both physicians and health plans can (fail to) exhibit appropriate expertise, thus defined.

1. Physicians

Illness and injury, or even the prospect of them, can produce a distinctive vulnerability. Reasonably good health is a precondition for most people to be able to attain many of their life goals, yet most people lack the knowledge and skills to treat themselves, and those who have the knowledge may be too incapacitated to use it when ill or injured. Hence, when physicians as professionals "profess"[6] to be able to help, they invite trust from people who have little choice but to rely on that expertise.

In the classic statement, the physician's expertise duty requires the physician to possess and utilize "the knowledge, skill and care usually had and exercised by physicians in his community or medical specialty."[7] That duty of care encompasses not just the internist's knowledge of how to sort out a diagnosis amidst complex symptoms and history, or the surgeon's skill to make careful incisions that correct the problem while avoiding damage to nearby tissues, but also knowledge about appropriate use of resources—knowledge about when to refer patients to specialists or to recommend sophisticated technologies, even those that may not be financially covered by the patient's health plan.[8] Expertise also includes personal effort. It does little good to know how to perform a complex surgical intervention if the surgeon is unwilling to take the time to do it properly. Failures of expertise thus include "poor technique . . ., sloppiness, inadvertence, and other forms of human error."[9] As elaborated in Chapter 7, these duties can also include advocacy, such as efforts to help patients gain access to resources that are controlled by other parties.

2. Health Plans

If clinical expertise is the province of physicians, administrative expertise and health services expertise are the province of health plans. Health plans in essence are corporate persons, and, just like physicians, they can exhibit or fail to exhibit the requisite knowledge, skill, judgment, and effort as they carry out their duties. As proposed in Chapter 5, many of those duties concern ordinary business administration, such as keeping track of who the plan's members are and which subscribers are eligible for which benefits.

In *Nealy v. U.S. Healthcare HMO,*[10] for instance, an HMO failed to give a patient proper identification.[11] As a result, the patient was not permitted to see the plan's physician for his angina and was unable to obtain the required referral to continue receiving care from his original physicians, as previously promised by the plan. In addition, although the HMO's physician renewed the patient's drug prescriptions, the patient was unable to fill them because the information provided to the pharmacy was invalid. Here, at least on the face of it, the key problem was not some sort of deliberate attempt to deny resources. Rather, it was a clumsy, ineffective attempt to provide them.

In *Jones v. Chicago HMO*[12] the mother of a three-month-old infant phoned her primary care physician's office, describing symptoms of fever, constipation, and overall illness. The assistant suggested using caster oil, and when Mrs. Jones insisted on speaking with the doctor, the assistant told her that the physician was unavailable but would return her call. Dr. Robert Jordan phoned Mrs. Jones late that evening, also recommending castor oil. By the time the infant was taken to a hospital emergency room the next day, her bacterial meningitis was so advanced that, even with aggressive treatment, she was left permanently disabled.

Among other findings, the Illinois Supreme Court held that the HMO could potentially be at fault for "institutional negligence," a form of direct corporate negligence, for assigning too many patients to one primary care physician. The court observed that this claim "involves an administrative or managerial action by Chicago HMO, not the professional conduct of its physicians."[13] Noting that an HMO "must act as would a 'reasonably careful' HMO under the circumstances," the court held that "[p]ublic policy would not be well served by allowing HMOs to assign an excessive number of patients to a primary care physician and then 'wash their hands' of the matter. The central consequence of placing this burden on HMOs is HMO accountability for their own actions."[14] Here, too, the problem was a failure to use adequate knowledge, judgment, and effort, rather than a failure, per se, to produce resources.

In *Payton v. Aetna*,[15] a 42-year-old man, after nearly dying from a drug overdose, sought coverage for treatment of substance abuse. After a series of administrative gaffes the health plan did eventually approve coverage, but, unfortunately, not until eight days after the plaintiff's death from a second overdose.[16] In permitting tort claims to go forward, Judge Herman Cahn found that unwarranted delay and confusion in processing requests for coverage can give rise to liability for negligence on the part of a health plan. Although not stated precisely in the terminology of this book, Judge Cahn offered a good description of what it is for a health plan to have and breach duties of expertise:

> In the context of a consumer who has purchased a 'health care' policy with an HMO, and who then finds himself or herself requiring treatment, the HMO should be held to a high standard in the manner in which it executes its contractual obligations. Decisions on applications should be expeditiously made, and reviews of those decisions on internal appeal should be resolved quickly. This is especially so, because the consumer, as occurred here, often needs immediate hospitalization or admission to a medical or rehabilitative facility.[17]

In some cases expertise duties require the plan to have a working knowledge of medicine, not just diligence in discharging the usual insurance functions of determining eligibility and benefits. As noted in Chapter 5, plans may sometimes practice medicine via their obligation to promulgate medically reasonable guidelines or to monitor quality of care delivered under their auspices. In *Crum v. Health Alliance Midwest, Inc.*,[18] for example, a 42-year-old man with a history of heart disease was experiencing agitation, nausea, and other symptoms. His wife telephoned their health plan's advisory nurse, who indicated that the problem was merely excess stomach acid. When the patient's wife called again a short time later reporting that her husband was now experiencing chest pain, the nurse suggested sitting at a 40-degree angle and drinking milk, reassuring them that he would be fine in the morning. An hour after the first call, as Mrs. Crum drove her husband to the nearest emergency room, he became unresponsive. Resuscitative efforts failed to save his life.

This case did not directly address tort claims because its central question was whether federal ERISA law preempts this sort of litigation to federal courts.[19] However, en route to remanding the case to state court, the federal district court observed that the problem in this case was not a failure to provide benefits. Rather, the plan provided poor-quality medical advice. In the terms of this book, the HMO's alleged failure was not a denial of resources. Rather, it was a breach of the expertise duty to choose medically credible guidelines for its nurses to use in advising enrollees.[20]

Plans can also owe expertise duties to their providers, not just to patients. In *Sanus/New York v. Dube-Seybold-Sutherland*[21] a dental HMO failed to provide dentists with up-to-date lists of enrollees. The plan was capitated, and providers needed that information in order to know which patients they were obligated to serve, to know how much capitation they were owed, and to manage their budgets appropriately. The dentists had no alternate means of verifying which of their patients were enrolled, and although the plan knew that to be the case, it persisted in providing incorrect information. Accordingly, the Texas appellate court found that the health plan had violated a special duty of good faith and fair dealing.

Health plans' duties of expertise can range broadly, including not only the kinds of duty cited above, but also duties to use due care in the utilization review process,[22] in credentialing and retaining physician staff, and the like.[23] A failure regarding credentialing can arise, for instance, if a plan fails to make adequate efforts to check physicians' backgrounds or if an administrator doesn't understand what qualifications to look for in a physician.[24]

Some commentators have opined that plans' errors of expertise are sometimes deliberate, even malicious.[25] That may be true. However, as observed in some of the cases above, many mix-ups and failures are simply the product of incompetence or inefficiency combined with the complexity of the task. Health plans, like physicians, are struggling to adapt to enormous changes throughout the health care sector. When they fail to have the requisite level of knowledge or fail to exercise adequate diligence, they, like physicians, may breach their expertise duties.

B. RESOURCES

As with expertise, plans and physicians alike can have resource duties.

1. Health Plans

Health plans' resource duties depend on the nature of the plan. Commercial health plans such as HMOs and indemnity insurers are largely defined by contract. Typically, these plans promise to provide or indemnify medically necessary care within whatever categories of care are covered,[26] then identify various exclusions and enumerate subscribers' responsibilities.[27] Another kind of health coverage arises through a self-insuring corporation that, as governed by ERISA, can choose whatever level of benefits it wants to provide for its workers. It can change those benefits at will so long as it complies with the relevant rules of notification and does not intentionally discriminate against any particular group.[28] Sometimes a company will contract directly with providers and administer the plan in-house,[29] while in other instances it may hire a third-party administrator to run the plan. In a third genre, benefits in government-sponsored health plans such as Medicare are outlined by legislation and specified by administrative regulation. These plans, like commercial and corporate plans, are usually defined in terms of coverage categories, medically necessary care within those categories, and various specified exclusions. Government-created resource entitlements, like others, can change over time as legislatures or regulators see fit.[30] Whatever type of plan, the specific content of the duty to deliver resources is largely a function of what has been promised, whether by contract, employer promise, or statute and regulation.

2. Physicians

Physicians' resource duties depend on what sort of control they actually have over resources in a given situation. Three basic arrangements exist, each carrying rather different resource duties for physicians.

The first arrangement is the old "artesian well" paradigm, in which payors reimburse covered services with minimal argument except for clearly noncovered treatments. Here, physicians have considerable influence, if not outright control over resources and can ordinarily be expected to provide whatever care they believe their patients need. If the health plan does not choose to limit resources, it would ill-behoove the physician unilaterally to deny his patients beneficial care in order to save money for third parties who have not asked him to do so.[31] Though generous indemnity insurance is uncommon today, it has not disappeared.

In the second kind of arrangement, payors exert tight utilization management (UM) over a wide array of interventions. Physicians may be free to order inexpensive tests and treatments, but beyond this they may be required to secure authorization for a wide variety of products and services, such as hospital admission, specialist consults, durable medical equipment, and sophisticated tests and treatments.[32] Failure to secure preapproval can precipitate significant financial penalties, such as a large bill for the patient or even the physician's own dismissal from the plan if he commits too many infractions or contests too many denials.

Under this second arrangement, the physician should not be saddled with a legal duty to commandeer resources without the owners' consent. Rather, the physician's main resource duty should be to advocate for his patient. If resource rules require that the physician obtain prior authorization by telephone, then his job is to do so.[33] If the plan has denied authorization for a resource that the physician believes is clearly needed, the physician has some obligation to help the patient to appeal the denial.[34]

In the third basic type of arrangement, physicians are much more free from external micromanagement because they are placed under financial incentives or risk-sharing schemes that motivate them personally to conserve resources. Milder versions of incentives, for example, include bonus arrangements, such as when physicians in an HMO share any unused money in the funds designated for hospitalization, lab tests, or consultation.

Capitation arrangements pose more substantial risk sharing. In physician-level capitation, primary care physicians are paid a fixed monthly sum to provide a designated array of outpatient services, regardless of how (in)frequently the patient presents for care. Such arrangements often encompass a wide array of outpatient care, including outpatient laboratory, X-ray, and consultant services, while leaving the largest expenses, such as hospitalization, home nursing, and durable medical equipment, with the health plan. In one example, individual primary care physicians in an HMO received $28 per patient per month, from which they were expected either to provide or pay for a designated array of outpatient services, up to $5000 worth of each patient's care.[35] In this setting, every intervention of capitation-covered care—every lab test, every X-ray—thus poses a personal cost to the physician.

A more moderate version is group-level capitation, in which the health plan pays a group of physicians a monthly per-patient sum in exchange for providing enrollees with a designated array of services. The group, in turn, can pay its physicians as it wishes, whether by salary, fee-for-service, or physician-level capitation.[36] The format of group-level capitation can vary considerably. Sometimes it can be a fairly simple transaction in which the MCO hands over the designated sum of money and says "give care as you see fit, so long as you provide the full range of services listed in the agreement." Such arrangements are not the only kind, however. The MCO usually remains contractually obligated to ensure that its enrollees receive the designated level of service and quality, even if the physician group exhausts its capitated funds prematurely. Hence, when physicians are not experienced in managing financial risk, MCOs may continue to guide their physicians.[37] Whether at the level of individual physician or of group, these capitation arrangements essentially appoint physicians as subcontracted health plan administrators within whatever scope is set by the capitation agreement.

The broadest economic incentive, variously called *full risk, extreme risk,* or *global capitation,* arises when a group of providers accepts the entire premium and provides all covered services.[38] In some cases the group is comprised exclusively of physicians, while in other cases it includes hospitals or other providers. An example of a fully physician-owned plan comes from the case of *Pegram v. Herdrich,*[39] in which physicians of the Carle Clinic were owners of a health plan that provided the complete spectrum of care, largely at clinics and hospitals owned by the physician group. Whatever the exact structure, physicians in global capitation have much more complete control over resources but are subject to significant financial consequences for the group. To promote diversity of health plans in the marketplace, Congress recently expanded the opportunities for physicians, hospitals, and other providers to assume full risk by forming provider-sponsored organizations (PSOs).[40]

Across the spectrum of these incentive arrangements, the extent of a physician's control over and responsibility for resources is generally proportionate to the level of financial risk assumed. The relationship is not absolute, however. Sometimes when plans retain control via close utilization management, they use incentives to encourage physicians to adhere faithfully to guidelines rather than attempting to subvert them. In other cases, however, the incentives do lead to a reduction of external oversight. It is also worth noting that some physicians work under mixed systems that combine incentives with some level of utilization supervision. Those incentives, in turn, can also be mixed. Some systems, especially some California independent practice associations (IPAs), have developed innovative physician payment systems designed "to balance the objectives of encouraging individual productivity and clinical cooperation. . . [by] blending elements of fee-for-service and capitation."[41] Such mixed compensation systems aim, among other things, to spread insurance risk, mitigate risk selection, encourage quality of care, "motivate appropriate scope of practice, and focus attention on desired changes in practice patterns."[42]

As will be discussed in greater detail later, these three different approaches to resources pose interesting challenges regarding the content and limits of physicians' resource duties. For example, the second approach, featuring external UM, raises questions about how vigorously the physician should advocate on behalf of patients. Reasonable efforts to make the required phone calls and sign the necessary forms are surely required. However, when the plan's UM process is unduly slow and cumbersome or when the physician risks "deselection" from the plan if he contests the health plan too vigorously, advocacy duties are arguably limited by "reasonableness," however difficult that notion may be to define. Other challenges arise when physicians engage in dubious measures such as "gaming the system," which can include everything from exaggerating a patient's symptoms, to intimidating the health plan's UM clerks, to outright lying.[43] These issues will be discussed further in Chapter 7.

The third arrangement, in which physicians gain resource control by assuming financial risk, creates distinctive conflicts of interest by pitting patients' needs against physicians' personal finances. Full risk arrangements also present an added kind of conflict, namely conflict of obligation. These latter are marked not by conflicts between the physician's personal welfare and his duties to someone else, but rather by conflicts between what he owes to one party (the patient) and what he owes to another party (other people in the enrolled population).[44]

This is because with full risk the physician group has actually become a health plan and must use the collective funds to cover the health needs of all their patients, not just an individual physician's own patients. Here the physician cannot claim, as in the second arrangement, that others, rather than he, are responsible for any resource denials. After all, under full risk the physicians have complete resource control. Hence it may be a challenge to distinguish, in a given case, whether a denial of resources to a particular patient represents an abdication of fidelity or a faithfulness to the needs of others and to the legitimate limits of the plan.[45]

In sum, physicians' resource obligations depend very much on the sort of financial structure in which they operate. When they have little real control over resources, they owe not resources, but their own personal efforts to help the patient obtain whatever resources are due. This is an expertise duty, not a resource obligation. Reciprocally, the more authority they have to control resources, as through bearing financial risk, the more they take on the character of a health plan, with affirmative duties to produce fiscal and physical goods and services.

C. LITIGATING BREACHES OF DUTY: EXPERTISE VERSUS RESOURCES

Once the distinction between expertise and resources is drawn, and once it is clear that both kinds of duty can be owed by both health plans and physicians, we must next consider what sort of liability should apply to each sort of breach. This book proposes that expertise issues should be addressed under tort law, while resource issues should be addressed in contract.

1. Expertise and Tort

Expertise and failures thereof fall within classic tort concepts of a citizen's obligation to exercise due care in her personal actions and to compensate those whom she carelessly injures. As professionals, physicians claim to possess a special knowledge, skill, and judgment. The emphasis on personal faculties such as these is evident in classic tort definitions of the medical standard of care, captured over a century ago. The physician

> is never considered as warranting a cure, unless under a special contract for that purpose; but his contract, as implied in law, is that he possesses that reasonable degree of learning, skill, and experience which is ordinarily possessed by others of his profession; that he will use reasonable and ordinary care and diligence in the treatment of the case which he undertakes; and that he will use his best judgment in all cases of doubt as to the proper course of treatment. He is not responsible for want of success, unless it is shown to result from a want of ordinary skill and learning, and such as is ordinarily possessed by others of his profession; or from want of ordinary care and attention.[46]

The theme is echoed throughout contemporary tort law.[47] Although tort expectations have sometimes come de facto to include costly technologies, as noted in Chapter 2, actual statements of physicians' obligations attend exclusively to faculties of mind as they emanate in personal conduct.

Some of the most powerful reasons for keeping expertise within the ambit of tort emerge when we consider the alternative—the idea of using contract, rather than tort, to govern expertise. Some authors have proposed that virtually every aspect of health care should be opened to contractual bargaining between consumers and providers, including "the quantity and quality of services."[48] On this view, consumers might bargain not only over modes for resolving disputes, such as arbitrarion, or over the size of recoveries if a patient is injured; they "might also agree to changes in the substantive obligations of providers, substituting a contractual standard of care for the common law standard of care applicable in a suit for damages."[49]

Chapter 9 will argue that patients should have considerable contractual freedom to make choices regarding the level of resources. However, although resource issues are excellent candidates for negogiation and choice, it makes much less sense for courts to accept a contract permitting a surgeon to make careless incisions, or an internist to recommend treatment without bothering to examine a patient or think carefully about his diagnosis. Almost all patients come to the health care setting with a significant deficit of information that leaves them poorly positioned to determine, for themselves, whether their physicians actually know what they are doing. At some point, patients need to have someone they can trust. Even conceding that not all physicians are equally gifted, a person in abject need of help for her illness or injury needs to be assured she will receive at least some reasonable level of skill and knowledge. Moreover, even if her health plan doesn't cover every potentially helpful intervention, she still needs someone who can reliably tell her what further care may be of use if she wishes to purchase it out of pocket. Moreover, if patients are to make intelligent decisions regarding which health plan to buy in the first place, they need reliable information that can help them determine not just what a plan offers, but how a proposed plan might affect their own personal well-being. Physicians should surely be one important source of this information, and patients should be able to count on a reasonable level of quality in their knowledge and services.

Just as patients should be able to expect at least some reasonable level of expertise from their physicians, so should they be able to count on adequate expertise from health plans, meaning at least some modicum of efficiency and effectiveness in that plan's administration and in its approach to arranging for care. Indeed, administrative expertise is, in essence, the concept of "good faith" already embedded in insurance tort law. Health plans might legitimately vary along a number of parameters, from their coverage of costy new technologies, to the ways in which subscribers will address alleged mismanagement (as by agreeing to arbitration), and the like. But it is difficult even to fathom a contract that expressly permits administrators to be careless and inaccurate when they make coverage determinations—that is, to breach their duties of administrative expertise. A "contract" permitting such poor performance would, in effect, deny the enrollee the benefit of his own bargain. This is illogical at best, and surely not likely to be upheld by courts.

2. Resources and Contract

In contrast to the intimate connection between expertise and tort, agreements about what kinds and levels of resources a plan will provide are natural candidates for contract law. Contract is the law of resource exchange, the law governing agreements to transfer goods and services in exchange for consideration. By definition it is the appropriate venue for resource issues.

Here, too, an important argument comes from entertaining the alternative—in this case by hypothesizing that we should adjudicate resource issues by tort. Because tort is the law that governs the interactions of strangers who cannot agree, in advance, on how they shall resolve mishaps, tort requires a single standard of care—

ordinary and reasonable conduct owed by all equally to all.[50] To address resource issues under tort law would presuppose that there is only one standard of (resource) care that all plans uniformly owe to everyone, with only limited room for variation around the margins. Everyone must receive—and that usually means purchase—the same level of resources, regardless of their preferences. As will be argued in Chapter 9, health care incorporates too many deeply personal values, admitting of legitimately wide variation, to mandate such uniformity.

In contrast, a contract approach to resources can permit citizens the freedom to choose what goals they want to reach through health care and how much to spend on what sorts of products and services toward achieving those goals. At the same time, clear contracts permit health plans and corporations to function with a level of economic predictability that is essential if they are to meet their obligations within a limited budget. This is because although they owe their subscribers what they have promised in the agreement, they cannot be compelled under ordinary contract law to provide more than was promised. Moreover, when health plans and consumers are willing to make their contracts considerably more explicit than they are at present— to meet the conditions for effective contracting—courts have become increasingly willing to enforce them, as will be shown in Chapter 10.

As a final argument, this expertise/tort, and resources/contract alignment can promote fairness and consistency. As matters currently stand, physicians may potentially be held liable in tort for failing to use a resource (e.g., hospitalization), while a judge deciding a contract claim in the very same case might excuse the health plan from making that same resource available to the patient on the ground that the contract did not require it.[51] Clearly, it makes no sense to find that the physician owed the care (because it is what other physicians would provide), even though the health plan did not owe it (because the contract excluded it). And yet this odd result is precisely what can happen if resource litigation against physicians is addressed in tort, while resource claims against health plans reside mainly in contract.[52]

The remedy must begin by making the expectations we place on providers and plans clearer and basing them on the specific functions that providers and plans respectively should fulfill. At that point, claims of a given type, whether expertise or resources, should be litigated under the same rules—tort or contract, respectively— whether the claims are brought against physicians or against health plans.[53] When that clarity has been achieved, each party has a better opportunity to conduct its affairs productively and properly, with considerably less fear of unfair and inappropriate liability. And patients will be able to bring clearer, more enforceable expectations to the encounter.

The next three chapters will explore these points in greater detail. Chapter 7 focuses on physicians' duties, both expertise and resources, while Chapters 8 and 9 focus on health plans. Chapter 8 considers plans' expertise duties and the tort liability to which they should be subject, while Chapter 9 considers contract issues regarding plans' resource duties.

7

RESHAPING LIABILITY FOR PHYSICIANS

A. PHYSICIANS AND EXPERTISE

From the discussion in Chapter 5 about which domains of health care should be controlled, respectively, by physicians and by health plans, and from the discussion in Chapter 6 about the distinction between expertise and resources, it is clear that physicians' most traditional, familiar responsibilities are duties of expertise. They must examine patients, form diagnostic hypotheses, explore those hypotheses, discuss treatment options and their likely benefits and risks, build trusting relationships and, in many cases, undertake tests and treatments requiring considerable training and experience. As noted in Chapter 5, physicians also have an important responsibility to recognize when patients do not fit the health plan's guidelines and to pursue reasonable alternatives. Further, physicians should critique the guidelines themselves, helping health plans to improve or replace them as necessary.[1]

As suggested in Chapter 6, physicians' obligations of knowledge, skill, judgment, and effort should be established according to existing tort traditions, which defer to the profession's prevailing practices. The reasons are familiar: the practice of medicine requires esoteric knowledge and clinical experience that cannot usually be judged well by ordinary laymen; the medical science in journals and textbooks must be tested against the realities of daily clinical practice to determine what actually works; medical wisdom needs freedom to improve and evolve over time as professional consensus shifts. Chapter 2 pointed out a few caveats to the traditional rationale for the custom-based standard of care. For instance, a simplistic empirical appeal to what physicians actually do may not be as reliable a way to identify what physicians believe is best as an "accepted practices" or "reasonable physician" approach. Still, for purely medical questions, such as whether a particular intervention is safe and effective, some sort of appeal to physicians' collective judgment should take the lead in setting standards.

Likewise, it makes sense to retain the established tort precept that, at least within a given specialty, physicians should possess roughly the same knowledge and skill. Medical education and training have become remarkably standardized across the nation in the past few decades, and courts have largely replaced locality-based training standards with national standards.[2] At the same time, traditional room for diversity via reputable minorities and differing schools of thought likewise remains viable. If medical knowledge is to grow and improve over time, physicians must be allowed to vary from the mainstream.[3]

Finally, and still in keeping with tort traditions, it also is appropriate to ignore finances so long as the issues are strictly limited to expertise—the knowledge, judgment, skills, and diligence that a physician individually possesses and exercises. If a physician accepts a patient for care, he makes a personal, professional commitment to use his own best efforts to help that patient, even if he cannot promise to commandeer other people's money and property in the process. Thus, the physician should not undertake a hasty physical examination or be sloppy and rushed in performing procedures just because the patient is poor. If the physician does not wish to care for the poor, it is better not to accept such a patient in the first place than to accept and then mistreat him.

B. PHYSICIANS AND RESOURCES

Holding physicians accountable for resource use is more complex, largely because physicians hold such varying kinds and levels of resource control. The bulk of the discussion regarding health care resources will appear in Chapter 9 because, for the present at least, health plans still have predominant responsibility. Still, physicians have an important and rapidly changing role in resource allocation. Few physicians still enjoy the old "artesian" option of ordering whatever they want and ignoring the cost. Rather, as noted in the previous chapter, physicians generally can have two basic relationships with resources. Sometimes they lack significant control and are required to secure utilization authorization from health plans at various junctures. Alternatively, they may hold substantial control via financial risk-sharing that places them at personal risk for the economic consequences of their medical/resource decisions. Each of these will be considered separately.

1. Physicians Lacking Resource Control

When physicians substantially lack resource control, as when they must secure approval from the health plan for a test, treatment, consult, or hospitalization, their principal duty will be patient advocacy, a duty classified under expertise because it involves the physician's personal effort and diligence. Some courts are willing to recognize an obligation to help patients gain access to rightful resources, particularly when the physician is in a unique position to help, such as by providing documentation that only physicians can provide. Often those duties will be technical requirements, for instance, to phone for authorization or fill out paperwork. The case of *Chew v. Meyer*[4] illustrates these issues.

Herbert Chew, a steel company worker who had undergone surgery, asked his surgeon, Dr. Meyer, to document for his employer that Chew's absence from work was medically necessary. Meyer agreed to direct his secretary to complete the necessary forms but, despite several inquiries and proddings from Chew, did not, in fact, send the forms until after Chew had been fired from his job for failure to furnish that very documentation. The Maryland Court of Special Appeals noted that the physician's promise constituted an undertaking that carried a duty to discharge the promise in a proper and timely manner. The court also found another basis for liability. In earlier times, the court acknowledged, the plaintiff's claim

> might well have been summarily rejected, on the basis that a physician's obligation ordinarily did not extend beyond his duty to use his best efforts to treat and cure. The traditional scope of the contractual relationship between doctor and patient, however, has expanded over the years as a result of the proliferation of health and disability insurance, sick pay and other employment benefits. Today, the patient commonly, and necessarily, enlists the aid of his or her physician in preparing claims forms for health and disability benefits. Such forms ordinarily require information possessed solely by the treating physician as well as the physician's signature attesting to the bona fides of that medical information. Consequently, appellant's assertion that the services Dr. Meyer contracted to perform for Mr. Chew included the completion and submission of insurance forms in addition to the surgery he performed, combined with an allegation that the doctor failed to complete and submit the document in question in a proper, *i.e.*, timely, manner states a plausible cause of action for breach of contract.[5]

Similarly, in *Murphy v. Godwin,* Mr. and Mrs. Murphy had requested their family physician to fill out some medical forms required for them to purchase a health insurance policy. When the pregnant Mrs. Murphy subsequently delivered twins with congenital illnesses, it was discovered that their physician had never sent the necessary insurance forms, despite several reminders. A Delaware superior court found that, when a physician-patient relationship exists, the physician's failure to fill out forms in cases such as this could constitute negligent nonfeasance.

> Although it is well known that physicians usually accommodate patients by filling in the forms required by them for various reasons connected with insurance, the question of a doctor's legal duty toward his patients with respect to completing insurance forms is apparently novel. The existence of such a duty may be found, however, by reference to established tort theory and recognized incidents of the doctor–patient relationship.[6]

The duties of advocacy go beyond filling out forms and making phone calls. Physicians should also inform patients about limits or obstacles to important treatments and about reasonable alternatives to noncovered interventions so that patients can choose whether to contest a denial or purchase extra care on their own. Part of a physician's expertise duty, after all, is to know which interventions might help a patient, regardless of whether the health plan is contractually obligated to fund them. Such duties are a major reason why physicians and other commentators objected so vigorously to the nondisparagement, or so-called "gag," clauses that allegedly appeared in many managed care contracts and that were said to inhibit physicians from discussing the limitations that plans imposed on treatment options.[7]

In a related vein, physicians also have an ethical, and perhaps also a legal, obligation to disclose the financial incentives that may interfere with their treatment decisions. Until it was overturned, an Illinois appellate court held that failure to disclose such incentives may constitute a breach of fiduciary duties,[8] and a federal circuit court found in another case that ERISA does not preempt such claims, even when the plaintiff has failed to establish that the physician committed malpractice.[9]

The situations discussed here do not invoke a physician's own contractual resource commitments since, ex hypothesi, physicians lack resource control. Rather, they involve judgments about the reasonableness of a physician's personal efforts and should be litigated as expertise issues under tort law. At the same time, while patients can rightly expect due diligence, they cannot demand unlimited effort, given that physicians usually have commitments to serve many other patients with a comparable measure of advocacy.[10] Hence, it is for the jury to determine how much effort was required and how much was given.

In a recent illustrative case, *Tabor v. Doctors Memorial Hospital,*[11] an emergency room physician diagnosed a patient as potentially suicidal and recommended psychiatric hospitalization. Upon learning that the family could not produce the required $400 deposit, the physician switched his recommendation to outpatient care. The patient committed suicide shortly thereafter. In this case, the physician could actually have waived the fee if he deemed the situation an emergency. Whether he failed to do so because he did not recognize the danger posed by the patient's combination of depression and drug use, or because he was unaware of the waiver option, or instead because he did not wish to complete the necessary paperwork, the physician's alleged failing appears to be a deficiency of expertise—a deficiency that, under the approach recommended here, might legitimately give rise to tort liability.

An important dimension in litigating physicians' advocacy responsibilities will be to distinguish between inadequate efforts by physicians and unruly obstacles imposed by health plans. For instance, if a physician simply fails to make a required phone call, then the blame for an inappropriate resource denial probably rests squarely on his shoulders. If the physician makes the call but is placed on hold for a long period of time because of the health plan's understaffing, then the plan begins to share responsibility. If the plan routinely makes such authorizations unreasonably difficult to obtain or if it commonly denies first-time requests and requires the physician to appeal in order to winnow out benefit claims, then the plan might be accused of "rationing through inconvenience."[12]

When the plan bears proportionately more responsibility, the physician bears less. Health plans' duties of expertise, including administrative efficiency, will be discussed further in Chapter 8. Suffice it to say here that in some cases the most powerful effect of utilization review may be to deter physicians from requesting authorization at all.[13] In complex cases like these, litigants may need to undertake extensive investigation to determine whose conduct carries greater liability, the physician who could have pressed for authorization but failed to do so or the plan that created such disincentives for physicians to request resources.[14] Such uncertainties, however, pose fact-finding tasks familiar in tort litigation.

2. Physicians with Resource Control

As discussed in Chapter 6, some physicians exercise significant resource control, usually by assuming financial risk.[15] Across a spectrum including physician-level, group-level, and global capitation, contract is the applicable body of law for resource denials, regardless of whether the specific resources in question were controlled by the health plan or by the physician. Accordingly, an important issue in litigation may be to determine which party actually owed which resources, because the contract claim should be lodged against the specific party who controlled and thereby owed the resources in question. Therefore, litigants will commonly need to examine two contracts: the one between the health plan and the patient, identifying the resources to which the patient is entitled; and the one between the health plan and the physician, describing how they have allocated resource control between them.

Although physicians should thus face standard contract liability when they deny resources they were contractually obligated to provide, they may also face another legal hazard. In a special twist, physicians in these risk-sharing arrangements can be fiduciaries in two different senses. First, they are fiduciaries of their patients in virtue of the traditionally confidential nature of the physician–patient relationship. And second, they may be fiduciaries, or at least have special obligations of good faith, in the same sense that any insurer has toward beneficiaries.

The law does not provide a clear notion of fiduciary relationships, but certain elements are salient.[16] An imbalance of power exists in which the weaker party must trust the stronger party to fulfill some important need. Reciprocally, the stronger party has superior power and information that could be used to exploit the weaker party.[17] The precise duties of the fiduciary cannot always be spelled out in advance, so in a given instance it can be difficult to tell whether the fiduciary is performing competently.[18] Because this difficulty presents further opportunities for exploitation of the vulnerable party, fiduciary law holds that the fiduciary must minimize the beneficiary's vulnerability by promoting the latter's interests above his own and by avoiding conflicts of interest.[19] When avoiding conflicts of interest is not possible, the fiduciary must inform the beneficiary and permit him to determine what will be done.[20]

Although it has been debated whether physicians are fiduciaries of their patients in the most technical legal sense,[21] courts nevertheless have freely described physicians as fiduciaries and assigned physicians the standard duties of fiduciary loyalty to patients.[22] The important point for present purposes is that when physicians bear substantial financial risk for the care they deliver, they are fiduciaries in a significant conflict of interest because they stand personally to win or lose as they make resource decisions for their patients.[23]

In financial risk-sharing arrangements, particularly global capitation, physicians enter the second kind of fiduciary, or quasi-fiduciary, relationship with respect to all the members of the plan. As noted in *Engalla v. Permanente Medical Group,* "[t]o the extent that it is an insurer, Kaiser [health plan] has a 'special relationship' with its insureds, . . . with heightened duties of good faith and fair dealing in the handling of claims for benefits under the contract of insurance."[24] Physicians under full risk share these heightened duties because they, like Kaiser, are a health plan.

To the extent that physicians are deemed fiduciaries in either setting, their conflicts of interest could pose several special legal risks. First, if those conflicts are not plainly disclosed to patients, they can substantially raise the physician's burden of proof in litigation. Although plaintiffs ordinarily must prove that the defendant owed and breached a duty, whether it be a tort-based standard of care or a contractual obligation, that burden is shifted when the defendant is a fiduciary who failed to disclose a conflict of interest.[25] In that situation, courts will presume that the fiduciary concealed his conflict in order to use his superior position to exploit the beneficiary. Accordingly, they will require the physician to prove he did not breach any duty toward his patient.[26] When physicians earn more money by providing less care, they may have an exceedingly difficult time proving that a denial of care was not tainted.[27]

Second, physicians in risk-bearing arrangements may be especially vulnerable to claims for bad faith breach of contract. Bad faith doctrine first arose in insurance law and is predicated on the fact that in certain kinds of contracts

[the] plaintiff seeks something more than commercial advantage or profit from the defendant. When dealing with an inn-keeper, a common carrier, a lawyer, a doctor or an insurer, the client/customer seeks service, security, peace of mind, protection or some other intangible. These types of contracts create special, partly noncommercial relationships, and when the provider of the service fails to provide the very item which was the implicit objective of the making of the contract, then contract damages are seldom adequate, and the cases have generally permitted the plaintiff to maintain an action in tort as well as in contract.[28]

The court goes on to note that

it is difficult to imagine a policy of insurance that is more important, where the insured seeks maximum security and protection, than the case of a major medical insurance policy to be used in paying for needed medical care that is usually beyond the economic ability of most people to cover without insurance. It is also difficult to imagine anyone who is in a weaker bargaining position than a person in need of major medical care as compared to his or her medical insurance company that has the power to deny benefits.[29]

To show bad faith a plaintiff must not just show that an alternate decision might have been justified, but that the denial of resources was without any reasonable basis and that the health plan knew, or recklessly disregarded, this lack of a reasonable basis for denying benefits.[30]

Clearly, bad faith doctrine poses a special challenge for physicians who have resource control via assuming a financial risk that, in turn, creates conflicts of interest. Physicians are traditionally expected not just to act in good faith, but to subordinate their own interests to their patients'. It is a central element of the trust inherent in that relationship.[31] Accordingly, when physicians have denied care that they arguably owed the patient in their capacity as controller of resources, and when they personally stood to profit from such a denial, the elements of bad faith—malice, oppression, or reckless indifference to the rights of subscribers—may be especially persuasive to a jury.[32]

The third special hazard is that remedies for breaches of fiduciary duty, even without bad faith, can reach beyond ordinary contract remedies to include punitive damages.[33] Though not invariably a feature of fiduciary law, "[p]unishment for breach of fiduciary duty through the use of punitive damages is increasingly common."[34]

These admittedly serious problems need not completely preclude physicians' assuming some financial risk if such risk is prerequisite to their holding clinical and resource control. First, arguably it is desirable for physicians to have a measure of resource control. As Chapter 5 suggested, health plans should not dictate all the daily details of care. Clinical guidelines are often based on little or no science; administrators do not always appreciate the clinical impact their guidelines can have; physicians can only provide adequate care if they have the freedom to develop a personal, trusting relationship with patients; that relationship, in turn, requires at least some measure of direct control over resources. If the "nouveau Golden Rule" is true—i.e., if "he who has the gold makes the rules" means that clinical control is now inevitably tied to financial responsibility—then no escape may exists from placing at least some consequences on physicians for their medical/spending decisions as the price for preserving an essential modicum of clinical autonomy.

Second, the hazards of incentives can be mitigated. Ideally, a well-designed incentive should create just enough hesitation for the physician to consider carefully whether a proposed intervention is genuinely desirable for the patient, but not enough to override good judgment. It should be enough to neutralize the incentives toward overservice that are embedded in traditional fee-for-service payment, but not enough to foster inappropriate skimping. Actual incentive arrangements vary widely along parameters such as whether the incentive is awarded on the basis of the entire group's performance or is tuned to each physician's spending; whether it involves a large or small portion of the physician's overall income; how frequently it is paid; and how directly it impinges on individual patient care decisions.[35] Incentives favoring cost containment can also be offset by incentives for quality improvement and patient satisfaction. They can even be complemented by incentives that motivate patients themselves to be cost conscious.[36]

Third, all health plans carry conflicts of interest and conflicts of obligation. No matter how a physician is paid, whether fee-for-service, capitation, or salary, exploitation opportunities can arise. And so long as the needs of enrollees exceed available resources, difficult decisions must be made regarding who shall receive how much of what. Some mechanism must be installed to ensure that resources are used wisely rather than poorly. In these decisions, fairness of the procedures by which decisions are made counts nearly as much as the adequacy of outcomes. Accordingly, those who hold resource control by assuming financial risk can address those conflicts by ensuring that their procedures for determining which patients should receive which kinds of care are carefully constructed, plainly disclosed, and meticulously implemented.[37] These points will be discussed further in Chapter 9, which explores health plans' contractual accountability.

8

RESHAPING LIABILITY FOR HEALTH PLANS: EXPERTISE AND TORT

As with physicians, health plans' expertise duties should be addressed in tort, while resource duties should be litigated under contract law. This chapter concerns the former, and Chapter 9 the latter. As noted in Chapter 3, tort allegations against health plans are not novel. Suits have been brought for a variety of claims, such as direct liability for negligent credentialing and indirect liability for staff physicians' malpractice.[1] The special contribution of this discussion is to place these cases in their proper context as allegations of failed expertise on the part of health plans, and to distinguish them from contractual failures to meet resource obligations.

First, this chapter will describe the duties of care health plans owe their enrollees. In accordance with the standard elements of tort, these are the duties that, when breached, can justify liability and damages if that breach has proximately caused the patient an injury. Chapter 5 proposed four domains of expertise that ideally ought to be under plans' control: (1) tending to business and administrative tasks, (2) identifying and encouraging adherence to patterns of good care, (3) identifying and remedying patterns of poor care, and (4) practicing medicine in certain circumstances. The first three require only brief discussion. The fourth requires considerably more attention because we need to find an adequate general definition of practicing medicine before we can determine specifically whether a health plan can practice medicine. Once that is done, it will be possible to describe a health plan's duty of care under tort when that plan is practicing medicine.

An important extension of this discussion will be to propose, in part B of this chapter, that health plans currently practice medicine far more often than they should. Because most contracts base benefits determinations on "medical necessity," most plans practice medicine routinely rather than rarely. This long-standing but deeply flawed tradition should be changed, as the arguments will show.

Once health plans' duties of care are outlined and appropriately circumscribed, it will be possible in part C of this chapter to discuss just how tort litigation against health plans should proceed when they are alleged to have breached their duties of expertise. We begin, then, by exploring how plans can be accountable in tort for breaches of their four kinds of expertise duties.

A. DUTIES OF EXPERTISE IN FOUR DOMAINS

1. Business Duties

Business duties concern efficient, effective administration of the plan so that subscribers can receive the reimbursements or direct care to which they are entitled. Often, of course, a failure to provide reimbursements or care will involve breach of contract, a topic reserved for Chapter 9. However, when such breaches result from a deficiency of the requisite knowledge, skill, judgment, or effort in the business of administering the plan, there should be a cognizable claim in tort. Although expertise and resource issues can be closely connected, there is nevertheless a genuine distinction. Not all careless or inefficient administration leads to a breach of contract-based resource duties. The inefficiency might cause only annoyance as resources are produced (perhaps even in excess) by routes and for reasons mysterious to the rational beholder.

The experience of Tennessee's TennCare program illustrates. In 1994, almost overnight, the state went from a conventional indemnity Medicaid plan to a managed competition model in which MCOs were to compete for this population. Of the dozen MCOs that received approval to provide care, ten of them were newly established for this program, and many of these had little prior experience in providing managed care.[2] Particularly at the outset, patients did not always know from whom to seek care, and providers did not always know by what rules to provide it. It was not uncommon for physicians and hospitals to see no payments for long periods of time, then suddenly receive substantial checks—with no indication of what they were for.[3]

Reciprocally, some breaches of contract involve no tort. If an insurer denies payment as a result of careful factual investigation and close scrutiny of the enrollee's policy, then even if a court later determines that the insurer wrongly denied the claim and thus breached the contract, there is no tort. Tort would only arise if the plan were culpably careless or inefficient in the process. In extreme cases, if the plan's tortious inexpertise is characterized by malice, oppression, or reckless indifference to the subscriber's rights, bad faith allegations might also be appropriate.[4]

2. Patterns of Care

Health plans' second domain of control is to establish and encourage adherence to good care guidelines. Such guides serve two main functions. In part, guidelines help to specify more precisely what the enrollee is entitled to receive under the contract. They should also, however, help physicians deliver the best possible care within the limits of that contract. As noted in Chapter 5, health plans can provide an important service by continually evaluating new information about which interventions are effective for which problems and by creating protocols and computer-based reminder systems to help physicians implement the best practices. These may concern the appropriate use of aspirin and beta-blockers for patients recovering from heart attack, for instance, or the criteria for when to use which antibiotics.[5]

As discussed in further detail below, these guidelines must be medically credible even if they may also be lean and cost-effective. Some familiar cases support this idea. Probably the most widely cited case is *Wickline v. State of California,*[6] in which a California appellate court held that a utilization review (UR) entity can be liable in tort for defects in the design, not just the implementation, of its UR process.[7] Although disagreeing with some aspects of *Wickline,* the same court later echoed this important conclusion in *Wilson v. Blue Cross of Southern Cal.,* finding that a health plan or UR entity can be liable if its deficient UR process is a "substantial factor" in causing a patient's injuries.[8] In *Thompson v. Nason Hosp.,*[9] the Supreme Court of Pennsylvania held that hospitals have a "duty to formulate, adopt and enforce *adequate* rules and policies to ensure quality care for patients."[10] That court extended this duty to health plans in *Shannon v. McNulty.*[11]

As noted in Chapter 5, many of the guidelines currently used are hardly paragons of credibility. They may be the product of inadequate science, bias or self-interest, haste, or a host of other flaws.[12] Health plans need to ensure that they choose, create, and adapt their guidelines with reasonable care, that they update and reevaluate them, and that they listen carefully and respond appropriately when their physician staff identify problems in those guides.

3. Surveillance for Inadequate Care

Health plans' third domain likewise requires considerable knowledge, judgment, and effort. The plan needs to understand what good medical care is in order to identify poor care. Like hospitals with medical staff committees, health plans will typically delegate such tasks to physicians who have the requisite medical expertise. Such delegation requires the plan to ensure that these peer review physicians themselves have adequate knowledge and judgment, and to give them the time, information sources, and whatever other support is necessary to exercise due care in these surveillance tasks.

Plans also have well-recognized duties to monitor and supervise their nonphysician staff, of course, from nurses to respiratory therapists to other clinical staff they may hire. Because these duties and plans' corresponding vicarious liabilities are well established, they will not receive further attention here.

Of note, an important literature is emerging on safety in health care. Much of it emphasizes that health plans should focus not so much on pointing fingers of blame at those who may have committed isolated errors, but on systems-oriented approaches conducive to quality improvement.[13]

This does not obviate the occasional need to focus on an individual problematic clinician, but it can place a positive, productive orientation on the health plan's need to identify and correct the quality defects that occur within its sphere.

4. Practicing Medicine

In the fourth domain, Chapter 5 proposed that health plans must sometimes, quite literally, practice medicine. When they do, they should be liable for traditional tort claims of medical malpractice—of the very same sort to which physicians are subject—and not just to the indirect liability they currently more typically bear. The claim that a plan can practice medicine deserves closer scrutiny, because it is the subject of intense debate.

a. The Debate

On the one hand, many physicians and other commentators have pointed out that MCOs' economic judgments have an enormous impact on the care that patients receive. In contrast to the "artesian" days of unlimited retrospective fee-for-service reimbursements, most health plans now limit closely which tests and treatments they cover. Given the enormous cost of care, denials of coverage are often tantamount to denials of care.[14] Coupled with this, the reasons underlying coverage denials may be intensely matters of medical judgment. Hence, when MCOs thereby change or significantly influence the patient's clinical care, these commentators conclude that the health plan is practicing medicine.

For example, in *Murphy v. Board of Medical Examiners,*[15] a physician performing utilization review on behalf of an MCO denied authorization for gallbladder surgery by pointing to medical evidence that indicated a different problem.[16] The Arizona Board of Medical Examiners (BOMEX) noted that in cases such as this, UR physicians' decisions "could adversely affect the health of a patient"[17] and concluded that because this UR physician had indeed practiced medicine, the board had jurisdiction over the quality of his practice. The Arizona appellate court agreed.

> Although Dr. Murphy is not engaged in the traditional practice of medicine, to the extent that he renders medical decisions his conduct is reviewable by BOMEX. Here, Dr. Murphy evaluated information provided by both the patient's primary physician and her surgeon. He disagreed with their decision that gallbladder surgery would alleviate her ongoing symptoms. S.B.'s doctors diagnosed a medical condition and proposed a nonexperimental course of treatment. Dr. Murphy substituted his medical judgment for theirs and determined that the surgery was 'not medically necessary.' There is no other way to characterize Dr. Murphy's decision: it was a 'medical' decision.[18]

Similarly, in *Morris v. Dist. of Col. Bd. of Medicine*,[19] the District of Columbia Board of Medicine found that a physician employed as medical director for a Blue Cross plan did indeed practice medicine in his utilization review capacities. His actions could reasonably be expected, as a practical effect,

> 'to influence the course of treatment of individual patients and, hence, to "treat" them within the meaning of the Act'. . . . Although he 'may not have treated or diagnosed patients directly, he had a considerable influence'—a 'substantial impact'—'on the treatment of patients insured by Blue Cross,' since 'if health insurance is not available, a procedure very well might not be performed.'[20]

In *Brandon v. Aetna Services, Inc.*,[21] a patient with severe anxiety disorder and substance abuse problems alleged that, in denying coverage for requested inpatient treatment and other care, the health plan "committed malpractice by engaging in the practice of medicine or psychiatry 'by undertaking to make decisions about what psychiatric and psychological treatment was and was not appropriate for Mr. Brandon,' and then failing to exercise the degree and skill ordinarily exercised by psychiatrists and psychologists. . . ."[22]

On the other side, MCOs generally insist that they do not practice medicine. Even when they engage in very detailed UR, MCOs argue that they are simply interpreting contracts and making coverage decisions.[23] Physicians and other providers remain free to treat patients as they wish, even when the plan declines to finance that care.

For example, in *Adnan Varol, M.D. v. Blue Cross & Blue Shield*,[24] a group of psychiatrists sued a health plan on the grounds that, as its UR interfered with their medical practice, the plan thereby engaged in unauthorized practice of medicine. The court rejected the argument, pointing out that health plans' decisions about medical necessity are no more the practice of medicine when undertaken prospectively than when undertaken in the traditional retrospective mode.

In *Assn. of Am. Physicians and Surgeons v. Weinberger*,[25] a physician organization alleged that federal regulations mandating utilization review had a chilling effect on medical practice. The district court disagreed, holding that there is no interference so long as the criteria acknowledge that a range of treatments and methods can be consistent with professionally accepted patterns of care.[26] Moreover, the court held that "[t]he 'Professional Standards Review' Law does not prohibit a physician from performing any surgical operations he deems necessary in the exercise of his professional skill and judgment. It merely provides that if a practitioner wishes to be compensated for his services by the federal government, he is required to comply with certain guidelines and procedures enumerated in the statute."[27]

In a similar vein, several courts have held that because corporate practice is illegal (i.e., corporations cannot employ physicians) and because the hallmark of employment is control over the employee's conduct, then a corporation such as an MCO cannot possibly be guilty of practicing medicine because it could not have exercised the requisite degree of control over the physician.[28]

States' medical licensure and practice acts also seem to support this view. Typically, to practice medicine is to "'diagnose, treat, operate or prescribe for any human disease, pain, injury, deformity or physical condition.'"[29] Clearly, an MCO cannot physically examine, treat, prescribe for, or operate on a patient in the literal sense portrayed in these statutes.[30] Only individual persons are capable of doing these things—as the old corporate practice case law pointed out.[31] Moreover, a number of states have declared, either by statute or via opinions of attorneys general, that UR does not constitute the practice of medicine.[32] Thus, on this view, someone who only evaluates information for financial purposes and does not actively provide medical care for patients is not practicing medicine.[33]

The debate is captured well in the case of *Corcoran v. United Healthcare, Inc.*[34] A physician had recommended inpatient care for a woman with a high-risk pregnancy, but her MCO decided that ten hours of home nursing care each day would be sufficient. When the fetus went into distress and died after the nurse had left for the day, the family sued for wrongful death and other torts. En route to its finding that all claims were preempted by ERISA, the Fifth Circuit discussed the question of whether the plan's utilization review and denial of hospitalization constituted a medical decision or a benefits decision.

The MCO argued that the denial "was a decision made in its capacity as a plan fiduciary about what benefits were authorized under the Plan. All it did, it argues, was to determine whether Mrs. Corcoran qualified for the benefits provided by the plan by applying previously established eligibility criteria."[35] The benefits decisions were based on medical information, but the basic activity was an administrative claims handling.

The plaintiffs, in contrast, argued that the MCO was clearly making medical decisions when it determined that the patient did not need continuous hospitalization but could do as well with limited home nursing. The utilization review process is rife with medical decisions, they pointed out, as the plan decides such questions as whether a surgery is necessary, how long a patient should be hospitalized, and which prescriptions and treatments are more appropriate than others.[36]

The Fifth Circuit could not "fully agree with either United or the Corcorans."[37] While it was true that medical decisions were ultimately left up to the beneficiary and her physician, that the MCO–beneficiary relationship was not precisely a physician–patient relationship, and that the MCO had contractually reserved the right to make benefits decisions on the basis of medical information, the court pointed out that prospective UR decisions have a powerful influence on treatment decisions, since beneficiaries may be far less inclined to pursue treatments that they already know will not be paid for. Indeed, the very purpose of prospective UR is to influence treatment decisions in just this way.[38]

Nevertheless, the court concluded in favor of the MCO. "Ultimately, we conclude that United makes medical decisions—indeed, United gives medical advice—but it does so in the context of making a determination about the availability of benefits under the plan. Accordingly, we hold that the Louisiana tort action asserted by the Corcorans for the wrongful death of their child allegedly resulting from United's erroneous medical decision is pre-empted by ERISA."[39]

b. The Resolution

Thus goes the debate over whether MCOs literally practice medicine. Preparatory to resolving the issue, three inadequate approaches must be reviewed and discarded.

First, the bare fact that an MCO's denial of resources has a significant impact does not entail that the denial was a medical decision or, beyond this, that it constituted the practice of medicine. Suppose, for instance, that the MCO's contract covers only thirty days of inpatient psychiatric care.[40] A patient who has reached this limit and whose MCO denies further funding might be promptly discharged by the hospital as a direct consequence, perhaps to her medical detriment. However, whatever harms result from that discharge cannot be attributed to the MCO.[41] The limits of coverage in such a case are clear and nonmedical, and the health plan is straightforwardly applying the contract language to the facts of the case. The plan's refusal to provide coverage that it plainly does not owe can, of course, affect subsequent treatment decisions and thereby the patient's medical outcome. But that refusal is no different than the refusal of the patient's next-door-neighbor, who also does not owe her any such funds and who also declines to provide them gratis. Accordingly, plaintiffs cannot claim that MCOs practice medicine on the sole ground that their coverage decisions affect patients' medical care and outcomes.[42]

This conclusion is echoed in *Morris v. Dist. of Col. Bd. of Medicine,*[43] discussed just above, in which the District of Columbia Medical Board found that a health plan's medical director was guilty of practicing medicine without a license on the ground that he could influence clinical decisions.[44] The appellate court overturned this decision:

> This definition of 'treatment' is so open-ended that it cannot reasonably be squared with the statutory term. In normal medical usage, 'treat' means 'to care for . . . medically or surgically: deal with by medical or surgical means.' . . . Conduct that merely '[a]ffects,' 'influences,' or 'substantially impact[s]' on the course of such care by others cannot itself be treatment without converting a major part of the business of health insurers such as Blue Cross into the 'practice of medicine.' Equating 'treat[ment]' with any conduct that 'practically [a]ffect[s]' it, in ways potentially involving no exercise of medical judgment, is contrary to any sensible interpretation of the statute.[45]

The second inadequate answer emerges from health plans when they presume that, so long as their activities involve interpreting the contract and making coverage decisions, they cannot also at the same time be practicing medicine. In contrast to the example of straightforward contractual caps on dollars or inpatient days,[46] many of health plans' benefits decisions are based on judgments about whether the care in question is "medically necessary." As the *Corcoran* court observed, in these cases the plan makes a medical decision in order to make its benefits decision. Such medically based decisions permeate benefit determinations because the concept of medical necessity serves as the contractual cornerstone defining benefits in most health plans.[47] The simple fact that the MCO points to a contract does not, of itself, preclude the possibility that it is practicing medicine in the context of making bene-fits decisions.

In the third inadequate answer, health plans suggest that they are incapable of practicing medicine because they cannot physically examine patients, perform surgi-cal or diagnostic procedures, and the like. However, this is a misunderstanding of the essence of practicing medicine. Arguably, the most central element in clinical medicine is not the hands-on skills of examining patients and performing pro-cedures. In many cases, lesser-trained personnel can master these tasks with consid-erable facility.

Rather, the heart and soul of medicine as a learned profession is judgment. Thus, in many cases the surgeon's most crucial contribution is a series of judgments: whether this patient presents a surgical or nonsurgical problem and, if surgical, which particular procedure, using what specific implants or devices, would be most suitable. During surgery further judgments are required about what to do if the patient has atypical anatomy or, even more importantly, what to do if things go wrong. The skills of cutting and suturing are obviously important and require signif-icant training and experience, but these activities are not the hallmark of being a physician.

Similarly, the internist must gather history, symptoms, and signs and make judg-ments about which diagnoses are most plausible, which further tests are likely to yield useful information at what risk, and how to weigh those risks against the hoped-for information. For therapy, additional judgments weigh the likelihoods of success for various treatments against their possible harms. The act of writing the orders or even performing a diagnostic or therapeutic intervention is often the least demanding use of their expertise.

Throughout, uncertainties pepper the process. The judgments require empirical estimations of likelihoods and normative evaluations about merits, which collec-tively are based on scientific literature, consensus, and the practitioner's own clini-cal experience. Interestingly, some courts have begun to embrace the notion that judgment is the central element of practicing medicine, for instance in settings such as telemedicine, in which there is no physical contact whatsoever between physician and patient.[48]

Having discarded these three errant views, it is now possible to develop a clearer concept of what it is to practice medicine, whether by a physician or by a corpora-tion. Two elements are necessary, yet neither alone is sufficient: making a medical judgment and significantly influencing care.

(1) Making a medical judgment

In light of the foregoing, the first element is the exercise of medical judgment—the formulation of observations and opinions based on the esoteric, highly technical knowledge base that is distinctive to medicine as a profession. Two kinds of judging typically are involved.

First, there are empirical judgments about what is going on. These are typically made by gathering diagnostic information about the patient and then combining these individualized observations with broader scientific knowledge about which diseases or injuries are usually associated with this patient's signs and symptoms. In the *Murphy*[49] case discussed above, the dispute between the health plan and the treating physician concerned whether the patient's rather vague abdominal symptoms did or did not indicate the presence of gall bladder disease.

Second, there are normative judgments about what ought to be done. These involve estimations about the likelihood, magnitude, and value of the benefits and harms that a given intervention might pose for a given patient. Again, the esoteric knowledge is both general and specific. One must scientifically understand the general risk–benefit profile of a particular test or treatment, but it is also essential to determine how closely that broad picture applies to an individual patient. An exploratory surgery may be desirable for a young, otherwise healthy person but unduly risky for a frail elderly person. In the *Corcoran*[50] case the medical debate concerned the circumstances under which a woman with a high-risk pregnancy should be placed in continuous hospitalization.

Bona fide medical judgments thus involve issues that go beyond the health knowledge of ordinary folk. It does not take a brain surgeon to know that a patient need not be hospitalized to remove an ordinary small splinter from the tip of the finger,[51] and when a health plan denies funding for that sort of care the plan is not making a medical judgment. Likewise, a difference exists between medical judgments and the legal judgments or language analyses that are also sometimes required to interpret key elements of a contract. Thus, a health plan does not make a medical judgment when it determines, for example, that an aesthetic rhinoplasty is a noncovered "cosmetic" surgery rather than a reimburseable "corrective" or "reconstructive" procedure (assuming the patient has no history of traumatic accident or disfiguring birth defect and no impediment to breathing). Ordinary language, not sophisticated medical examinations, will suffice to determine that for this patient the procedure does not serve distinctly health-oriented goals. Admittedly, borderline cases will be plentiful and difficult.[52] The point here is simply that not all contractual interpretations and not all judgments about the nature of an enrollee's problem and its remedies require judgments of esoteric medical science.

(2) Significantly influencing care

Making a medical judgment does not, by itself, constitute the practice of medicine. A person sitting at a distance, merely contemplating someone's medical condition as an intellectual exercise, may be making medical judgments but obviously is not practicing medicine. To constitute practice, a medical judgment must in some sense be carried out—put into practice. It must be used to determine or at least significantly influence which care will be provided to a particular patient. This is the second element of practicing medicine.

The notion of "significantly influencing" must be included alongside "determining" the patient's care, because even physicians do not always determine their patients' care. The patient, after all, has some say in the matter. He can decline what is offered, request an alternative approach, or ostensibly agree with what is proposed and then fail to adhere. From a legal standpoint the inquiry into whether the MCO exerted the requisite level of influence should most plausibly be understood in classic causality terms, as the question of whether the MCO's coverage decision was a "substantial factor" in bringing about the treatment decision and thereafter the patient's outcome.[53]

The notion of "substantial factor" can be elusive to define, but in this context it might best be thought of along two dimensions. First, it must be the case that the MCO actually does owe (coverage for) the medical service in question. As noted above, when the MCO does not owe, for example, more than thirty days of inpatient care, then its refusal to provide coverage beyond that cannot possibly be "the cause" of the patient's hospital discharge, any more than a similar refusal by a neighbor who lives across the street.[54] The patient's lack of money will clearly be a factor in her decision to forego care, but because the health plan did not owe the coverage, then the patient's lack of money is an unfortunate fact of life that is not attributable to the MCO.[55]

Of course, cases will arise in which it is initially unclear whether the health plan owes coverage. In such instances it may be necessary to explore contractual questions before it can be ultimately determined whether the MCO practiced medicine in the two-pronged sense of making a medical judgment plus significantly influencing care.

Sometimes these contract questions can bring us right back into medical territory, as, for example, when the relevant contract clause is a requirement that the proposed intervention be "medically necessary." In these cases the health plan can be contractually correct only if first it is medically correct. Thus, if a proposed intervention was clearly "necessary" by any reasonable medical judgment, then a health plan denying that care has made a bad medical judgment and denied care that it in fact owed. In other cases the medical judgments will not be so clear. However, if the medical question is even seriously debatable, then once again we must conclude that the plan owes the care. After all, per Chapter 4's discussion of *contra proferentem,* contractual ambiguities (here, the ambiguity of "medically necessary") must ordinarily be construed against the drafter—the health plan. Thus, when a medical necessity judgment is the key to contract interpretation, a health plan's denial of coverage should only prevail if its medical judgment is clearly correct. Below we will explore further the problems that arise when health plans base contractual coverage decisions on medical necessity judgments.

The second dimension in determining whether an MCO's denial of coverage is a "substantial factor" in a treatment decision is the question of whether the denial was "material" to the decision. Materiality, a notion adapted here from the law of informed consent,[56] refers to information and decisional factors that are important enough, at least potentially, to sway a decision one way or another. As physicians decide what interventions to offer, or as patients decide what sort of treatment to undergo, they will consider a number of factors. In many cases a denial of funding will be decisive. Because medicine is often very expensive and because alternate sources of care or funding are increasingly difficult to obtain, sometimes either providers will refuse to offer it or the patient will decline the intervention because he cannot afford to pay for it.[57] In other cases, however, a health plan's decision may not be so crucial. The patient may have to pay only slightly more out of pocket, or providers may be willing to waive their charges, or other sources of funding may be readily available. In these cases the health plan's causal role may be substantially less.[58] One way or another, the question of materiality is fact-specific and can only be answered by examining the details of each case.[59]

In this context it is important to draw a distinction. It is one thing to determine whether an MCO's medical judgment substantially influenced the decisions made regarding a patient's care—that is, whether the MCO has practiced medicine—and quite another to discern whether those treatment decisions, in turn, were the cause of the patient's final outcome. For example, an MCO's decision not to cover bone marrow transplant for breast cancer may well have been pivotal in determining whether the patient ultimately received the transplant. It is another thing entirely to decide whether the lack of that treatment was the ultimate cause of this patient's death or whether, instead, the death was simply the product of an incurable disease. At that point the discussion has entered the realm of standard tort litigation in which four elements must be satisfied: duty of care, breach of duty, injury, and causation. Those questions, central to any finding that medical malpractice has been committed, can arise only after it is established whether the health plan was practicing medicine in the first place.

With the foregoing explication of the four domains of expertise that health plans owe their enrollees, it is now possible to discuss how tort litigation should proceed when plans are alleged to have breached those duties. That question will be explored in Section C of this chapter. However, an important intermediate step should be taken first. As proposed in Chapter 5, a major goal in adjusting health law to current economic and social realities is to assign tort and contract liabilities appropriately between plans and providers. That allocation, in turn, should be based on an appropriate division of control over various aspects of delivering health care. Doctors should do what they do best, as should health plans. As further argued in Chapter 5, MCOs should practice medicine sparingly rather than routinely because their major focus should concern patterns of care, not over-the-shoulder micromanagement. If so, then an important task in establishing the appropriate scope of tort liability for health plans will be to consider how much, when, and why MCOs currently practice medicine. As the following discussion proposes, health plans currently practice medicine far more than they should. Important reforms in this situation will be recommended before we then discuss how tort litigation should proceed when a health plan breaches its duty of expertise.

B. REDUCING CORPORATIONS' PRACTICE OF MEDICINE

A primary source of plans' practicing of medicine stems from the fact that health care contracts are standardly based on the concept of medical necessity. So long as health plans must first decide whether an intervention is medically necessary (thereby making a medical judgment) before they can make their coverage determination and so long as that financial coverage is prerequisite to receiving care for so many patients (thereby leading these medical judgments to have a significant impact on patients' treatments and outcomes), plans will continue to practice medicine routinely rather than sparingly. For many reasons, this arrangement needs to change.[60]

As noted in Chapter 4, although virtually all health plans now define their benefits in terms of medical necessity, this has not always been the case. For many years health plans covered almost any service that a physician chose to order until it became evident that some physician services were extravagent, untested, exclusively for convenience, or dubious in a host of other ways. However, not until the 1960s, in an attempt to curb costs, did health plans begin seriously to restrict what they would cover by introducing the rubric of "medical necessity." As further noted in Chapter 4, however, courts have often declined to to enforce plans' denials of coverage because the term was so vague. Over time plans attempted to carve out more explicit exclusions, such as for experimental or cosmetic care. Except for those, medical necessity has remained the fulcrum of health care contracts.[61]

To be precise, most health plans do not actually contain language stating an express promise to cover all medically necessary health care. Rather, contracts typically identify the categories of services they cover, such as inpatient care and outpatient care (including hospital and health professional services for both emergency and nonemergency situations); care for mental illness and substance abuse; prescription drugs; laboratory, radiology, and diagnostic services; home health care and hospice services; durable medical equipment; rehabilitation; and the like.[62] Not all plans cover all categories and, for care within the accepted categories, plans typically carve out exceptions. Common exclusions are for services that are "not medically necessary," "experimental," or "innovative." By implication, however, so long as a service is within an accepted category and is deemed medically necessary, it is covered.[63] One would be hard-pressed to find a health plan contract that explicitly denies services that fall within a covered category and that the plan acknowledges to be "medically necessary."

Note further that this implicit promise to cover all necessary services within the accepted categories is not limited to indemnity plans that govern resources via financial reimbursements and explicit utilization review. The promise also applies to capitated and other risk-sharing plans. An MCO might contract with primary care physicians (PCPs) under a capitation agreement, for instance, requiring them to provide primary care and a spectrum of laboratory, radiology, and specialist services.[64] Although such arrangements leave physicians considerable freedom to deliver care as they deem appropriate, in fact the contract the patient signs with the health plan will still contain the familiar categories of services, the same exclusions for experimental and medically unnecessary services, and the same implicit promise that, if a service within those categories is necessary, it will be covered. Moreover, the MCO's contract with PCPs will ordinarily list the kinds of services that physicians must cover in exchange for that capitated sum.[65] However specific or general that list may be and however free these physicians may be to deliver extra care, they must at least provide medically necessary services of the covered types. Hence, the plan's promise to the patient is the same no matter how it pays its physicians.

If health plans clearly owe their beneficiaries medically necessary care, however, it is not at all clear what medical necessity is. The term is notoriously difficult, if not impossible, to define. At one extreme, an intervention is only called "necessary" if it is " '*essential* to reach a goal of improving or curing a *disease.*' "[66] In principle, this minimalist definition could preempt many interventions currently deemed standard—in principle, even such mundane things as anesthesia for painful procedures. In contrast, Medicare's definition of "reasonable and necessary" inquires whether the intervention is " 'safe and effective, not experimental, and appropriate' " as defined by the Food, Drug, and Cosmetic Act of 1938.[67] On this much broader approach, an intervention is necessary if it "works."[68] In another common definition, medical necessity means "sufficiently accepted within the medical community to be covered as acceptable medical care."[69] Middle-ground definitions have begun to add the caveat that a service is only "necessary" if there is no comparable service that is "more conservative or less costly."[70]

Historically, health plans have tended to operationalize medical necessity by deferring to the collective judgments of the profession.[71] However, in light of the term's vagueness and the difficulty of enforcing benefit limits, plans have increasingly felt compelled to adopt clinical guidelines by which they then tell physicians, rather than ask them, which care is necessary and which is not. Many plans have also added specific procedures for determining the necessity of new technologies and innovative procedures.[72]

The problems with using "medical necessity" as the contractual cornerstone of health care benefits go far deeper than familiar complaints about meddling. Three major problems arise that, collectively, constitute sufficient reason to discard the concept entirely in favor of an alternative—namely, guidelines-based contracting, to be discussed further in Chapter 9.

The problems of contractual reliance on "medical necessity" affect everyone— plans, physicians, and patients. (1) The vagueness of "medical necessity" makes it very difficult for health plans to enforce denials of coverage, a problem that, in turn, makes it very difficult for plans to control their costs and thereby their premium price. (2) The concept does not fit the clinical realities of medicine and, as a benefits standard, it requires continual second-guessing of and interference with physicians. (3) The necessity standard mistreats patients in several ways: by decreasing their benefits as "medical necessity" is quietly redefined; by cultivating over-expectations through the promise of sameness among various health plans that, in fact, deliver very different levels of benefits; and by removing choices legitimately left to patients via the imperative of "necessary."

1. Problems of "Medical Necessity" for Health Plans

From health plans' perspective, perhaps the biggest drawback to the medical necessity criterion is the fact that its vagueness renders benefit denials difficult to defend in court. As a general principle of contract law, courts routinely construe ambiguities against contracts' drafters.[73] As explained in Chapter 4, this doctrine of *contra proferentem* is based on the fairness principle that because the party writing the agreement had the opportunity to make the wording clear, its failure to do so should not work against the party who lacked this opportunity.[74]

Given the obvious vagueness of the medical necessity concept, courts have often overturned health plans' denials of benefits on this familiar contractual ground. In *Van Vactor v. Blue Cross Ass'n*[75] the Illinois Supreme Court held that because "medically necessary" was ambiguous and contract disputes must be construed in favor of the insured, the patient should receive coverage for inpatient removal of impacted wisdom teeth. In *McLaughlin v. Connecticut General Life Ins. Co.*[76] the California Supreme Court likewise cited *contra proferentem* to hold that a Bahamas medical clinic's immunoaugmentive therapy should be covered for terminal lung cancer. In *Ex Parte Blue Cross-Blue Shield of Ala.*[77] the Alabama Supreme Court mandated coverage for inpatient care of osteoporosis-related fractures, while in *Group Hospitalization, Inc. v. Levin*[78] the District of Columbia appellate court awarded inpatient care for back pain. Many more cases could be cited,[79] but the upshot is clear. So long as health plans invoke the ambiguous concept of medical necessity to guide benefits decisions and so long as courts honor *contra proferentem,* plans can expect to lose frequently when their denials are challenged.[80]

This need not happen. Many recent court decisions have upheld benefits denials when the contracts are clear, a subject to which we will return in Chapter 11.[81] Suffice it here to say that because courts balk when the only basis for benefits denial is a fuzzy claim that "we deem this medically unnecessary" and because reciprocally they are quite willing to uphold clear contracts,[82] a health plan that wants to enforce limits on its expenditures effectively should abjure the medical necessity tradition in favor of considerably more explicit contracts.

2. Problems of "Medical Necessity" for Clinical Medicine

The ill fit between "necessity" and ordinary medical care is immediately obvious in the question facetiously bandied about when health plans first considered what to do about a newly approved drug for male impotence: how often per month (per week? per day?) is drug-assisted sexual intercourse "medically necessary"? Most medical decisions do not post clear choices of life versus death nor juxtapose complete cures against pure quackery. Rather, the daily stuff of medicine is a continuum requiring a constant weighing of uncertainties and values.[83] One antibiotic regimen may be medically comparable to and much less expensive than another but with slightly higher risks of damage to hearing or to organs such as kidneys or livers. For a patient needing hip replacement, one prosthetic joint may be longer-lasting but far costlier than an alternative. Of two equally effective drugs for hypertension, the costlier one may be more palatable because it has fewer side effects and a convenient once-a-day dosage.

Across such choices it is artificial precision to say that one option is "necessary," with the usual connotation of "essential" or "indispensable," while the other is "unnecessary," with the usual connotation of "superfluous" or "pointless." Various options have merits, and often no single approach is clearly *the* "correct" choice. A given option might be better described as "a good idea in this case," "reasonable given the cost of the alternative," "probably better than the alternative, if X rather than Y is the goal," "about as good as anything else," or "not quite ideal, but still acceptable." In many cases the real question is whether a particular medical risk or monetary cost is worth incurring in order to achieve a desired level of symptomatic relief or functional improvement or to reduce by some increment the risk of an adverse outcome or a missed diagnosis. A huge array of treatments fit this description: more or less worthwhile, but not (un)necessary in any ordinary sense. The patient will not die without it, and alternatives can be reasonable even if each has its drawbacks.

More broadly, concepts like necessity, appropriateness, and effectiveness can be defined only relative to a goal.[84] Antibiotics are not "effective" per se. They are effective against bacteria but, barring the placebo effect, ineffective against viruses. Hence, it makes no sense for a physician to prescribe antibiotics if the goal is to eradicate a viral infection. But if the goal is to placate a relentlessly demanding patient who insists on antibiotics for his viral infection, the prescription may indeed serve this latter aim—which is why so many physicians write so many antibiotic prescriptions for viral illnesses.[85] Choices in this realm require a level of clinical complexity that is not reflected in simplistic notions like necessity and that should not be hidden under blanket categories connoting a façade of precision.[86] It would be far better to acknowledge that, across a broad spectrum of such choices and trade-offs, it is legitimate for people to come to different conclusions about what sort of price is worth paying, medically and financially, to achieve what kinds of goals. To presume that a medical intervention is objectively either necessary or unnecessary belies the legitimacy of such variation in human goals and values.

The problem marches from the conceptual drawing board right into the clinical setting. As health plans try to apply this ill-fitting notion to actual medical decisions, their routine second-guessing and intrusions into the clinical setting are disruptive to provider–patient relationships and often are counterproductive. A considerably less intrusive approach, guidelines-based contracting, as outlined below, would have plans identify far more directly and specifically what they do and do not cover, with no implication that this or that alternative is categorically "unnecessary."

3. Problems of "Medical Necessity" for Patients

Patients can be harmed in several ways when benefits are allocated according to medical necessity. In the first place, the concept invites enrollees to entertain high, uniform expectations. So long as virtually every plan implicitly appears to promise all "necessary" care within the covered categories and so long as a person assumes (as many laymen do) that medicine is highly scientific and precise, then it is reasonable for health plan subscribers to expect that all plans based on medical necessity will provide the same benefits, aside from whatever explicit exceptions may differentiate them. And if, beyond this, subscribers invoke the most common conception of medical necessity—the definition requires only that an intervention be safe, effective, and appropriate in order to be "necessary"—then enrollees will believe they are entitled to receive "everything that works," regardless of the price of their plan. Indeed, the very notion of medical necessity implies a thoroughly scientific, medicine-based evaluation to which economic and other normative considerations are irrelevant.[87]

This bright promise of high, uniform benefits could hardly be farther from reality. As pointed out above, "medical necessity" can be defined very differently from one health plan to the next, ranging narrowly from only those interventions that will diagnose or cure disease to broad versions encompassing virtually everything that works. Even a uniform definition would not solve the problem. The federal Medicare program for the elderly and disabled, for example, ostensibly provides a uniform set of benefits to all enrollees, even though various insurers act as the plan's fiscal intermediaries. Yet in a study conducted by the General Accounting Office, Medicare payment for a chest X-ray was 451 times more likely to be denied in Illinois than in South Carolina; payment for a physician office visit was almost 10 times more likely to be denied in Wisconsin than in California; and payment for real-time echocardiography was nearly 100 times more likely to be denied by Transamerica Occidental than by Blue Shield of California.[88]

Just as the definition and practical implementation of medical necessity can vary widely from one plan or geographic region to another, so can implementation change quickly and quietly even within a plan. One area in which an erosion of benefits is particularly disturbing concerns interventions that mainly restore or preserve quality of life.[89] These are the interventions that provide comfort and function, as distinct from more dramatic life-and-death treatments. People do not often die from untreated cataracts, for instance, even if their lives are considerably disrupted by an inability to see well enough to read or drive. Yet patients in some prepaid health plans are significantly less likely to have cataract extraction than patients in fee-for-service (FFS) plans.[90]

Similarly, rehabilitation once deemed standard is also becoming scarcer.[91] Patients with stroke may be discharged to nursing homes rather than to rehabilitation facilities, with potentially less opportunity for improved function.[92] A plan may decide that epidural anesthesia is unnecessary for normal vaginal childbirth since, after all, the pain is only transient.[93] In some cases, entire medical disciplines are under economic pressure because they focus mainly on quality of life. These range from dermatology and mental health care to ophthalmology, orthopedics, reconstructive plastic surgery, and end-of-life care.[94] Less care does not necessarily mean worse care, of course, because the "artesian" fee-for-service system rewarded excesses that can sometimes harm more than help. But at some point, less is worse.

As a health plan's (usually undisclosed) guidelines and thus its specific benefits shift underneath the vaguely worded contract, the result can be a steady erosion, an undertow right underfoot, in that plan's actual coverage. A subscriber cannot know, up front, precisely what he has purchased in a health plan nor be sure later that he owns what he originally (thought he) bought. It may cover much less than he thinks if administrators flesh out the slippery "necessity" concept differently than he expects. When necessity is defined according to physician acceptance, the iteration of what "works" can change as fleetingly as the fashions of consensus.[95] And because the vague concept of "necessary" does not fit quality-of-life–oriented interventions very well, it is easy for health plans to dub these interventions discretionary, hence unnecessary, and therefore eminently eliminable.

Of note, when health plans shrink their iteration of necessary services, patients do not often enjoy financial savings. Everyone but the patient seems to benefit as health plans, employers, and governments pocket the savings while patients endure greater discomfort, reduced function, or even a diminished chance for survival. Unfortunately, so long as the deleted interventions are dubbed "unnecessary," ostensibly patients are not being deprived of anything important, and the underlying, value-laden trade-offs remain unrecognized. Even when the benefit cuts serve mainly to avert cost increases, patients rarely have the opportunity to participate in decisions about which of the benefits financed by their own money should be cut and which retained.[96]

In this sense, the notion of necessity also preempts choice. "Necessary" is an imperative. As defined by an Ohio appellate court borrowing from *Webster's Dictionary,* it means: essential, inevitable, inescapable, predetermined, compulsory, absolutely needed, required.[97] The general tenor is that the thing is indispensable. In medicine people other than the patient make most of the important decisions regarding what should be covered and what should not. Up to a point this reasoning is valid. If the fundamental objectives of health care are to save lives and preserve capacities for function, medical science has much to say regarding which sorts of care are essential, which are marginal, and which are actually harmful toward those goals. But that is hardly the final word. Necessity and effectiveness, as noted, can only be defined relative to a goal.[98] And the principle of informed consent holds that the patient, not the health plan or even the physician, should ordinarily choose the goals and, within certain parameters, also the means of treatment.[99]

Calling an intervention "necessary" usually means the health plan must cover it and thus that subscribers must pay for it in the purchase price. When "necessity" is defined as "everything that works," people can be forced to pay for care that many might deem excessive.[100] Combine these features with the fact that it is virtually impossible to know in advance what a necessity-based plan includes, and it becomes comparably impossible to select a plan on the basis of what it does and does not cover. Consumers have little or no control over what they buy.

Other commentators have also questioned medical necessity as the fulcrum for benefits decisions.[101] However, for the most part those observers, noting that the concept is vague, propose that we need a more uniform way to identify which interventions are "truly necessary" and which are not.[102] However, as should by now be evident, the real problems run far deeper than these previous discussions suggest. The very idea of trying to classify each intervention as somehow intrinsically "necessary" or not, and thereby of trying to assemble a single set of standards identifying "the" appropriate care in each situation, is inherently misguided.

C. TORT LITIGATION FOR BREACH OF EXPERTISE DUTIES

1. Torts Regarding Administration and Guidelines

At this point we can discuss how tort litigation against health plans should proceed when plans have allegedly violated their duties of expertise. As a prefatory note it may be recalled from Chapter 6 that health plans' breaches of expertise often will be associated with breaches of resource duties—though not necessarily, because the two are distinct. Breaches of contract, as wrongful denials of reimbursements or health care, will be discussed in the next chapter. Meanwhile, expertise duties, which concern the process more than the outcome of decision making, should be addressed in tort.

In any given case one of the first and often most difficult issues will be to determine whether the problem is one of contract, or tort, or both, and whether the breach was committed by the physician(s), the health plan(s), or both. Resolving such questions requires careful factual investigation. The case of *Ouellette v. Christ Hosp.*[103] highlights the challenges. A woman was hospitalized for removal of her ovaries. Allegedly, her HMO's guidelines required that patients should be discharged within two days after this procedure. Although Ms. Ouelette was experiencing pain, fever, and blood clots in her urine on the second day of hospitalization, a hospital nurse informed her she must leave by 6:00 pm. The patient's physician stated that, had the nurse informed him of the patient's late deterioration, he would not have discharged her.

ERISA preemption issues were resolved by remanding the case to state courts, at which juncture some interesting factual questions might arise regarding who breached which duties. If the HMO actually did mandate, with no flexibility, that patients must be discharged two days after this type of surgery, one might challenge the medical credibility of its guidelines—potentially a problem of HMO expertise. However, it is quite possible that the HMO guidelines actually stated the two-day time frame as only a goal, to be revised if medical circumstances require it. In that case, other scenarios are possible. Perhaps an HMO representative, inadequately informed about the guidelines, wrongly informed the hospital that the guidelines were not as flexible as they in fact were—another problem of HMO expertise, if it did not properly train and supervise its representatives.

Alternatively, perhaps the problem came from the hospital, which allegedly was under an incentive scheme from the HMO. In this scenario, perhaps the hospital influenced its staff to discharge patients too promptly—another expertise problem, but this time from the provider side rather than from the HMO (unless the incentive scheme itself was so overbearing that it created an undue influence on providers, another allegation the plaintiff made in this case). Or perhaps the nurse simply took matters too much into her own hands. This would again represent a problem of provider expertise if the hospital inadequately selected, trained, and supervised its nursing staff.

In yet another scenario, perhaps the guideline was not actually misapplied in this case, so that there was no breach of expertise at all. Many patients are now discharged earlier than they might have been under past practices because home care and other support services have made it possible to treat many more conditions on an outpatient basis. If the discharge itself was reasonable but the HMO failed to provide appropriate outpatient support services, then there may be a breach of contract as well as of expertise. Or if the discharge and its follow-up were done in a medically reasonable way, there may have been no breach of any duties at all.

Indeed, the court does not describe any actual physical injury the patient suffered, only discomfort and anxiety: Ms Ouellette "continued to suffer from the after-effects of surgery."[104]

Numerous scenarios are possible, and the determination of who erred in what ways and whether the problems represented errors of expertise, of resources, or both can be made only with detailed investigation. Such situations do not challenge the basic analysis presented in this book. They simply present complex factual questions of the sort that juries are routinely asked to answer.

We may proceed, then, to consider how health plans' breaches of expertise should be litigated in tort. Just as with physicians' expertise breaches, these suits should follow standard tort requirements: a duty of care, a breach of that duty, and an injury proximately caused by the breach. Such breaches could occur in any of a health plan's four domains of expertise: business administration, promoting patterns of good care, monitoring for patterns of poor care, and practicing medicine. The first three will be briefly examined here before focusing on MCOs' practice of medicine.

a. Business Administration

The duty of care governing business activities should be established in fairly traditional ways, such as by examining the industry's own routines and collective experience in this very complex enterprise. Just as physicians can best judge whether a fellow physician properly sutured a wound, experienced health plan administrators have crucial insights about what constitutes efficiency and accuracy in delivering goods, services, and payments when and where they are supposed to go. Accordingly, expert witnesses can comment on what sorts of behavior are within the normal range of industry (in)efficiency and which ones fall outside the bounds of acceptability. Industry customs might also be supplemented by respected treatises and by the guidelines or recommendations of reputable industry organizations. Additionally, consumers, with their considerable experience on the receiving end of health plans' administrative successes and mix-ups, also have an important perspective on what level of ineptitude is reasonable to expect within the normal, acceptable range of inefficiency. This input will mainly come from juries of laypeople.

Also important is the concept that just as the law has never demanded that physicians practice error-free, a certain amount of imperfection in plans' business decisions must be accepted as inevitable. As noted by one court: "'A doctor is not negligent simply because his or her efforts prove unsuccessful. The fact a doctor may have chosen a method of treatment that later proves to be unsuccessful is not negligence if the treatment chosen was an accepted treatment on the basis of the information available to the doctor at the time a choice had to be made; a doctor must, however, use reasonable care to obtain the information needed to exercise his or her professional judgment, and an unsuccessful method of treatment chosen because of a failure to use such reasonable care would be negligence.'"[105]

Analogously, the Business Judgment Rule is a "judicial doctrine that protects directors from liability for mistakes in judgment exercised in good faith, without divided loyalty, with appropriate inquiry, and with the rational belief that the decision is in the best interest of the corporation" (or, in this case, of the health plan and its beneficiaries).[106] "The rationale for the Rule is that it encourages rational risk-taking and innovation, limits litigation and unfair liability exposure, encourages service by competent directors, and limits judicial intrusiveness into the affairs of the corporation."[107]

The Seventh Circuit likewise embraced some leeway for error in *Frahm v. Equitable Life Assur. Soc. of U.S.*[108] The court noted that health plan administrators who function as fiduciaries in ERISA plans have a duty of care, but that duty does not require them to produce ideal results. They are expected only to exercise the "care, skill, prudence, and diligence under the circumstances then prevailing that a prudent man acting in a like capacity and familiar with such matters would use in conduct of like enterprise."[109]

These sources for establishing plans' duties of business expertise are summarized in *Jones v. Chicago HMO.*, in which the Illinois Supreme Court found that tort suits against HMOs can appropriately use the same sorts of evidence appropriate to make a tort claim against a hospital: "the standard of care required of a hospital in a case of institutional negligence may be shown by a wide variety of evidence, including, but not limited to, expert testimony, hospital bylaws, statutes, accreditation standards, custom and community practice. . . . [T]his variety of evidence is appropriate given the inherent diversity in hospital administrative and managerial actions, only a portion of which involves the exercise of medical judgment."[110]

b. Guidelines for Good Care, Surveillance for Poor Care

Clinical practice guidelines and the guidelines by which plans monitor physicians' performance quality[111]—plans' second and third domains of expertise—likewise must measure up to a standard of care. MCOs must bring good medical reasoning to the process whereby they select and modify their guidelines over time because those guidelines will significantly influence plans' practice of medicine and the ways in which their physicians practice.

Case law supports the point. *Wickline v. State of California*[112] opined that defects in design of utilization review, which obviously can encompass medically unreasonable guidelines, can warrant tort liability. In *Shannon v. McNulty*[113] a Pennsylvania superior court noted that

> [t]hese decisions may, among others, limit the length of hospital stays, restrict the use of specialists, prohibit or limit post hospital care, restrict access to therapy, or prevent rendering of emergency room care. While all of these efforts are for the laudatory purpose of containing health care costs, when decisions are made to limit a subscriber's access to treatment, that decision *must pass the test of medical reasonableness*. To hold otherwise would be to deny the true effect of the provider's actions, namely, dictating and directing the subscriber's medical care.[114]

The court went on to note that the health plan "was under a duty to oversee that the dispensing of advice by its telephone-nurses would be performed *in a medically reasonable manner*.[115]

The state of Washington requires in its patient protection legislation that utilization review criteria be based on reasonable medical evidence.[116] Similarly, in *Crum v. Health Alliance Midwest, Inc.*[117] a man with a history of heart disease experiencing agitation, nausea, and symptoms classic for heart attack was told by a telephone advisory nurse that he had excess stomach acid. If the guidelines the MCO provided for those nurses truly identified indigestion as the only plausible diagnosis, it would be difficult to call them medically credible. In sum, plans' creation, selection, and adaptation of clinical guidelines and of physician-profiling instruments should reflect sound medical judgment.[118]

At the same time, the complexities inherent in assessing guidelines' medical credibility must be appreciated. As detailed in Chapter 5, a dearth of scientific research makes guideline construction precarious, although outcomes research is growing steadily and solid techniques for crafting reliable guides are emerging. Quite likely courts adjudicating challenges to the scientific merits of guidelines will need, at certain points, to implement a *Daubert*[119] type of process to appraise the credibility of testimony on the scientific worth or this or that guideline.[120] Havighurst suggests that in this process, a court

> might consider whether the drafters consulted with objective sources and medical experts, expressly considered trade-offs from a consumer perspective, and disclosed the economizing nature of the exercise to the insureds and anyone acting on their behalf. It might also credit an insurer's reliance on objective medical advice in implementing exclusions from coverage, its willingness to consult with the treating doctor in difficult cases, and its use of reasonable procedures for finally resolving close questions. If a court could be satisfied on these scores, there is every likelihood that health care 'rationing' that accorded reasonably with contractual language would be permitted to proceed.[121]

Two additional caveats are also important. One is the need for courts to accept flexibility and a diversity of approaches when no decisive reason exists to adopt any one particular approach. It is the guidelines-equivalent of the "two schools of thought" rule by which tort law permits physicians' practices to vary.

The other caveat is that this diversity can legitimately be shaped by cost considerations. As discussed in the next chapter, there are many legitimate ways to make the risk–benefit and cost–value trade-offs implicit throughout medical decision making, and people should have the freedom to make choices about how much they are willing to spend for what level of health care resources.[122] The bare fact that a health plan does not cover an intervention that science shows to be of value does not, ipso facto, permit a conclusion that the guideline is inadequate. Rather, the evaluation should consider whether the plan's cost–value trade-offs have been made clear to enrollees and whether they fit within a reasonable rationale in the context of the plan's overall resource constraints.

Accordingly, tort evaluation in this area should focus largely on procedures. Relevant questions include how the MCO chose or developed the guideline in question—what scientific basis it has, whether qualified physicians were invited to comment on it, and how readily the plan makes changes if clinical experience shows the guideline to be flawed.

Across these first three of health plans' expertise domains—business administration, guidelines of good care, surveillance for poor care—the foregoing discussion addresses the most challenging aspect of litigating health plans' duties of expertise: establishing what standard of care the plan owes the enrollee in each of these domains and what sort of evidence is needed to determine whether that duty has been met or breached. Of course, two other elements of tort remain, namely the existence of an injury and a causal relation between a breach and the injury. These should be established in tort law's usual ways, although causality issues merit a special comment. As noted in the definition of what it is for a health plan to practice medicine, a plan cannot be said to be a "substantial factor" in causing a patient's course of care or outcome if, in fact, the plan did not owe the treatment in question. In this sense, part of the tort causality question requires examining the contract.

Also important to consider is that the bare fact that a patient has an unfortunate outcome does not mean that her condition is different from what it would have been had she been treated differently. Some illnesses are not easily treated, and a health plan's refusal to provide this or that intervention does not necessarily mean that the patient's subsequent poor outcome is due to the lack of that treatment. For example, over the past decade a number of courts have found MCOs at fault for wrongful death by denying autologous bone marrow transplant (ABMT) for women with breast cancer. Recent studies, however, indicate that the treatment is no more effective than conventional chemotherapy.[123] Therefore, even if the health plan might have had some contractual obligation to provide the treatment, or even if its administration breached expertise duties,[124] a plan that denies the treatment should not be fingered as the cause of a woman's poor outcome once science has published a clear conclusion.[125]

2. Tort Claims When Health Plans Practice Medicine

It is time now to consider those cases in which the health plan has allegedly practiced medicine and gone beyond merely being careless in its administrative and supervisory tasks. As noted in Chapter 3, health plans have long been subject to tort claims of direct liability for corporate negligence and vicarious liability for the actions of their employees or ostensible agents. In many cases these claims are called "medical malpractice," but to be precise, as yet few claims have been made for classic medical malpractice—practicing medicine below the standard of care—because it has been controversial whether and under what definition a health plan can literally practice medicine.[126] As argued above, this book holds that health plans can, do, and sometimes must practice medicine. And so it becomes appropriate to consider the conditions under which they can rightly be held at fault for classic medical malpractice.

As a prefatory point it is useful to note that if health plans renounce traditional contractual reliance on "medical necessity" in favor of explicit guidelines-based contracting (to be discussed further in Chapter 9), they will have vastly reduced the extent to which they practice medicine and thereby reduced the extent to which they are vulnerable to this particular tort claim. Under guidelines-based contracting the plan points to its detailed guidelines and says "if you purchase this plan, here is precisely what you get. . . ." Immediately, most of the instances in which health plans are currently practicing medicine by making medical judgments about "necessity" will be transformed into fairly straightforward matters of contract interpretation. Administrators will look at the relevant part of the plan's guidelines and conclude: "see, here it is—you do not get that in this plan." When this is the case, so long as the administrators exercise due care in coming to their conclusions, their decision is subject to standard contract law but not to malpractice tort law. When a plan has wrongly but non-negligently failed to provide what it was obligated to cover, contract law can provide surprisingly adequate remedies (more on this in Chapter 10).

Admittedly, not all guidelines-based contract interpretations will be clear and straightforward. Even the best clinical guidelines cannot cover every possible scenario. Sometimes they will be unclear about the case at hand, and in other cases they may fail to take into account a patient's atypical presentation or unusual clinical condition and will require a legitimate exception. These scenarios are probably the leading instances in which an MCO will practice medicine and thereby potentially be subject to malpractice liability.[127]

On whatever grounds it is made, a malpractice claim against a health plan cannot succeed unless the plaintiff first shows that the MCO was actually practicing medicine. To recall the definition above, practicing medicine involves two dimensions: (a) making a medical judgment that (b) has a significant impact on the patient's care and outcome. Both these dimensions require elaboration.

a. Making Medical Judgments

Clear guidelines that apply clearly to a particular situation do not require an MCO to make medical judgments. If an otherwise healthy adult bumps his head but experiences no dizziness or loss of consciousness, a guideline might suggest a brief period of observation followed by instructions for rest and for reexamination if symptoms change. If such a patient nevertheless demands a CT scan just to be sure his headache does not signify terrible trauma or a sudden onset of brain cancer, the MCO can point to the guideline and declare "see—here it is: you do not get that in this situation."

A well-crafted guideline will also provide alternate options for common variations of the situation, as, for example, when someone has experienced loss of consciousness, double vision, or the like. More broadly, within these various scenarios, guidelines commonly offer an array of options, not just one-size-fits-all mandates.[128] Well-constructed, flexible guides are usually able to address the great majority of routine situations, and routine situations, by definition, represent the great majority of cases.[129] When guidelines are sufficiently clear and applicable to the particular patient, there should be little need for discussion.[130]

Note that in cases in which a guideline clearly permits a particular service or product and the MCO nevertheless wrongfully denies it, the plan is engaging in straightforward breach of contract, not the practice of medicine. For instance, if an MCO's drug formulary includes a particular medication the patient prefers, but a

UR clerk mistakenly says that drug is not on the list, then the problem is simple breach of contract. An expertise-tort involving sloppy business practices might be alleged, but it will not be a tort of classic medical malpractice.

At the same time, even the best guidelines will not cover every scenario. If the head-bumping patient is a child who also happens to have gobbled up the anti-coagulent (blood-thinner) pills prescribed for her grandmother, the standard guidelines may be inapplicable because in this unusual scenario there is an increased danger of intracranial hemorrhage or other complications atypical of ordinary head bumps. In exceptional situations the MCO must combine two sorts of reasoning.

1. When the "letter" of the guideline is insufficient, the MCO must interpolate the "spirit" of the contract to apply to the instant situation. This periodic need to interpolate is common throughout contracts and contract law. If the contract is generous, the MCO might have to approve whatever interventions would maximize the health and safety of the patient, regardless of cost. But if the plan generally restricts enrollees to the most cost-effective interventions, the options will be more limited. It is one thing for the patient to request a flexibility that can be legitimately encompassed within the overall resource philosophy and limits of the plan, and quite another to ask for a clearly higher level of care. In this process, the MCO is not necessarily making medical judgments. These decisions are often more akin to interpretations about the logical and conceptual fit between a proposed treatment and the kinds of treatments generally encompassed within the plan.

2. A different sort of reasoning requires the MCO to discern, as it evaluates requests for care outside the guidelines, whether the proposed care is likely to help the patient or whether some alternative would be as good or better. For these judgments the MCO must know what the patient's current condition is, which kinds of interventions have what probabilities of helping, with what risks, and the like. A request for a costly drug that is not on the formulary, for instance, will require information about what side-effects the patient has experienced with the approved drugs, or what contraindications the patient's condition may present, how likely the requested drug will be to avoid side-effects, and so forth. In such situations the MCO is making medical judgments. These medical judgments can be made well or poorly, with adequate or inadequate information, and with a good or poor understanding of the clinical realities of diagnosis and treatment for people in this patient's situation. In this context MCOs should be held to a medical standard of care for the adequacy of the factual and medical basis on which they make their medical judgments.

b. Affecting Patient Care

Aside from making medical judgments, practicing medicine requires that the judgment be implemented. As observed previously, two elements are important.

First, the denied intervention must be owed by the MCO to the enrollee. When it is not owed, then even if the lack of coverage prompts a denial of care and ultimately an adverse outcome, that outcome is not attributable to the plan. The MCO is no more responsible than any other bystander who also did not owe the intervention.[131] Undoubtedly, a significant area for litigation will focus on the ambiguous cases in which coverage is unclear. But if contracts are based on reasonably clear guidelines instead of fuzzy "medical necessity," these instances should be far fewer than is currently the case. Indeed, the prospect of reducing their susceptibility to medical malpractice claims should be an incentive for MCOs to move away from medical necessity–based contracts toward guidelines-based contracting.

Second, the denial of resources must have a significant impact on decision making. The actual impact of a denial can vary from case to case. In many instances, given the high cost of care, a denial of coverage will obviously qualify as "significantly affecting patient care." Even a rather minor impact on care could warrant a finding that the health plan practiced medicine, albeit with a recognition that the plan will have a lesser responsibility for the outcome when its denial was less material to the patient's care and outcome. In many jurisdictions the health plan's actual level of responsibility can be analyzed in terms of proportionate (comparative) fault.[132] Other times the denial may mean only a limited increase in the patient's copayment, as when the plan covers 80% instead of 90%.[133] The patient may be affluent, or the service may be inexpensive, or other sources of funding may conveniently be found, or providers may offer free care.

These analyses will most likely be case-specific, perhaps inquiring how easily that individual could have gotten treatment despite the denial of coverage, or perhaps inquiring more broadly whether the "reasonable person" would have deemed the influence significant. But again, the court need only inquire into this issue if it finds that the health plan did owe the patient the coverage in question. If coverage was not owed, then obviously its denial could not have been a "substantial factor" in causing the treatment decision, no matter how badly the patient needed the treatment or the money. And the plan will not have practiced medicine.

3. Holding Health Plans Liable for Medical Malpractice

At this point, a claim that might earlier have seemed a bit outlandish should seem fairly self-evident. Health plans can practice medicine, quite literally. And when they do, they should be susceptible to claims of medical malpractice, of the same sort for which physicians have traditionally been held liable. When an MCO has practiced medicine, the usual tort criteria of duty of care, breach, injury, and causation will apply. Injury and causation will be established in the usual ways, as discussed above regarding plans' expertise duties for administration and guidelines.

For technical reasons, the duty of care governing a health plan's practice of medicine will be a bit different from that governing a physician. A physician's expertise duties include, for example, the obligation to examine the patient carefully, to listen carefully and knowledgeably to heart sounds, or to use a scalpel with precision so as to avoid damaging nearby tissue. Obviously an organization cannot literally perform such hands-on functions nor engage in reasoning as an individual human does. An organization must therefore achieve the equivalent of such reasoning and hands-on examination by seeking information and advice from persons who can. In doing this the MCO's duty of care will be to obtain sufficient input from people who are qualified to give it. The MCO must obtain an adequate, accurate, factual picture from those who examine the patient[134] and must then assess that information with the aid of qualified advice. For example, it should not ask a dermatologist about appropriate care for a child in pediatric intensive care or draw conclusions about the effectiveness of lung reduction surgery for emphysema by asking a general pediatrician.[135]

Thus, when health plans practice medicine, tort litigation will focus heavily on the quality of evidence and the quality of reasoning behind the plan's decision. Because these cases lie at the borderline between individuals' needs and those of the broader population of the plan's members, or at the fuzzy edges of contract language, the emphasis is on procedure. Courts should look not so much at the substantive decision the health plan makes as at the procedures through which it was decided.

Peregrine and Schwartz offer a useful analogue from the business setting. The determination of whether a business judgment is reasonable and adequately informed "will likely include (i) the importance of the business judgment to be made; (ii) the time available for obtaining information; (iii) the costs related to obtaining information; (iv) the director's confidence in those who reviewed a matter and those making related presentations; and (v) the condition of the corporation's business at the time and the nature of competing demands for the Board's attention."[136] Adapting this approach to health plans' decision making, item (iv) would focus on the qualifications of the physicians and other experts who provide specific information about the particular patient, general information about that patient's illness or condition, and the reasonable approaches to its treatment. Item (v) legitimizes the need to acknowledge the competing demands for the health plan's funding as well as the spirit by which the guidelines direct resources for enrollees' care.[137]

This chapter has opened the door to tort liability for MCOs on a wide range of grounds, from administrative carelessness to classic medical malpractice. As noted at several points, however, health plans could significantly limit their exposure to malpractice tort by changing significantly the way in which they contract. It is to contract law that we now turn.

9

RESHAPING LIABILITY FOR HEALTH PLANS: RESOURCES AND CONTRACT

Chapter 6 proposed that contract rather than tort should be the primary legal avenue for addressing resource issues in health care. As noted there, tort law mandates a single, uniform standard of care—a uniformity now far more illusory than real. Moreover, as pointed out in Chapter 2, when resource requirements are incorporated into a tort standard of care that physicians owe all their patients, physicians are granted too much power to determine how much money other people must spend for what kind of health care. Such choices should instead belong mainly to the people who receive and who directly or indirectly pay for care. Contract law governs people who come together to work out their own agreements. It thus provides the better vehicle for providing citizens with the freedom to decide what level of health care resources to purchase in what sort of delivery system.[1]

However, Chapter 4 observed that the conditions for effective, enforceable contracting are not well met in the current health care environment. Contracts are often ambiguous and adhesory, and benefits determinations made under these conditions can seem or be arbitrary. As a result, courts are frequently obligated to favor the patient over the health plan, thereby potentially impeding plans' ability to manage resources effectively.

As Chapter 8 then explained, a major source of this vagueness is health plans' reliance on "medical necessity" as the cornerstone of their contracts. Basing benefits determinations on medical necessity creates serious problems for plans, providers, and patients alike. The term's vagueness must commonly be construed against plans, making it difficult for them to enforce even reasonable limits on their re-

126

sources and thereby also difficult to plan for all enrollees' care within a limited budget. For physicians "medically necessary" simply does not fit the nuances of clinical reality. And because it requires health plans to make medical judgments as part of their benefits determinations, plans must routinely second-guess clinical decisions, a move that often locks physicians in combat with plans and even with their own patients. For patients "all medically necessary care" promises uniform, generous benefits. Yet actual benefits vary widely and are steadily eroding as health plans cut back on "unnecessary" benefits. Medical necessity thus perpetuates the myth of consistent, ample benefits even while its vagueness is the very tool used to undercut patients' care. Conversely, "necessary" also sometimes functions as an imperative mandating costly benefits, raising premium prices, and preempting legitimate patient choice.

All this suggests that substantial change is needed before contract law can fulfill its promise as the best forum in which to account for health care resources. Contrary to the usual contract paradigm in which two or more parties have relatively equal bargaining power to create an exchange designed to maximize the welfare of each, health care contracts will not be fully effective until the conditions for enforceable contracting are met: choice, information, and bargaining power.[2] Those conditions are the focus of this chapter.

A. CONDITIONS FOR EFFECTIVE CONTRACTING

1. Choice

Ideally, health care contracts should offer real options that permit people to place their own value on health care services and let those values be reflected in the scope and cost of the health plans they purchase. However, there is a caveat. Because people place differing values on health care relative to alternative expenditures they might make with the same funds, permitting genuine choice means permitting diversity among health plans, which is tantamount to inequality of entitlements to receive care. In a society that has traditionally prized egalitarian health care (at least in principle if not in reality), it will be important to discuss the justifications for openly accepting such inequality.

a. The Ideal

As argued previously, different people can have widely differing views about what goals are important to achieve in health care and what risks and costs are worth paying to reach those goals. If so, then bona fide choices among health plans should present real differences regarding the amounts and kinds of services available at what cost. In effect, patients should be able to choose among varying tiers of care. Tiered health care has been proposed by this author[3] and by others[4] and need not be elaborated in detail here. A variety of reasonable approaches have been described, and it is not the purpose of this book to provide a definitive analysis. Hence, the following is offered as just one plausible possibility.[5]

"Basic" care, the kind to which all citizens should have assured access, should encompass interventions that are clearly effective in promoting the central goals of medicine: preserving life; preventing illness, injury, and premature death; relieving unnecessary pain and suffering; preserving or improving function for major life activities; and ameliorating disabling conditions.[6] When only one intervention exists that can reliably achieve such a goal, it should ordinarily be considered basic. If more than one treatment is available with roughly comparable effectiveness, then basic care might include only the less costly.

Tiers of care that exceed this basic level might differ in various ways. First, plans could differ on the threshold of evidence required before a test or treatment is deemed sufficiently "safe and effective" to warrant inclusion in the plan's benefits. As noted in Chapter 5, the strength and quality of scientific evidence on behalf of such conclusions can vary considerably. David Hadorn identifies several possible standards of proof: (1) "[r]easonably expected to provide significant net health benefit;" (2) "[r]easonably well demonstrated to provide significant net health benefit;" and (3) "[c]learly demonstrated to provide significant net health benefit."[7] On such a scheme, leaner plans might demand a stronger burden of proof before adding a new intervention, while a richer plan might accept any intervention that is reasonably promising until and unless evidence shows it to be ineffective.[8] An innovative multi-organ transplant, for instance, might be excluded by a basic plan if it showed less than a fifty percent chance of one-year survival.[9] Leaner plans might also exclude treatments that are not clearly intended for a medical problem, such as growth hormone for children who have no deficiency of growth hormone or other specific medical indication.[10]

Second, plans could vary regarding interventions that are only marginally different in their effectiveness and safety. If a costly new drug adds only a small benefit, such as an improved success rate of two percent or less, a leaner plan might presume to use the less costly version and restrict the new one, perhaps for limited indications or only with special justification. Or, as emerging science permits diagnosis of genetic predispositions toward diseases such as breast cancer, leaner plans might demand a great rather than small likelihood that a trait would produce disease before covering prophylactic treatment.[11]

Third, health plans might differ on matters of transient comfort and convenience (as distinct from long-term function and quality of life). Thus, richer plans could include the convenience of costlier, once-a-day drugs,[12] while leaner ones might emphasize generics.[13]

Fourth, plans might vary in the extent to which they offer access to research trials. Although health plans would help themselves as well as their members by contributing more support to carefully selected research protocols,[14] basic plans might limit their participation to the most promising trials and permit only a limited number of patients to enroll in a given trial at any one time. Costlier plans might offer broader access to approved trials, and still richer plans might permit access to trials that are based more on theoretical promise than on research-based evidence. Thus, novel surgical procedures might be found only in the richer plans until they have a reliable track record.

While offering genuine diversity, such a tiered approach need not involve a large, confusing smorgasbord of choices with endless combinations and permutations of benefits. For most people a few basic plan types would be far easier to learn about and choose among. Human autonomy is often better enhanced by a limited range of real choices than by an endless array of minutiae.[15] Therefore, instead of having each health plan create its own guidelines, as is often currently the case, one might envision just a few tiers, perhaps four or five, with each tier's level and kinds of care nationally standardized from plan to plan.[16]

At that point, various insurers and MCOs could choose at what levels they wish to offer health plans. One company might want to offer plans at just the first level or two, another might want to focus on upper-end plans, and another might offer a plan at every level. At any given tier consumers might find a number of insurers and MCOs offering plans from which to choose. Competition among plans would then focus not on the level of benefits offered (since these would be explicit and standardized at each tier), but on the quality of their providers, the convenience of their facilities, their premium costs and copays, and the like. Various plans might also provide ways to enhance enrollees' choices, for example, by offering access to off-plan providers, tests, and treatments through cost-sharing.[17]

Such a move has precedent. Recognizing that excessive variety can become confusing if not paralyzing to intelligent choice,[18] the federal government made basic changes several years ago in the so-called "MediGap" insurance that many older citizens buy to cover expenses not covered by Medicare. These plans had become so numerous and varied so widely that comparison shopping was virtually impossible. Accordingly, federal legislation limited insurers to just ten levels of MediGap insurance. A given insurer might offer all ten or only a few selected levels, but each of the ten coverage levels must be the same, no matter which insurer offers it. Plans then compete on other factors, such as quality of service and cost.[19]

If applied throughout health care, the proposed four or five tiers would probably have greater credibility if their respective guidelines were constructed not by MCOs, employers, or proprietary organizations,[20] as is currently the case, but rather by an independent entity whose purpose is to study health care interventions and outcomes and to create appropriate clinical protocols. Such an agency could be government sponsored, or perhaps better, it might be a private, nonprofit entity funded by contributions.[21] Indeed, if guidelines were produced by an independent agency, then a nagging legal problem would be signicantly ameliorated. When health plans construct their own guidelines, courts must continue to construe the ambiguities against the plans, *contra proferentem*. In contrast, if standardized guideline tiers were designed by an independent entity, their ambiguities could no longer be construed against the health plan because the plan did not write them. Litigation against the plan would instead focus on whether its agents interpreted the guidelines fairly and in a manner consistent with the overall spirit of that tier's resource philosophy.[22]

At any rate, once such options are established, each person should be able make his or her own choice. The point may seem self-evident, but it deserves notice. When patients have the power to choose, plans have a powerful incentive to please them rather than an employer whose values and objectives may be very different from their employees'. Further, the power of choice provides a motive to learn more about what each plan offers and to hold the plan accountable, through the power of exit, for the quality of care it actually provides. Employers might still play a role, because group purchasers usually enjoy lower premium costs, but patients should have considerably greater choice than most do at present.

Ideally, choices should also exist within plans, not just between them, to permit opportunities to fine-tune one's coverage. Lower-cost health plans could permit subscribers to upgrade their coverage at various junctures for an extra fee; reciprocally, a more lavish, everything-included plan could offer rebates to those who opt to forego discretionary interventions.

b. The Caveat

Real choices among health plans presuppose real differences among plans. That means differences in people's entitlements to care and, consequently, inequality of care. One person will receive a given service while someone else in the same situation will not. That sort of inequality makes some observers deeply uneasy, yet good reasons exist to believe that diversity of resource entitlements should be openly accepted, even embraced.

This book takes as a given the idea that, in an affluent society with a commitment to treating all citizens with respect, a universal assurance of some basic level of health care seems imperative. However, a uniform minumum does not entail uniformity at all levels for several reasons.

The first reason is practical. Although mandating uniformity may be attractive for its appearance of social equity, the reality is virtually impossible to achieve. As noted in Chapter 8, even in the Medicare program, which purports to provide a single, uniform set of benefits for all enrollees, intermediary payors vary tremendously in their actual implementation of these benefit standards.[23] So long as health care is as complex as it is and so long as human beings must administer programs to meet those complex needs, human judgments will vary.

In addition, absolute equality would not be advisable even if achievable. As noted by Blumstein and Sloan,

> equality of access may be an unattainable and even undesirable goal. Leveling up would require such a staggering commitment of resources that other public priorities would unduly suffer; leveling down would promote gross inefficiency, lower quality, achieve a dubious sort of equity in which waiting time would be the main resource allocator, and threaten fundamental precepts of freedom by barring individual expenditures for health above some arbitrary limit set by government. Indeed, as a practical matter, it is doubtful that any such government program could be enforced at all.[24]

Siliciano makes the further point that so long as physicians and other providers have the contractual freedom to refuse to care for any patient for any reason, including indigence, then tort law's current demand of a unitary standard of high-tech care for all patients they accept has the perverse result that the indigent have ever-diminishing access to care.[25] "By mandating a unitary standard of care that is more expensive than some patients can afford and that other actors in the health care system are increasingly unwilling to subsidize, tort law effectively encourages providers to choose the liability-free option of declining to treat a significant minority of the medically underprivileged population."[26]

Beyond this, people can legitimately differ on the value they place on the various goals that health care can achieve, from reducing their risk of undetected illness, to increasing their comfort during medical procedures, to improving their ability to function in the daily tasks of life, to making extra-sure (at extra-high cost) that an infection is eliminated a little sooner rather than a little later. By the same token, legitimate choices exist between health care and the world outside. Elsewhere in life people forego many products and services they deem not to be worth the cost, even though the items may be clearly useful in their own right. People buy cheaper, older cars that are less crash-worthy than new ones,[27] and many buy a good restaurant meal before boosting their retirement fund. On the whole, the freedom to make such quality-of-life choices is vital. It is the currency of human autonomy that permits each individual to be the kind of persons he wants to be and to live as he sees fit.[28] Only if they have at least some opportunity to choose among health plans and levels of care can patients meaningfully act on these values in the important setting of personal health care.[29]

If the foregoing arguments are correct, it is time to jettison the pretense of uniformity and acknowledge that it is legitimate for some people to want (and pay for) more health care, while others put their priorities elsewhere. And if it is imperative for us as a nation to fund a basic level of care for the uninsured, it is also legitimate to circumscribe that level to save funds for other national priorities.

c. The Realities

At present, ideals and realities do not entirely match. Most people have little or no selection among health plans. One study found that eighty-four percent of employers only offer one health plan.[30] Another study concluded that seventy-eight percent of firms offer just one plan, although often with multiple products, such as a POS version of an HMO (point-of-service, permitting expanded choices for added fees).[31]

And yet the situation is changing. Many large corporations already offer a number of health plans for employees' selection. Many more firms, both large and small, have joined their economic power in purchasing pools that lower costs via group leverage, thus permitting employees a far wider array of plans than any one firm could provide on its own.[32] With suitable legislation, such purchasing pools can proliferate.[33]

Moreover, within individual plans, opportunities for in-plan "upgrades" to fine-tune one's coverage are already fairly common. Point-of-service plans permit patients, for an additional payment, to select a provider not on that plan's panel. Likewise, copays on discretionary interventions can permit patients who want the extra care to obtain it without burdening everyone else by mandating those services universally and adding them to the premium price.[34] Similarly, medical savings accounts (MSAs), properly crafted, can provide greater options by permitting people to pay for routine expenses out of dedicated savings accounts while buying cata-strophic policies to cover higher expenses. When the individual is paying for these low-end services, there is little need for intrusive, over-the-shoulder utilization man-agement.[35]

2. Information

a. The Ideal

The best arguments supporting greater specificity and clarity in health plan contracts are the problems of vagueness and covertness. So long as health plans, including commercial insurers and HMOs, self-insured plans, and even government programs, give only vague promises in exchange for large amounts of money; so long as these plans commonly keep secret the guidelines by which they award benefits; so long as the actual benefits people receive within a particular plan keep fluctuating under the rubric that "we have decided that service is (no longer) necessary"; and so long as different plans make widely differing judgments under the very same benefits lan-guage, it will be difficult for us as a nation, and for health plans individually, to serve populations well while treating individual patients fairly. Moreover, without clarity it will remain difficult for patients to make intelligent decisions about their own health care purchases and resource utilization and to ensure they receive the value they paid for.

Accordingly, the second essential element of effective, enforceable contracting is information. People signing onto a health plan deserve to know what they will receive for their money and to be able to discern whether they have received what they were promised. To be sure, the sheer complexity of medicine and of health care systems probably precludes the thoroughgoing "meeting of the minds"[36] envisioned in standard texts on contracting. Still, the situation could be improved considerably. For fair, effective, enforceable contracting, the guidelines describing each tier—or, in today's world, the actual guidelines to which a given health plan refers in making its benefits decisions—should be open to current and prospective enrollees, thereby eliminating the secrecy that now predominates.

This does not mean that prospective plan subscribers must understand and affirm every clause of every guideline before the contract is valid.[37] Such detailed compre-hension is not required for valid contracting in health care, any more than a contract to buy an automobile requires the buyer to understand how the car is put together in every mechanical respect. Rather, subscribers should receive a general outline of the health plan's general resource philosophy,[38] perhaps supplemented by case illustra-tions showing how the plan implements that philosophy, plus information about how to inspect the complete guidelines.[39] A Website might meet the latter need well.[40] Such openness would also expose guidelines to examination, critique, and improve-ment from physicians and the public alike.

The proposal is best called "guidelines-based contracting." Instead of writing contracts in vague terms and then fleshing them out with a set of covert, detailed (but quietly changeable) clinical guidelines, health plans should simply drop the notion of medical necessity, open their guidelines to inspection,[41] describe the procedures by which they adjudicate disputes, and make these guidelines and procedures the explicit basis on which they contract with enrollees. The health plan states to the enrollee, "if you buy this plan, here is what you get:. . . ."[42] Whether through the several-tiered hypothetical system described above, or simply through plans' opening their existing guidelines and procedures as the contractual basis for coverage, guidelines-based contracting would permit better information and accountability for patients and clearer rules for providers, while permitting plans to enjoy markedly stronger contract enforcement and thus considerably improved financial stability.

b. The Caveats and Realities

As pointed out earlier, ideals do not match realities. Health plans thus far have shown little inclination toward the openness recommended here. In addition, a potentially significant barrier to opening guidelines is the fact that some are commercially proprietary, requiring that the plans using them to avoid disclosing their contents. If guidelines-based contracting is to become the norm, some resolution, perhaps a broad-based buy-out, must be found for this problem.[43]

Here, too, however, the situation is hardly static or finalized. Health care is in a period of extraordinary turbulence. Although efforts toward cost containment have been underway for many years, the period of greatest transition did not begin until the early 1990s, when managed care finally began to stem the relentless rise of premium prices.[44] During this time a huge variety of arrangements has come and gone as plans and providers try to rewrite health care on a radically different economic basis. Plans and providers are learning from encounters with each other, with patients, and with their accountants that some of the arrangements they have tried do not work very well. Intensive utilization management and gatekeeping systems have risen, and then given way to broader profiling of providers and practices; incentives are moving from crude, physician-level capitation to more sophisticated mixes rewarding productivity, quality, cost-consciousness, and other improved practices.[45]

Plans are also beginning to learn through harsh experience with the courts that little point remains in continuing to rely on vague language they know will be construed against them; they are learning that the more specifically they write their exclusions and other provisions, the more likely they are to be enforced.[46] Reciprocally, concealment of important provisions is beginning to cause major trouble. The incentive schemes by which plans encourage providers to cut costs are prompting judicial scrutiny as some courts find health plans and physicians alike may have breached fiduciary duties by failing to disclose such incentives.[47]

Further, there is movement toward less proprietary secrecy for clinical guidelines. New Jersey, for instance, effectively precludes such secrecy by requiring that health plans permit their participating providers "an opportunity to review and comment on all medical and surgical . . . protocols . . . of the carrier."[48] Washington state has a similar provision.[49] Elsewhere, health plans in particular geographic regions such as Minnesota and New Mexico have begun to agree on uniform treatment guidelines for common conditions, a step that requires those guidelines to be open for physicians to follow.[50] In addition, some health plans now encourage providers to pattern their practice on guidelines that are already published in books and on the Internet.

3. Bargaining Power

Standard descriptions of contracts portray two parties of roughly equal power, each of whom is reasonably capable of looking out for his own interests. As many commentators have observed, patients do not usually enjoy that sort of parity. Indeed, their vulnerability is the trait that renders the physician–patient relationship, and likewise the insurer–insured relationship, essentially fiduciary.[51]

Nevertheless, much of that vulnerability can be ameliorated, even if not entirely eliminated. As described above, real choices among and within health plans and adequate information about those options can go a long way toward empowering patients to look out for their own interests. Unlike the setting in which a patient desperate for care is asked to sign an exculpatory agreement as a prerequisite for treatment,[52] choices among health plans are usually made at a time when consumers have the opportunity to seek information, ask questions, and reflect on their decisions.[53] Moreover, many enrollees have an annual opportunity to switch to a different plan if dissatisfied with what they have chosen. Additionally, people who obtain their health plans through their employment or through other groups often have bargaining agents who can negotiate on their behalf and who can insist on quality as well as price. Some employer coalitions, for instance, have used their purchasing power to mandate quality standards. One such coalition, the Pacific Business Group on Health, has required its health plans to meet specified quality parameters and has published patient-reported data on the quality of physicians' care.[54]

In fact, courts are willing to honor the terms of health plan contracts that were chosen by subscribers who had real choices, information, and bargaining power.[55] In *Madden v. Kaiser Found. Hosps.*,[56] for instance, the California Supreme Court was willing to hold an enrollee to the terms of the plan's arbitration requirement. The court reasoned that the plaintiff, a state employee, had a powerful bargaining agent, namely the state of California, that had assembled several plan choices, some of which did not include the arbitration requirement. An employee who wanted to avoid arbitration could have choosen another plan. Hence, when vulnerability is markedly diminished by adequate information and choice, courts are prepared to enforce consumers' decisions.[57]

B. GUIDELINES-BASED CONTRACTING: CHOOSING AND ENFORCING RESOURCE ENTITLEMENTS AND RESOURCE LIMITS

There are good reasons to believe that guidelines-based contracting and contract law can serve well as the focus for accountability regarding health care resources. Chapter 10 will explore the issue in depth, but a few comments can be offered here. On the one hand, guidelines-based contracting permits much greater opportunity for patients to choose the resource level they want to purchase for their health care and to hold health plans to account when they do not deliver. At the same time, it permits health plans to circumscribe much more clearly what they do and do not cover and to enforce those limits in an above-board spirit of fairness to all. And with greater predictability in their obligations and expenses, MCOs can plan more effectively for meeting diverse needs of a population within a defined budget. For physicians the enhanced openness and clarity of guidelines-based contracting could relieve much of the rancor and gamesmanship that currently drains the joy from clinical practice. If physicians know, rather than having to guess or argue about, what a plan covers, if the "sunshine" of open guidelines prompts plans to enforce their resource limits more evenly than they do at present, and if physicians have some assurance that the patient has chosen his plan voluntarily and knowledgeably, then physicians could more easily work within the parameters of that plan, even if it does not cover every intervention that might ideally benefit the patient.

Many of the disputes that surround health care resources are already, of necessity, addressed in contract. Chapter 4 identified three major scenarios in which patients typically contest health plans' refusals to provide a benefit. The first is prospective: the patient believes he needs a particular treatment, the health plan denies it, and the patient asks the court for an injunction to mandate financial coverage or, in the case of an HMO, the care itself. Such cases are almost always resolved on the basis of contract, as the judge examines the agreement to see whether the disputed service is covered. When patients are desperate and treatments are "last hope," judges sometimes interpret that contract rather liberally. But even then the issue is still settled by examining the contract.[58]

The second scenario is retrospective: the health plan denied coverage but the patient received timely treatment anyway, and now either the patient or his providers sue for financial coverage. These, clearly, are also contract cases.

The third scenario is also retrospective, but with an unhappy outcome: the health plan's refusal of coverage caused a delay or denial of treatment that, in turn, allegedly caused an injury. These cases are likely to prompt tort suits, yet even here traditional contract law figures prominently. As noted in Chapter 8, the health plan could not have "caused" the adverse outcome[59] if it did not contractually owe the coverage in question. Thus, the typical tort action against an MCO will also involve questions about contract.[60]

In the final analysis, fundamental improvements in contracting and in the contract enforcement process seem essential. Only if contractual limits are enforced can MCOs keep their expenses predictable and controllable, and only if that happens can they make rational, forward-looking business plans for the best care of large populations within limited budgets. Perhaps even more important, only if contractual entitlements in health care become considerably clearer and more reliable can patients use them to implement important priority choices about how much they value what kinds of health care relative to other goods. If patients consistently receive more than they are entitled to, such as via judge-made insurance, premium costs must inevitably rise, forcing choices between health care and other important goods. Reciprocally, if patients consistently receive less than they are entitled to, for example, as benefits covertly erode under the rubric of "unnecessary," the important values patients sought to achieve through purchasing the health plan will not be reached.

From any perspective, solving the problems will require effective, enforceable contracting. Plans need to say "you get this, but not that" and make it stand. And consumers need to be able say "I bought specifically this, and you must provide it."

To be sure, it can be difficult to live with the human consequences when plans say "no, you may not have this intervention because you did not buy it." A society accustomed to an "artesian well of money" that mandates the latest and greatest technologies will surely take offense at some of those denials. But there is no reasonable alternative. Endless expenditures that proliferate untested treatments and costs must now give way to a sober recognition of limits. Just as important, an acceptance of those limits will affirmatively give us the freedom, both as a society and as individuals, to decide with a clearer and more thoughtful mind what we value in health care.

III

ASSESSING THE PROPOSED APPROACH: PROSPECTS FOR JUDICIAL ACCEPTANCE

10

JUDICIAL ACCEPTABILITY

Part III begins by recapping a few important points. The economics of medicine have fundamentally, irrevocably changed. Gone are the days in which physicians and patients could enjoy an essentially dyadic relationship, free to choose whatever treatments they wanted. Before World War II that dyadic relationship was possible because physicians had so little to offer that medical care was affordable; later it was sustainable because of generous, relatively unquestioning third-party payment. That "artesian well" lasted only a few decades, until exploding health care costs in the 1970s and 1980s finally gave way to serious cost constraints in the 1990s.[1]

In this setting several things have become about as certain as death and taxes. Health care is now highly technological, enormously expensive, and likely to remain so as long as the nation is affluent. Few people of ordinary means can afford to pay for the care of a major illness or injury directly out of pocket, thus ensuring that spreading of risk, with third-party financing, will likewise continue.

This situation, in turn, triggers further consequences for the financing and delivery of care. When where one party must pay large amounts of money to cover someone else's decisions, as in health care, that payor will not ordinarily permit that "someone else"—here, providers and patients—to generate unlimited expenditures. Either the payor will tell the spenders specifically what they can and cannot buy, or the payor will limit its financial risk by transferring the economic consequences of medical choices to the people who make the spending decisions. In health care the former approach is utilization (micro)management, while the latter prompts incentive arrangements such as capitation, financial bonuses, penalties, and risk pools to ensure that physicians personally pay the consequences of "excessive" care.[2]

Current legal doctrines are not entirely prepared to cope with such a radical transformation in health care financing and delivery. Chapter 2 noted that physicians stand to be held liable in tort for resource deficiencies that may be completely outside their control. Familiar doctrines like the locality rule, prevailing custom, and reputable minorities allow for flexibility among physicians' practices, but only so long as those variations stem from medical or scientific disagreements. Diversity based on economic considerations is not envisioned because those doctrines are founded on the standard tort requirement that physicians owe an essentially equal quality of care to every patient without regard to costs. In light of current realities, it is time to abandon the traditional physician-set, cost-indifferent standard of care.

Chapter 3 observed that tort law also has a troubled relationship with health plans. In an ironic similarity to physicians, MCOs stand to be held liable in clinical practice areas over which they have no real control—and which they should not control if we do not want MCOs intrusively second-guessing physicians. While plans can reasonably be expected to monitor their physician staff for patterns of poor care or for the most obvious breaches of good practice, it is both impossible and undesirable for them to supervise literally every physician move. Yet current expansions of direct and indirect liability invite inappropriate MCO conduct by imposing inappropriate legal liability.

Even in the domains that health plans should control, such as overall resource management for a population of subscribers, tort accountability tends to focus too much on individual bad outcomes with too little interest in whether the policies that led to those outcomes were carefully constructed and fairly administered. In some instances ascriptions of tort liability can actually punish health plans for doing good work because even the best policies will occasionally work adversely for individuals. MCOs thus stand to be penalized for doing the right thing. Once again, it is evident that health law needs an overhaul.

Chapter 4 pointed out that contract law likewise poses problems because the conditions for effective contracting are not well met in the health care setting. Most plans write their contracts in the hopelessly vague language of medical necessity, which in turn means that courts often apply *contra proferentem* and rule against them when benefits decisions are disputed. Arbitrariness and adhesion further impede contract enforcement. Even when contract language is clear, some courts have permitted desperate patients' pleas to prevail over contract terms. One result has been a spiraling circus of gaming and subterfuge in which health plans feel impelled to resort to inconvenience as a covert means of drawing limits they cannot enforce overtly. Physicians often respond with gaming of their own, while patients find their coverage steadily eroding.

This book then suggested how law should regard the obligations and liabilities of health care plans and providers. As a policy matter, society must first decide who should be controlling which aspects of health care before it can appropriately assign legal duties and liabilities. Chapter 5 suggested that health plans should focus on resource policies and on patterns of care, while physicians should provide individualized care, fine-tuning the clinical implications of the plan's overall resource policies.

Once it is agreed who should control what in health care, it is possible to adjust legal duties and liabilities to the new economic realities of health care. As domains of control are sorted out, Chapter 6 showed that it is crucial to distinguish between two very different kinds of duty that plans or providers can owe to patients: expertise obligations versus resource obligations. Expertise questions should be addressed via tort law, and resource disputes should be resolved in contract because the level of resources a health plan owes a subscriber should depend on what level that person bought, not on what physicians customarily do. Chapters 7, 8, and 9 then discussed how tort and contract law can adjudicate the conduct of physicians and health plans with respect to their exercises of expertise and their allocations of resources.

Ostensibly, this book proposes significant changes in the way courts currently address health care litigation. It requires courts to invoke a conceptual distinction—expertise versus resources—that is not currently built into the language of adjudication. It also requires courts to attend more carefully to the factual nuances of complicated cases.

The alternative, however, is to fail to attend to these clinical and economic realities, a failure that can lead the judiciary to make badly misguided decisions. Indeed, recent case law bears ample evidence of cases in which courts simply do not understand the actual financial structures by which care has been delivered or important clinical features that medically distinguish one case from another.[3] Ill-informed courts can unfairly penalize plans and physicians who may have been acting properly and, perhaps even worse, they can exacerbate the turbulence in this difficult transition time by giving conflicting messages to plans, providers, and patients about what is expected of them.

A recommendation for change, however, needs some proposal as to how that change should be accomplished. Legislation outlining plans' and physicians' respective domains of control and liability is one option, although, as always with legislative reforms, the familiar danger exists that the "sausage-making" process will produce a product that looks disconcertingly different from the original intent. Moreover, whatever we may think about the desirability of legislation, ultimately the allocation and character of tort and contract liabilities will be fleshed out by the judiciary. Given the chaotic scene now pervading the common law of health care, we will at least need a clearly focused evolution in the common law toward a more coherent, consistent, reality-based approach than we currently see.

Fortunately, that evolution is already under way. In this chapter a closer examination of basic tort and contract concepts, as evidenced in case law trends, will suggest that the U.S. legal system is surprisingly well prepared to adopt the approach offered here. This is especially evident regarding physicians' duties but is also true regarding health plans' proposed liabilities in both tort and contract. Indeed, the approach presented in this book does little more than draw on long-standing common law traditions, albeit with a distinctive conceptual underpinning that will lend coherence and focus to future case adjudication. The compatibility between existing doctrines and the proposed approach can even embrace ERISA, as discussed in Chapter 11.

A. PHYSICIANS' LIABILITIES

Chapter 7 suggested that existing tort doctrines and case law should largely be preserved when plaintiffs allege that physicians have violated duties of expertise. Hence, this book's proposals pose no disruption to the status quo in that area.

When physicians have apparently failed in resource duties, Chapter 7 requires a factual inquiry into whether the physician actually controlled the resources in question. When the physician had little or no control, as when the health plan exercised close utilization management, the allegation amounts to a deficiency of effort and advocacy—a failure of expertise—and the case remains in tort. Again, the proposed approach fits well with existing doctrine.[4]

As briefly noted in Chapter 7, some courts have expanded physicians' advocacy duties to include an obligation to disclose important financial arrangements. In *Neade v. Portes* an HMO physician declined on several occasions to order further diagnostic evaluation of chest pain in a 37-year-old man with numerous risk factors for heart disease. Noting that the physician failed to disclose incentives that encouraged him to restrain care, an Illinois district court held that the plaintiff had a cause of action for breach of fiduciary duty against the physician, separate from his cause for medical malpractice. The decision, however, was reversed on appeal.[5]

More recently, in a case with remarkably similar medical facts, the Eighth Circuit held that ERISA does not preempt a cause of action against a physician for failing to disclose incentives.[6] When remanded for further proceedings, however, a state appellate court determined that the trial court had acted appropriately when it excluded information about managed care incentives as beng irrelevant and potentially confusing, misleading, and prejudicial under the facts of that case.[7] Courts' views differ,[8] and this area of litigation is very new. Still, it would not be surprising to find more courts expecting physicians not just to disclose incentive arrangements, but to defend patients' interests in at least some kinds of scuffles with health plans.[9]

In contrast, when physicians exercise personal control over resources, as with various capitation arrangements,[10] then the physicians are acting either as a complete health plan or as subcontracted administrators over a portion of the plan, and the case should be resolved under contract, as discussed below.

B. HEALTH PLANS' LIABILITIES: EXPERTISE AND TORT

This book's most distinctive recommendations concern health plans. We turn first to tort. As discussed in Chapter 5, health plans' proposed duties of expertise, to be governed under tort, are: (1) business administration, (2) setting and overseeing patterns of good care, (3) identifying and responding to patterns of poor care, and (4), in selected circumstances, practicing medicine. Emerging case law is quite consistent with finding torts in this area (see Chapters 3 and 8).[11] A few points can be added here.

1. Business Duties

As previously noted, courts have willingly assigned tort liability when health plans have been careless regarding business and administrative activities.[12] By extension from cases governing hospitals, health plans now have a recognized duty to ensure that personnel, including medical staff, function properly and effectively.[13] Failure to review claims carefully, including failure to seek adequate information on which to make a fair decision, is a classic scenario prompting tort liability. In *Wickline v. State of California*,[14] a California Court of Appeal stated in dicta that "[t]hird party payors of health care services can be held legally accountable when medically inappropriate decisions result from defects in the design or implementation of cost containment mechanisms."[15]

In *Wilson v. Blue Cross of Southern Cal.*, the same court held that utliization review entities can be held jointly liable for tortious conduct. The court pointed to the *Restatement of Torts 2d* "which provides, 'The actor's negligent conduct is a legal cause of harm to another if (a) his [or her] conduct is a substantial factor in bringing about the harm, and, (b) there is no rule of law relieving the actor from liability. . . .' "[16] Other courts have agreed that health plans' failure to design and implement utilization control systems can result in liability under direct corporate negligence.[17] Reciprocally, adequate, appropriately implemented procedures can ward off liability.[18] When an MCO's administrative carelessness is deemed to rise to the level of outrageousness, malice, oppression, or reckless indifference to the rights of subscribers, courts have also been willing to recognize the tort of bad faith, as noted in Chapter 8.[19]

Recent cases also have challenged incentive arrangements that reward physicians for cost consciousness. According to plaintiffs, plans create incentives as a business maneuver to cut costs without regard to quality. Some of these suits challenge the very existence of risk sharing. Illinois courts, for instance, have acknowledged that a jury might take a capitation system into account in evaluating the quality of the patient's care. In *Petrovich v. Share Health Plan*, the HMO's "use of the capitation system could lead to the reasonable inference that Share's method of compensation to its participating physicians created a disincentive to order tests or make referrals and thus exerted control over its physicians' medical decisions. Here, plaintiff testified at her deposition that Dr. Kowalski told her that Share would not pay for more tests. This evidence was relevant to whether plaintiff was led to believe that Dr. Kowalski was controlled by [the HMO]."[20] In *Herdrich v. Pegram*[21] the Seventh Circuit held that capitation arrangements in ERISA cases can prompt physicians to skimp on care, breaching their ERISA fiduciary duty to beneficiaries.[22] On appeal, however, the U.S. Supreme Court found that incentive arrangements do not in themselves constitute a breach of ERISA fiduciary duty.[23]

A related group of cases focuses on health plans' failures to disclose incentives, analogous to claims against physicians for their failures to disclose incentives, as discussed just above. In *Shea v. Esensten,* for instance, a primary care physician told a 40-year-old man that his chest pains and other symptoms did not warrant a cardiology consult. As the patient's symptoms continued he offered to pay for the visit himself but was still told it was unnecessary. When the patient died shortly thereafter, his estate sued on a variety of causes, including the MCO's failure to disclose the physician's financial incentives. Such knowledge, the plaintiff argued, would have prompted the patient to seek care on his own. The Eighth Circuit held that the failure to disclose was a breach of the ERISA plan administrator's fiduciary duty.[24] Not all courts agree with this analysis, and the issue is sure to be a future bone of contention.[25] In any event, as these cases arise more frequently regarding ERISA plans, they may well encourage or facilitate tort actions for nondisclosure in the non-ERISA setting.

2. Patterns of Care

Health plans' second proposed expertise duty is to create and implement patterns of good care. As argued in this book, (1) plans' guidelines should be medically credible; (2) courts should recognize that plans have an important duty to promote the welfare of all their enrollees, not just this or that individual; and therefore (3) courts should evaluate plans' performance by examining their policies and implementation, rather than simply looking at individual plaintiffs' outcomes.

(1). Several courts have explicitly expected medical credibility. As noted in Chapter 8,[26] *Thompson v. Nason* found that hospitals have a "duty to formulate, adopt and enforce *adequate* rules and policies to ensure quality care for patients,"[27] a duty extended to health plans in *Shannon v. McNulty.*[28] The latter court emphasized that because health plans' policies and guidelines can significantly affect care, they must be medically reasonable.[29] Other courts agree.[30]

(2). Although plans are expected to exercise due care in choosing guidelines, a number of courts have also recognized that trade-offs between individual and group welfare are inevitable. In *Creason v. Department of Health Services*[31] a state disease screening program for newborns happened to miss a particular infant's illness. The California Supreme Court refused to fault the program simply because its chosen methods of gathering and interpreting data fell short in this instance. In his concurring opinion Justice Kennard opined that "to impose civil liability on the Department here and in any similar future case may well threaten the continuation of a generally beneficial statewide program that has screened millions of California babies for disabling congenital disorders. . . . 'Far more persons would suffer if government did not perform these functions at all than would be benefitted by permitting recovery in those cases where the government is shown to have performed inadequately.' . . . The facts of this case are heartrending, and the desire to afford the stricken child and her parents some measure of comfort and financial assistance is strong. But these considerations alone cannot dictate the outcome in this case."[32]

In *Doe v. Southeastern Penn. Transp. Auth. (SEPTA)*[33] a self-insured public employer happened to learn through its program for monitoring drug costs that an employee had AIDS. The Third Circuit held on various grounds that the employee's privacy had not been violated. The court particularly pointed to the employer's need to track its drug costs, to ensure that drugs are provided only to those authorized to receive them, and to contain costs by requiring generic drugs whenever feasible. "Employers have a legitimate need for monitoring the costs and uses of their employee benefit program, especially employers who have fiscal responsibilities, as does SEPTA, to the public. As health care costs rise, as they have in recent years, and employers become obligated to expand employee coverage with greater protection for more illnesses and health conditions, health care costs become a major concern for employers as well as for Congress."[34]

Another case openly acknowledged resource scarcity as it upheld a denial of benefits. In *Barnett* v. *Kaiser Foundation Health Plan, Inc.,*[35] the Ninth Circuit upheld Kaiser Permanente's denial of liver transplant for a man with hepatitis B, which had been made on the ground that the man's disease was of a type that would soon reinfect any new liver. Kaiser's medical criteria deemed this complication to be an absolute contraindication to liver transplant, an exclusion criterion based largely on the shortage of livers for transplant.[36] Though accepting the policy, the court hastened to add that acknowledging an organ shortage was not equivalent to endorsing decisions based on financial savings to the health plan.[37] However, by openly considering the impact that one patient's care can have on other patients competing for the same resources, the decision opens the door to more overtly financial reasoning in future cases. Other courts echo the theme, willing to find that the interests of broader populations can legitimately win over the needs of individuals.[38]

Similar observations note a classic dilemma for ERISA plan administrators. As the Ninth Circuit observed: "Plan trustees are required to discharge their duties 'solely in the interest of the participants and beneficiaries.' . . . At the same time, however, they have a duty to keep the Fund financially stable. '[T]he purpose of a Fund is to provide benefits to as many intended beneficiaries as is economically possible while protecting the financial stability of the Fund.' "[39] In *Ricci v. Gooberman,* a New Jersey district court rejected ostensible agency theory for ERISA HMO plans expressly because of such broader concerns. If HMOs were held liable for the actions of their independent physicians, they would have to carry liability insurance to cover the same acts of these providers, "resulting in higher costs that certainly trickle down to the plan beneficiaries."[40] Likewise, the U.S. Supreme Court has noted that greater exposures to liability tend to create higher costs for those who deal with health plans and thereby for the plans themselves. "There is, in other words, a 'tension between the primary [ERISA] goal of benefitting employees and the subsidiary goal of containing pension costs.' "[41] Compromises must sometimes be made if employees are to have benefit plans at all.[42]

(3). Consistent with the idea that plans' accountability should emphasize policies and implementation rather than individual outcomes, one state's highest court emphasized that it is a mistake to hold an institution such as a hospital liable simply because a particular patient had an adverse outcome at the hands of its staff physicians. In *Baptist Memorial Hosp. System v. Sampson,*[43] the Texas Supreme Court overturned an appellate court's holding that a hospital would be liable for the mal-practice of its emergency room physicians regardless of whether they are indepen-dent contractors and regardless of whether the patient had any good reason to think they were agents of the hospital.[44] The court rejected the idea that a hospital should bear "a nondelegable duty . . . solely because it opens its doors for business."[45] Such a duty need not be imposed in order to safeguard patients because "[a] patient injured by a physician's malpractice is not without remedy. The injured patient ordinarily has a cause of action against the negligent physician, and may retain a direct cause of action against the hospital if the hospital was negligent in the perfor-mance of a duty owed directly to the patient."[46] In other words, the institution should be held liable only for failures of its own duties, not for failures of others who are neither under its control nor represented to be such. Other courts have reached similar conclusions.[47]

In sum, courts seem increasingly willing to evaluate plans on the basis of whether their conduct was reasonable and prudent, and no longer just simplistically on the basis of whether they produced the favored result for the plaintiff. Just as physicians are not obligated to guarantee a good result, but only to use reasonable knowledge and skill,[48] so should health plans be obligated not to produce the best outcome for each enrollee, but rather to exercise good faith and adequate expertise in carrying out their commitments under the contract.

3. Surveillance for Inadequate Care

Health plans' third expertise duty is to monitor providers and staff for the quality and adequacy of their services to patients. Here, too, little needs to be said beyond the discussion in Chapters 3 and 8, which establishes that health plans' duties to enrollees include credentialing and monitoring staff, dereliction of which can consti-tute direct corporate negligence.[49]

As the Texas Supreme Court pointed out in *Baptist Memorial Hosp. System v. Sampson*,[50] this should not be seen as a duty to prevent every instance of poor care. Even attempting to do so would be cumbersome and would intrude on distinctively clinical responsibilities that can only be properly carried out by individual clinicians working with individual patients in a trusting personal relationship.

An apt illustration of the problems inherent in expecting play-by-play "supervi-sion" comes from *Charter Peachford Behavioral v. Kohout*,[51] in which a team of psychiatrists and psychologists allegedly misdiagnosed the patient as suffering from multiple personality disorder and from a history of sexual abuse in satanic rituals, then allegedly used inappropriate treatments to help the patient "recover" her "mem-ory" of these events. Although the decision focused on the definitions of "em-ployee" versus "independent contractor," an important lesson can be gleaned from thinking about what a hospital would need to do in order to catch or prevent such diagnostic and treatment errors. Unless these doctors displayed a pattern of poor diagnostic decisions across other patients' care, realistically the only way the hospi-tal could be guilty of failing to "supervise" its medical staff adequately is to suppose that supervision must include reading each patient's chart frequently, independently examining patients (also frequently), and potentially arriving at competing diagnoses and treatment plans.[52] Shy of duplicating physicians' care—for all patients, not just this or that one, if all errors are to be prevented—the institution could not reasonably have averted this error.

Accordingly, rather than averting every adverse event, the health plan's duty must be to institute mechanisms whereby patterns of poor care are reasonably likely to come to its attention. These mechanisms will ordinarily resemble the peer review and quality assurance committes that are commonplace in hospitals.[53] As noted by Chittenden, the real question is not whether a duty exists for health plans to investigate their providers (of course they must), "but how to define the standard of care MCOs must meet to satisfy their duty. . . . If an MCO can show that the physician would have been accepted as a panel member even with exercise of reasonable care in selection, obviously no liability would attach."[54]

4. Practicing Medicine

Earlier it was noted that although tort suits against health plans often raise claims in the name of medical malpractice, until recently these did not ordinarily allege medical malpractice in the classic sense of literally practicing medicine below the standard of care.[55] Rather, the claims have been mainly for corporate negligence or for vicarious liability. This situation is changing, however, as more suits allege bona fide medical malpractice[56] and as some states specify by statute that health plans do practice medicine and can be held liable for medical malpractice. Texas' law is the first and best known. The statute first defines the way MCOs can practice medicine: "'Health care treatment decision' means a determination made when medical services are actually provided by the health care plan and a decision which affects the quality of the diagnosis, care, or treatment provided to the plan's insureds or enrollees."[57]

The statute goes on to apply the definition: "A health insurance carrier, health maintenance organization, or other managed care entity for a health care plan has the duty to exercise ordinary care when making health care treatment decisions and is liable for damages for harm to an insured or enrollee proximately caused by its failure to exercise such ordinary care."[58]

Of note, this Texas statute was challenged on ERISA grounds. Although several other features of the statute were held to be preempted by that federal law,[59] the Southern District of Texas Court held that ERISA does not preempt the so-called malpractice provision that permits health plans to be held liable for failing to exercise due care when making treatment decisions. These issues concern the quality of the care rendered, not the quantity.[60] On appeal the Fifth Circuit agreed with the district court on this central issue, namely that ERISA does not preempt the statute's imposition of liability for medical malpractice.[61] More will be said about ERISA in Chapter 11. Meanwhile, several other states have enacted similar measures.[62]

C. HEALTH PLANS' LIABILITIES: RESOURCES AND CONTRACT

The foregoing discussion suggests that much of current doctrine and case law seem comfortable with the idea of holding physicians liable, as is traditional, for their deficiencies of skill, knowledge, judgment, and effort. Likewise, there seems to be good fit with the idea of holding health plans liable in tort for their own acts of carelessness, culpable ignorance, or other deficiencies of expertise.

It remains now to consider whether courts will also embrace the idea of resolving resource issues strictly within contract law. After all, the rules of contract are somewhat less favorable than is tort toward injured patients, partly because damages are considerably more limited and partly because courts are obligated to uphold denials of resources, even to patients' potential detriment, so long as the contract is sufficiently clear.

We must also discuss whether courts will be comfortable with permitting patients to to receive different levels of care—acceptable within a contract framework but distinctly contrary to the tort notion of one-standard-fits-all. Whereas current tort-based common law might expect a physician to deliver a certain level of resources, the proposed approach would limit resource entitlements according to the patient's contract, regardless of physicians' preferred practices. For each of these two issues, we will find that judicial traditions and trends are remarkably compatible with this book's proposals. We turn first to the latter question.

1. Variations in Levels of Care

Courts have not always smiled on contracts that limit liability in the health care context. For instance, exculpatory agreements in which patients release health care providers from tort liability as a precondition for receiving care have been generally struck down as against public policy.[63] Even clauses mandating arbitration as an alternative to litigation have occasionally been nullified if courts felt that bargaining conditions were inequitable.[64]

Still, there is good reason to believe that courts can permit health plans to offer varying resource packages, so long as they provide a reasonable level of basic care. Indeed, judges have already done so in a variety of cases.[65] Many plans, for instance, require higher copayments for costlier drugs, while others enforce lifetime caps on all care, and some cover only limited mental health benefits. Plans also differ in coverage exclusions, and these exclusions have been upheld in many instances, based on the plain language of the contract.[66]

Similarly, federal ERISA law permits employers to provide whatever level of benefits they wish and to change those benefits virtually at will. "Health care benefits provided in employee benefit plan are not vested benefits; the employer may modify or withdraw such benefits at any time, provided the changes are made in compliance with ERISA and the terms of the plan.' "[67] "When setting and changing the terms of a plan, the employer may act to promote its own interests, just as it may do when setting wages."[68]

Government health plans, likewise, are hardly uniform.[69] Individual states' Medicaid plans vary widely in their eligibility requirements and benefits.[70] Even Medicare carriers that enact ostensibly the same benefit package can, in fact, adjudicate benefits very differently.[71]

Moreover, the Supreme Court has openly accepted such variations. When the state of Tennessee reduced the number of hospitalization days covered for Medicaid patients from twenty to fourteen, the Court upheld the reduction, noting that[72] "the benefit provided through Medicaid is a particular package of health care services, such as 14 days of inpatient coverage. That package of services has the general aim of assuring that individuals will receive necessary medical care, but the benefit provided remains the individual services offered—not 'adequate health care.' "[73] And in a different but somewhat analogous setting, the Court has acknowledged that indigents accused of a crime are entitled not to optimal counsel, but only to adequate opportunity to present their cases.[74]

Courts also accept some resource variation via their long-standing willingness to permit physicians' medical standards of care to vary. As noted in Chapter 2, there are the familiar allowances for reputable minorities, different specialities, and differing localties.[75] The latter includes a recognition that not all localities have access to the same levels of resources.[76] Further, a few states still honor doctrines of charitable and sovereign immunity, in which nonprofit providers, such as charity hospitals or the state itself, are largely exempted from liability for causing injury.[77] Other states expressly waive liability for physicians who provide medical care for the poor.[78] Furthermore, the state of Oregon in its 1989 Medicaid resource prioritization plan acknowledges that Medicaid recipients may be entitled to a reduced level of resources. The statute explicitly exempts physicians from tort liability when the plan's resource constraints send their care below prevailing practices.[79]

Clearly, courts permit health plans' resource packages to differ. The next question is how far they are actually willing to go to enforce the limits created by such packages. Chapter 4 observed that courts must often side with plaintiffs when the conditions of effective contracting are not met in health care. Nevertheless, it will be seen here that if contracts are written clearly enough, free of adhesion and not arbitrarily applied, courts are surprisingly willing to enforce them as written, even to patients' disadvantage.

2. Courts' Willingness to Enforce Contractual Limits

Courts have shown an increasing willingness to bind individuals to the terms of their health care contracts when basic conditions of enforceable contracting have been satisfied. In *Nazay v. Miller,* for example, the Third Circuit upheld an insurer's requirement that the patient pay thirty percent of his medical bills because he failed to secure advance approval for his care.[80] The patient knew at least a full day ahead of time that he would need to enter the hospital, thereby giving his wife an opportunity to phone for precertification well within the required time limit.[81] In addition, the patient presented the hospital admissions staff with an outdated insurance card that lacked proper precertification information.[82]

Analogously, in *Loyola University of Chicago v. Humana Ins. Co.*[83] surgeons per-

forming coronary bypass surgery responded to an intraoperative emergency by im-
planting an artificial heart as a bridge to the human heart transplant that was performed a month later. The insurer refused reimbursement for the artificial heart on
the ground that it was experimental and for the human heart transplant because the
patient failed to secure utilization review approval as required. The Seventh Circuit
upheld. "This is a contract case and the language of the benefit plan controls. Again,
Loyola and Mr. Via were certainly free to attempt these life-saving procedures, but
Humana is not required to pay for them."[84] The court continued:

> As the plan unambiguously states, no benefits are payable without prior approval. It
> is undisputed that necessary records on Mr. Via's condition were not sent by
> Loyola until after the heart transplant and that the records were not received by
> Humana until after Mr. Via's death. . . . Although it seems callous for Humana to
> deny coverage for a life-saving procedure and thereafter deny all subsequent hospi-
> tal expenses—in essence saying to Mr. Via 'we will not cover you because you
> should be dead'—Humana's humanity is not the issue here. This is a contract case
> and the language of the benefit plan controls.[85]

The Tenth Circuit echoed the theme in *McGee v. Equicor-Equitable HCA Corp.*,
upholding an HMO's refusal to pay for nursing home care for which prior UR
approval had not been sought as required. "We are mindful that the objective in
construing a health care agreement, as with general contract terms, is to ascertain
and carry out the true intention of the parties. However, we do so giving the language its common and ordinary meaning *as a reasonable person in the position of
the HMO participant,* not the actual participant, would have understood the words
to mean."[86] The court pointed out that "[w]hile it is readily apparent Mr. McGee
sought the best possible care for his daughter, he was still obligated to work within
the defined contractual borders of the HMO he elected to participate in."[87] These
borders may be especially important in managed care. "HMOs are not traditional
insurance companies designed to indemnify participants for services they unilaterally select at any geographic location. Instead, HMOs . . . provide comprehensive prepaid medical services within a defined geographic area, and with specific
exceptions, only by participating medical professionals and facilities."[88] Equicor, the
defendant HMO, had made rehabilitation benefits contingent on periodic determinations by the patient's physician, a requirement Mr. McGee knew about but chose not
to fulfill.

Across these cases and others[89] judges have emphasized that courts are not free to
rewrite clear contractual language. One of the strongest statements comes from a
Federal district court in Massachusetts: "This cause of action—that contractual
promises can be enforced in the courts—pre-dates the Magna Carta. It is the bed-
rock of our notion of individual autonomy and property rights. It was among the
first precepts of the common law to be recognized in the courts of the Common-
wealth and has been zealously guarded by the state judiciary from that day to this.
Our entire capitalist structure depends on it."[90] And the Seventh Circuit agreed,[91]
"'we are not permitted to allow our sympathies and desires to vitiate clear principles of contract and labor law, and in particular, we refuse to amend the clear terms

of the health and welfare benefits contained in the [agreement].' "[92] " 'In the absence of a clear, unequivocal and specific contractual requirement [placing a duty on a party,] we refuse to order the same. To hold otherwise and to impose such a requirement would, in effect, enlarge the terms of the policy beyond those clearly defined in the policy agreed to by the parties.' "[93] Many other recent cases likewise insist on faithfulness to contract language.[94]

3. Adequacy of Contract Remedies

If the arguments presented in Chapters 6 and 9 are correct, contract appears, at least theoretically, to be the best means for society and for health plans to meet the needs of populations while being fair to individuals and for people to make choices that best implement their own values. However, an important remaining question is whether contract law provides adequate remedies when health plans fail to meet their resource obligations—sometimes to patients' disastrous detriment. To be sure, many breaches of contract will also be accompanied by tort suits when the contract breach is the product of carelessness or other defect of expertise on the part of the plan. In those cases the full panoply of tort remedies will be available. Accordingly, this discussion inquires only about instances in which an honest, nonculpable breach of contract occurred, leaving contract remedies as the exclusive source of reparation for the patient. The following discussion will show that contract law, properly understood, can provide surprisingly adequate remedies.

Chapter 4 proposed that lawsuits claiming breach of contract will generally arise within one of three scenarios: (1) prospectively to secure (coverage for) a treatment when there is still time for the treatment to be effective, (2) retrospectively to obtain reimbursement after treatment has been timely obtained, and (3) retrospectively to claim damages after denial or delay of treatment has allegedly caused additional harms. Arguably, contract remedies can adequately address most cases in all three categories.

The first scenario can easily justify injunctions for specific relief. Contract remedies are either specific, requiring actual performance of the contract, or substitutional, mandating some other form of compensation, usually monetary damages.[95] In ordinary contract settings injunctions for specific performance are relatively rare, largely as a matter of efficiency.[96] This is because in typical business situations, if breaching a contract is to the advantage of one party, and if the other party can be fully compensated for any loss resulting from the breach, then permitting the breach, rather than compelling performance, may bring the greater benefit for everyone.[97] However, in cases in which monetary compensation would clearly be inadequate, the rules of equity permit courts to compel actual performance of the contract.[98] In health care it is well known that denials or delays of surgery, physical therapy, medications, or other important treatments can cause disability, serious pain and suffering, and even death. In these cases assuring treatment when it can still be effective is usually preferable to setting monetary compensation after the harm is done. Thus, when the need for treatment is clear and the health plan does owe it, courts have no trouble mandating that actual treatment (for HMOs) or assured payment (for indemnity insurers) be provided.[99]

The second scenario, in which people merely want reimbursement for timely treatment already received, is equally amenable to traditional contract remedies. These cases do not even require that a distinction be drawn between specific performance and substitutional relief because the remedy requested is monetary. If a court finds that an insurer owes coverage, it simply requires payment. This precise scenario arises less often in an HMO, in which the health plan promises health care instead of financial reimbursement. Nevertheless, the issue can arise if, for instance, a subscriber pays out of pocket for denied treatment that he believes the HMO should cover and later requests reimbursement, or if the subscriber is traveling away from home and pays for care from an out-of-plan provider. These situations can lead the HMO member to sue for his costs.

The final scenario, in which harms have resulted from delay or denial of treatment, is plainly the most difficult because the injuries may be far more substantial than the cash value of the treatments the patient should have received. For example, in *Dearmas v. Av-Med, Inc.,*[100] a man's auto accident injuries were significantly exacerbated because his HMO sent him to four hospitals in three days, none of which provided an appropriate surgeon.[101] Such horror stories cry out for greater compensation than whatever actual dollar value would have been paid for specialist services, drugs, hospital care, and the like. Fortunately, contract remedies can be considerably broader than these direct dollar values.

In general, the purpose of damage awards under contract law is to place the individual "as nearly as possible in the position he would have been in had the contract been fully performed."[102] Three kinds of contract remedies are generally discussed. The prevailing form cites the injured party's *expectation interest,* in which the "court attempts to put the *promisee in the position in which the promisee would have been had the promise been performed* (i.e., had there been no breach)."[103] The two other types of remedy are *reliance interest* and *restitution interest.* Because these two offer smaller damages and apply to more purely commercial transactions that have limited relevance here, they will not be discussed.[104]

Expectation damages are calculated according to several factors. First, one must assess the *loss in value* that the promisee incurs from nonperformance or from defective performance.

> If, for example, the party in breach was to render services to the injured party and performed them deficiently, the *loss in value* equals the difference between the value to the injured party of the services that were to have been rendered and the value to that party of the services that were actually rendered. If no services at all were rendered, the *loss in value* is simply the value to the injured party of the services that were to have been rendered.[105]

Second, "other loss" includes incidental and consequential damages.

> Incidental damages include additional costs incurred after the breach in a reasonable attempt to avoid loss. . . . Consequential damages include such items as in-

jury to person or property caused by the breach. If, for example, services furnished to the injured party are defective and cause damage to that party's property, that loss is recoverable.[106]

Incidental damages will not figure prominently in health care suits because patients who lack medical expertise or are in need of urgent attention will not often be able to mitigate their own damages. However, consequential damages are obviously pertinent. For example, a failure to provide hospitalization or at least adequate home nursing services might cause fetal death in a high-risk pregnancy.[107] Similarly, harms caused by delays, even when treatment is ultimately rendered, can authorize additional damage awards.[108]

In health care the combined sum of loss in value plus consequential damages can be substantial. For instance, if a patient could have expected a full recovery from prompt and qualified care for broken vertebrae and if a lack of proper care caused him to become a paraplegic, then the combined value of his direct loss and the added consequential damages could produce a long list of damages, including current and future costs of special medical care, personal attendants, medical devices and other equipment, and lost employment or earning potential, among other costs and inconveniences.

Admittedly, it is commonly supposed that contract damages do not extend this far. Yet there are strong reasons to believe they can and should. After all, the limits currently found on contract remedies, such as the refusal to grant punitive damages in ordinary contract cases,[109] are mainly intended to ensure that someone does not end up in a better position than he would have enjoyed had the contract never been made.[110] But this limit does not require that an injured promisee must endure a substantially worse condition than he would have been in but for the breach. There is no way that money can restore sight when blindness follows the failure to provide adequate medical care, but that person should not shoulder myriad extra costs of living for which financial compensation could be given.

A number of commentators and judges support this broader view of contract remedies. Damages for emotional distress, for example, have already been allowed in cases in which such distress is a clearly foreseeable consequence of breaching the contract. These cases include "an innkeeper who wrongfully ejects guests amid streams of foul language and false accusations as to their morality; breach by a funeral parlor operator who furnished a leaky casket and vault; breach by the operator of a legal gambling parlor who for a monthly fee contracted with the husband not to permit the wife to continue her gambling which was destroying the family."[111]

In insurance cases, especially, emotional distress damages may be awarded when small claims and unsophisticated policyholders appear to prompt insurers to breach their duties too readily.[112] As the argument goes, "emotional distress resulting from an insurer's nonperformance is foreseeable at the time of contracting in many insurance transactions, and contract law is flexible enough, if properly applied, to provide a remedy for this kind of loss."[113]

Aside from emotional damages, a broad range of other kinds of losses that result from a contract breach should be compensable under the general principle that "all loss, however characterized, is recoverable."[114] This is particularly true in the context of insurance and health plans.

> Contract remedies are not inherently incapable of redressing the kinds of losses and injuries frequently suffered by insureds when insurers fail to perform their obligations. Insureds should be able to recover those extracontractual damages that naturally flow from the insurer's breach and are foreseeable at the time of contracting. . . . [M]ost insurance transactions are more than ordinary commercial transactions. . . . [C]ontract law has long recognized that some kinds of contracts are designed to protect peace of mind and that nonperformance can lead to serious mental anguish. In these areas, courts have expanded the range of foreseeability, permitting parties aggrieved by breaches to recover more than allowed under the traditional contract remedy.[115]

Thus, a broader recognition by courts of the many kinds of injuries that truly are foreseeable at the time of health plan contracting could credibly warrant a considerably broader range of remedies than is standardly recognized.[116] In the end, those who are injured should receive whatever compensation is necessary to place them, economically if not literally, in the position they should and would have occupied if the health plan had met its obligations. The extent of this compensability will be circumscribed by four traditional limits on contract remedies.

First, the injured party cannot recover for losses that reasonably could have been avoided.[117] As noted above, however, this caveat will not often apply in health care, where it is generally not reasonable to expect the ill or injured patient to fend for himself.

Second, the injury must have been foreseeable as a probable result of a breach at the time the contract was made.[118] This requirement is fairly specific. "It is not sufficient that the breaching party had reason to foresee that some damage would occur. The loss which actually occurred must have been foreseeable."[119] In other words, "foreseeable damages are limited to those which would follow from the breach in the ordinary course of events or which would ordinarily occur from circumstances about which the breaching party knew or should have known at the time the contract was made."[120]

In health care, this caveat will often be fairly easy to satisfy. It has already been noted that a failure to assure financial coverage can foreseeably result in a lack of treatment.[121] Moreover, failures to render timely and adequate treatment can yield quite predictable medical results. When the natural history of an illness or injury is fairly well known and when the typical results of adequate treatment likewise fall within a known range, it can be foreseen that a failure to treat properly will lead to a poorer outcome, within identifiable parameters, than would otherwise have been expected. For instance, if a particular type of cancer is virtually always completely curable when detected early, but the health plan fails to provide a promised level of screening that would almost certainly have detected such a cancer at that early stage, then advancement of the disease and the further problems that eventuate might be fairly attributed to the health plan's breach of contract.

In the third caveat, the damages themselves must be calculable with a reasonable level of certainty.[122] Highly speculative claims, such as that an infant who died from denial of treatment would surely have grown up to be President, will not be accepted because allowing such claims would not permit contracting parties to place reasonable limits and prices on the risks they assume.[123] This requirement for certainty of calculations can pose a significant challenge in health care litigation because many patients suffer not only from a primary illness or injury but also from assorted other comorbidities and biological idiosyncrasies that can complicate predictions. Still, medicine is based on science, and statistical and observational generalities can be applied in many cases. If someone's illness is aggravated because her treatment was delayed by resource denials, her extra hospital time, further treatment costs, requisite home health aids, and even lost wages are calculable within a reasonable range of certainty. Furthermore, as outcomes studies grow in prevalence and quality, it should be possible to predict with increasing reliability what a patient's condition might have been with appropriate treatment. In addition, courts tend to be more lenient with the certainty requirement when it appears that the contract breach was willfull.[124] Thus, in cases in which a health plan deliberately or recklessly denies benefits to contain its costs,[125] courts may be more inclined to give patients the benefit of the doubt.

Finally, in contract law as in tort law, there must be a demonstrable causal connection between the breach and the injury.[126] This challenge, too, can be formidable because of the many complexities and contingencies in health and health care. But such issues are familiar and manageable. They are the daily stuff of health care litigation.

If expectation damages are interpreted to include all of the foreseeable harms that can be quantified with reasonable certainty, then contract law is well-equipped to address health plans' breaches of contract in all three basic scenarios. Prospective requests for injunction can mandate actual treatment or assurance of coverage. Retrospective reimbursement for treatments already received can be monetarily compensated. And retrospective suits for the harms of treatments denied or delayed should be able to cover a wide variety of damages that scientific medicine renders foreseeable and measurable.

In sum, when no breach of expertise duties has occurred, contract damages are arguably able to provide adequate compensation, even without the greater damages allowed under tort. At the same time, even this broader reading of contract remedies would not hold health plans to an unreasonable standard, such as to foresee the results of denying treatments that were not available at the time the patient was ill or that were not approved for general use at the time the patient signed on with the plan. Courts should refrain from finding excuses to add tort damages and instead should honor the terms of health care contracts and the good faith efforts of administrators to make necessary but inevitably difficult benefit determinations.

Perhaps the greatest argument on behalf of this strong reliance on contract and its allowable damages is that written contracts will not have force unless they are generally enforced as written. As shown in Chapters 4 and 9, absent solid contracts and good enforcement, people will have little opportunity to decide, on the basis of their own values and priorities, how much they want to spend on what sort of health care. When resource mishaps are addressed on the basis of outside standards rather than from within contractual terms, outsiders are imposing their own views about what health plans should cover. It may be appropriate for the nation to specify some basic level of benefits that all plans should provide,[127] but beyond that the great diversity of human values should have an opportunity to flourish.

Furthermore, post-hoc legal determinations that a plan should have provided more than it promised can adversely affect everyone else who purchased that plan with the hope of limiting their costs by limiting their benefits. Judicial awards, after all, do not affect just the case at bar. Once a court declares that a new test or treatment should have been provided to one patient, by implication every other patient in a similar situation should receive a similar level of care. And "similar" can be defined very broadly. For instance, if a health plan is forced to provide endless intensive care to an anencephalic infant,[128] then other patients in similarly dire straits wanting comparably heroic care must be comparably accommodated. Potentially, this could reach beyond other permanently unconscious patients to encompass patients with terminal or other serious illnesses who want costly but marginal treatments. These unanticipated expenditures will then affect all the people with ordinary needs who depend on the same pool of funds for their care. Reduced availability of nursing care, physical therapy, patient education, and similar types of less dramatic care is the likely result. In addition, the costs of widespread litigation can further threaten health plans' financial stability. The totality of implications is sobering for plans and for the people who depend on them.[129]

Accordingly, if the terms of the contract are clear, its limits should be enforced even if the subscriber later wishes he had purchased a more comprehensive plan. If the contract's implications for a particular case are unclear, then the principal question should not be whether the beneficiary wants or will benefit from the treatment in question nor what physicians customarily do in such a situation. Rather, the focus should be on whether plan administrators have faithfully and carefully implemented fair procedures for resolving ambiguities and disputes.[130]

D. IMPLICATIONS FOR LITIGATION

As argued here, existing case law, doctrines, and trends are surprisingly compatible with the proposal to distinguish between expertise and resources, addressing the former in tort and the latter in contract. Current law also supports permitting plans' resource packages to vary and expecting subscribers to abide by whatever limits they have chosen. Once such conceptual matters are clear, the main challenge in litigation will be to pursue factual questions carefully. Only with adequate fact finding will it be possible in complex cases to determine whether the patient's injury arose from defects of expertise, denials of resources, or both, and only then can courts determine when to invoke contract doctrines, and when to use tort.

Some recent case scenarios will help to illustrate these points. Suppose a woman with cancer claims that her HMO delayed her diagnosis and then treated her with atypical, ineffective chemotherapy.[131] Initially her primary care physician told her that the breast lumps she found were nothing to worry about. A year later, when she was referred for mammography, the radiologist read the results as normal, while the surgeon who subsequently examined her did not perform a biopsy.[132]

This brief sketch leaves the providers and MCO looking obviously culpable, yet in reality one cannot determine what sorts of claims, if any, are appropriate without further factual inquiry. Several scenarios are possible. Under one description, it is possible that no one erred. According to the patient's history and physical examination the mass may have been consistent with fibrocystic disease, thus warranting a careful watch-and-wait approach; the radiographic images may have been genuinely difficult to interpret (false negatives are not uncommon in mammography); and the surgeon's decision to defer biopsy may have been guided by sound criteria that normally work well. The bare fact that a patient's problem was not promptly diagnosed or that her treatment did not work well do not mean *ipso facto* that someone erred.

Under another description, deficiencies of medical expertise may have occurred. Perhaps the primary care physician did not know what signs to look for when evaluating a breast mass or what protocols to follow to ensure that fibrocystic lesions had not given way to malignant ones. Possibly the radiologist was not fully trained in reading mammography or maybe the surgeon overlooked some important features of this patient's case. If inexpertise played such roles, the issues would be tort claims against the physicians. At the same time, if the HMO had been taking adequate care to credential and monitor these physicians' performance, there would not necessarily be any tort cause against the HMO. After all, the health plan's job is not to prevent physicians from making any errors but rather to detect patterns of errors. On the other hand, if one or more of these physicians had been a consistently poor performer, then the plan may have failed to credential and monitor properly, thereby potentially indicating a deficiency of expertise on the part of the HMO.

In yet another scenario there might have been a resource problem. Suppose the MCO has a policy limiting specialist referrals or biopsies.[133] If the policy was applied incorrectly in this patient's case, a breach of contract may have occurred. If it was correctly applied and the patient unfortunately fell on the wrong side of such a cap, then perhaps there was no violation of resource duties. In either case, it would be appropriate to examine the guideline. If it is medically unreasonable, the MCO may be tortiously at fault for a breach of expertise duties. On the other hand, if the guide is medically acceptable as well as properly implemented, then there may be no cause of action against the health plan in either contract or tort. Only a close investigation can determine what the real facts, and thereby the real tort and/or contract issues, are.[134]

Such inquiries are often complex, partly because good medical care cannot ordinarily be provided without using resources, from routine laboratory tests to sophisticated radiographic imaging and from simple bandages to complex regimens of surgery and chemotherapy. As illustrated above, the bare fact that a resource was not provided does not entail that a resource was "denied." Only a detailed investigation can sort out what happened and why. As these factual complexities are pursued, a few rules of thumb may be useful.

If a medically important resource is not clearly excluded by a health plan's guidelines, or if the plan's explicit procedures for resolving uncertainties do not point to a reasonably clear exclusion, then it is plausible to presume that the resource should be provided. Granting the patient the benefit of the doubt is consistent with *contra proferentem* and would serve to encourage health plans to be clearer with their guidelines, more detailed in their procedures for resolving ambiguities, and, in general, more explicit about what they promise their enrollees.

When a patient does not receive a resource that arguably should have been covered, the factual inquiry to sort out tort and contract breaches must head in several directions, each of which pursues the question "why did this happen." The physician's reasoning is usually the first thing to consider. If she simply did not know that this was an appropriate resource to use, and that is why she did not order it, then the health plan is probably not implicated because it apparently did not "deny" the resource. However, there may be other reasons the physician did not use a particular resource. If the health plan put up major obstacles to discourage physicians from even attempting to secure resources, then the plan may share the responsibility. In either case, expertise issues would be at stake, whether on the part of the physician or on the part of the plan.

In a different scenario, if the physician actually tried to obtain the test or treatment in question and the health plan denied it, the issues obviously involve resources. However, further inquiry should still focus on "why did this happen." If the health plan was careful and conscientious—if it committed no error of expertise—but nevertheless made an error, then the case belongs strictly in contract. However, if the plan bungled by failing to look carefully at the patient's situation and the physician's request, then there may also be an expertise error to pursue in tort. Only a careful, factual investigation can determine why the denial occurred, and only with such information can it be determined what sort of claim, if any, the plaintiff may appropriately make against whom.

E. SUMMARY

In the final analysis, the law addressing patients' adverse outcomes in the context of health care should be and reasonably can be far better attuned to the profound changes in the ways health care is now financed and delivered. Courts need to inquire, up front, precisely who owed what to whom—whether the duty was one of expertise or of resources and whether it was owed by the health plan or by providers such as physicians.

As they undertake that inquiry, courts need to be clearer and more consistent in applying the appropriate body of legal doctrine, whether tort or contract. With the greater conceptual coherence and improved consistency recommended in this book, much of the unsettling unpredictability and even the periodic unfairness that now mark health care litigation could be considerably ameliorated. Existing doctrine and case law provide good foundations for such a transition. For the most part, all that is needed now is a focused, concept-driven implementation.

One major hitch exists, of course—ERISA. Whereas this book recommends that health plans should be accountable in tort for their breaches of expertise duties and in contract for their breaches of resource duties, ERISA tends to throw the proverbial monkey wrench into the works by preempting most of these causes of action. It is now time to undertake that important discussion.

11

SPECIAL ISSUES IN ERISA

This book does not offer an in-depth analysis of ERISA,[1] but a brief overview will provide necessary background to the discussion.[2] ERISA was born in a time of economic "stagflation"—a stagnant economy marked by high inflation.

> When Congress was considering ERISA in the early 1970's, there was great concern over the possibility of widespread termination of employee benefit plans. . . . In fact, it was becoming increasingly apparent that many long time employers might be unable to meet benefit obligations owed to aging work forces. . . . At the same time, Congress was concerned that the Social Security system, itself strained by the increasing demands made on it by retired workers, could not be relied upon to provide adequate retirement benefits for the vast majority of covered workers.[3]

Thus, ERISA was enacted partly to ensure that employee benefit plans are established on financially sound principles, but also partly to ease costs and administrative burdens, particularly for multistate corporations that had to fit their benefits to as many as fifty different sets of laws.[4] If the costs of benefit plans could thereby be made more predictable and more clearly circumscribed, it was hoped that firms would continue to offer such plans, thus removing from Congress the potential onus of having to meet huge burdens through federal programs.[5]

Accordingly, the statute established a quid pro quo: in exchange for requiring that pension plans be funded and vested under federal specifications, all benefit plans (welfare benefits as well as pensions[6]) were placed under a uniform set of federal rules that would ease their administration and minimize unanticipated expenses. For

160

welfare benefits such as health plans no requirements were specified for vesting or funding. The main requirement is that the plan deliver what it promises. Employers can design their welfare benefit plans, including health care, however they wish and can change them virtually at will so long as they satisfy certain requirements such as notification. Indeed, ERISA statute and case law are quite emphatic that employers must not be required to provide any particular level or kind of benefits.[7]

Because ERISA applies strictly to businesses engaged in interstate commerce,[8] it does not cover every employment situation. It does not apply to government workers or church employees, for example. Other than these limited exceptions, however, almost all benefit plans that workers receive as part of their employment are governed by ERISA.

Several features are worth noting. The preemption of state law in favor of federal law[9] is pervasive. Within ERISA's ambit, all benefit plans are governed—pension plans, health care, and all other workplace benefits.[10] And where ERISA governs, state laws, including tort and contract, are generally preempted.[11] In health care, for instance, ERISA has largely shielded employment-based health plans from accountability for malpractice, wrongful death, breach of contract, fraud, intentional or negligent infliction of emotional distress, and the panoply of other state-based causes of action for which the health plans might otherwise have been liable.[12] Through this preemption, welfare benefit plans have been protected against lawsuits that could significantly complicate the plans' administration and potentially deplete their resources.[13] A serious drawback, however, is that plaintiffs are sometimes left with no remedy at all for an injury that otherwise would quite surely have been a tort permitting substantial damages.[14] This issue will be discussed further below.

There is an exception to this otherwise broad preemption. Per the so-called "savings" clause,[15] states are permitted to regulate the business of insurance. A state can require all commercial insurers to provide mental health care benefits[16] or to cover in vitro fertilization, for instance. However, in the so-called "deemer" clause, ERISA specifies that firms' self-funded plans are not deemed to be insurance and hence are not subject to states' insurance regulation. By implication, if an employer pays out of pocket for employees' health needs rather than buying a commercial insurance product, it can avoid costly lists of state-mandated benefits.[17] As a result, states cannot broaden their citizens' access to health care by mandating that businesses provide or enrich their health plans for employees.[18]

Remedies for breaches of duty within ERISA are, like causes of action, strictly limited by federal law. They include the monetary value of the wrongly denied benefit and sometimes attorney fees and certain forms of injunctive and other equitable relief.[19] Thus, in health care cases the patient can win an injunction requiring a test or treatment or, retrospectively, the monetary value of the health services that were denied, but not much more. The plaintiff cannot claim damages for the medical consequences of that denial, nor for pain and suffering, nor any other state-based remedy.

In applying ERISA over the years, courts have preempted a wide variety of tort claims against ERISA health plans, affording them a remarkable degree of protection against lawsuits. For example, in *Dearmass v. Av-Med,*[20] the plaintiff's auto accident injuries were significantly exacerbated because his HMO sent him to four hospitals in three days, not one of which provided a neurosurgeon. Because his HMO plan was an employment benefit, however, all tort claims, including negligence, "dumping," and loss of consortium, were preempted.[21] In *Kuhl v. Lincoln Nat. Health Plan*[22] a patient urgently needed heart surgery, including aneurysm repair. During a series of delays in authorizing the surgery and choosing the hospital, the patient's heart deteriorated so badly that the surgery could no longer be performed. He was placed on a list for transplant but died before a donor heart became available. The patient's estate sued his HMO for medical malpractice, tortious interference with the physician–patient relationship, emotional distress, and breach of contract, but ERISA preempted all claims. A host of claims have been similarly preempted in other suits.[23]

Even while upholding ERISA's preemption, however, some courts have expressed concern. Benefit plans are protected, but individuals with ostensibly legitimate causes of action can be left completely without remedy. In *Corcoran v. United HealthCare, Inc.*, a newborn infant died after an insurer denied both hospitalization and twenty-four-hour home nursing for the mother's high-risk pregnancy, opting instead for more limited home nursing services. Preempting tort claims for wrongful death, emotional distress, negligence, and medical malpractice, the Fifth Circuit lamented:

> The result ERISA compels us to reach means that the Corcorans have no remedy, state or federal, for what may have been a serious mistake. This is troubling for several reasons. First, it eliminates an important check on thousands of medical decisions routinely made in the burgeoning utilization review system. With liability rules generally inapplicable, there is theoretically less deterrence of substandard medical decisionmaking. Moreover, if the cost of compliance with the standard of care (reflected either in the cost of prevention or the cost of paying judgments) need not be factored into utilization review companies' cost of doing business, bad medical judgments will end up being cost-free to the plans that rely on these companies to contain medical costs. ERISA plans, in turn, will have one less incentive to seek out the companies that can deliver both high quality services and reasonable prices.[24]

Because ERISA's preemption of state-based tort and contract liability can significantly diminish injured patients' access to remedies, this law deserves a closer look. Chapter 11 offers three main observations.

First, recent ERISA case law has created an important distinction. In the interest of limiting ERISA's preemption and expanding patients' opportunities to bring state-based claims against health plans, many courts now distinguish between claims alleging that the plan has denied benefits it promised and claims alleging only that the care received was poor quality. They have concluded that while the former quantity-of-care claims are still preempted by ERISA, the latter, quality-oriented claims are not.

Second, the quality–quantity distinction strongly parallels, even if it does not precisely match, the expertise–resources distinction. More precisely, the courts' approach should be regarded as a flawed approximation of the expertise–resources distinction—that is, as a somewhat fumbling attempt to capture the conceptually clearer, more cleanly applicable ideas embedded in the notions of expertise and resources. Although courts' "quantity" notion tracks closely with "resources," their applications of the "quality" concept are seriously problematic. This is seen in a number of cases that courts have chosen to identify as "quality" claims, not so much because the court can point to a credible concept of "quality" to justify the label, but simply because the court would prefer to let an injured patient take his case to the more generous state courts. Such results-oriented rulings do not provide plausible justifications for their decisions nor clear, reliable guidance for future cases. The result is sometimes an aggravation of the confusion in this important area of ERISA litigation.

Third, the problem can be fixed because the ideas implicit in the quality–quantity motif are essentially, even if imperfectly, on the right track. If courts can shift their thinking just a bit, supplanting "quality" with the clearer, more circumscribed notion of "expertise," they will be able to bring a more coherent, conceptually intelligible approach to these difficult preemption cases. The overall result will match what most courts hope to achieve: a variety of cases will legitimately be remanded to state courts, while others will still be preempted by ERISA into federal courts. But the reasoning will be rationally more defensible and more consistent with the legitimate legislative objectives behind this complex law. Each of these observations is explored below.

A. QUALITY–QUANTITY: PARALLELING THE EXPERTISE–RESOURCE DISTINCTION

Haas v. Group Health Plan, Inc.,[25] is one of the earliest cases that began to capture the quality–quantity distinction. An HMO's nurse practitioner was negligent while removing impacted ear wax, damaging the patient's tympanic membrane. A federal district court found that although nearly all the plaintiff's tort claims against the ERISA plan were preempted, in this case a claim for vicarious liability was not. The court noted that although ERISA applies to adjudication of benefits, in this case no benefits were denied. The nurse practitioner delivered the benefits the plan owed but allegedly did so in a careless fashion. Since the nurse practitioner was the plan's employee, it followed that the plan had vicarious liability.[26]

In *Haas* the court seemed to make a strong, albeit implicit, distinction between resources and expertise. In this case, because the plan held itself out as the actual provider of care and this alleged wrong strictly concerned poor skill in providing that care—not any denial of specific benefits or rights under the plan—the court concluded that ERISA was not involved.

The same distinction emerges even more clearly in *Kearney v. U.S. Healthcare, Inc.*[27] The patient died of thrombotic thrombocytopenic purpura (a clotting disorder), allegedly because the primary care physician failed to diagnose the problem so that the patient could be referred for appropriate specialist care. The court noted that

ERISA preempted most of the plaintiff's claims, including misrepresentation, breach of contract, and an allegation that the plan restricted access to specialists, on the ground that such suits involve benefit determinations. However, when the plan holds itself out as the actual provider of care rather than merely paying or arranging for care, then its physicians' malpractice in failing to diagnose can be regarded as the plan's own malpractice. The claim for vicarious liability was thus not preempted. As the court observed, "a claim that one was denied a promised benefit is preempted. A claim that one received a promised service from a provider who performed that service negligently is another matter."[28] Again, a strong distinction is implied between expertise (the physician's knowledge and skill) and resources (promised benefits that are either provided or denied).[29]

Following these important precursors from district courts, the Third Circuit Court of Appeals in *Dukes v. U.S. Healthcare*[30] provided the seminal case on which the subsequent cases in this growing trend rely. In the process of caring for an ear problem, the plaintiff's physician ordered some blood tests, which the hospital refused to perform. Eventually the tests were done, revealing very high blood sugar, but by then the plaintiff's deterioration and death could not be averted. The court focused on the ERISA statute, Section 502, which states that federal preemption applies to suits "to recover benefits due . . . under the terms of [the] plan, to enforce. . . . rights under the terms of the plan, or to clarify . . . rights to future benefits under the terms of the plan."[31] In this case, the court noted,

> the plaintiffs' claims . . . merely attack the quality of the benefits they received. The plaintiffs here simply do not claim that the plans erroneously withheld benefits due. Nor do they ask the state courts to enforce their rights under the terms of their respective plans or to clarify their rights to future benefits. As a result, the plaintiffs' claims fall outside the scope of § 502(a)(1)(B).[32]

The court concluded that the plaintiff's quality-oriented case could be heard in state courts rather than being completely preempted to federal courts.[33]

A host of cases has followed closely on *Dukes'* heels. In *Herrera v. Lovelace Health Systems, Inc.,*[34] a physician allegedly botched the patient's vasectomy. The federal district court held that, since the question concerned whether the physician "'possessed and utilized the knowledge, skill and care usually had and exercised by physicians in his community or medical specialty,'"[35] it thereby raised issues of quality rather than quantity of care. Hence, ERISA did not preempt claims against the MCO for medical malpractice, negligence, corporate negligence, and intentional infliction of emotional distress. In *Crum v. Health Alliance-Midwest, Inc.,*[36] a forty-two-year-old man with a family history of heart disease, severe chest pain, and other symptoms consistent with heart attack was told by a telephone triage nurse that he was merely experiencing gastric upset. The federal district court held that this complaint did not concern any denial of benefits, but rather a poor quality of the benefits provided—here, nursing advice. A New York state court reached the same conclusion in *Tufino v. N.Y. Hotel & Motel Trades Council*[37] when physicians' failure to monitor a patient's postoperative anticoagulents led to a subdural hematoma (bleeding in the brain) and death.[38]

In a different but still consistent line of cases a number of courts have ruled that because the case at bar involved quantity-of-benefits (i.e., resource) issues, the ERISA preemption must apply. In *Tolton v. American Biodyne, Inc.,*[39] a psychiatric patient committed suicide after denial of hospital care. The Sixth Circuit preempted claims for bad faith, malpractice, and wrongful death, among others. "In the case at hand, plaintiffs' claims that arise from an allegedly improper denial of benefits to an beneficiary fall squarely within Section 502(a)."[40] *Turner v. Fallon Community Health Plan, Inc.*[41] followed Tolton's reasoning. A woman with breast cancer had requested bone marrow transplant. Because the cancer had metastasized to her bone marrow and because her health plan explicitly excluded that treatment for conditions like hers, the transplant was denied. The district court upheld the denial and preempted state-based claims for wrongful death, loss of consortium, and breach of contract, among others. The First Circuit affirmed.[42]

Similarly, in *Cannon v. Group Health Service*[43] an HMO initially denied, then granted approval of bone marrow transplant for acute myeloblastic leukemia. During the seven-week delay before the plan changed its ruling, however, the plaintiff's deterioration rendered her medically ineligible for the treatment. The Tenth Circuit, noting that the denial involved a benefits decision, ruled that ERISA preempted state-based claims such as negligence, bad faith, and breach of contract.[44] The plaintiff's lack of significant remedy within ERISA and the lack of an alternative remedy outside federal law did not change the legally inevitable ruling.[45]

A number of other courts have followed the *Dukes* distinction, and its line of reasoning has quickly built broad acceptance.[46] The fundamental trend appears sound. In principle, even if not always in application, the *Dukes* quality–quantity distinction parallels fairly well the expertise–resources distinction. On the one side, quality of benefits often concerns the level of knowledge, skill, and diligence with which care was provided. Cases such as a punctured tympanic membrane or a botched vasectomy do not fundamentally involve ERISA's primary concern, which is with breaking a promise to provide benefits. Except in cases in which the benefit provided is of such poor quality that it is equivalent to no benefit at all or in cases where the plan actually promises a certain quality of benefit,[47] deficiencies of expertise simply do not fit the picture of preemption intended by ERISA. As *Dukes* notes, "[w]e find nothing in the legislative history suggesting that Section 502 was intended as a part of a federal scheme to control the quality of the benefits received by plan participants."[48]

On the other side, quantity disputes inquire whether resources were provided as promised in the terms of the benefit plan. Although a prominent objective of ERISA is to ensure that employers deliver what they promise, the statute also specifies that they need not offer any particular kind or level of benefits. Hence, any attempt by states—or courts—to mandate that an ERISA plan cover this or that benefit must be promptly overridden.[49] Accordingly, insofar as ERISA was intended to apply to the kinds and amounts of benefits provided in the workplace, then purely qualitative, expertise-type issues are rightly winnowed out, just as the *Dukes* line suggests.

Reciprocally, any time a court might try to require that an ERISA plan cover some particular resource that it did not promise to cover, then that court would violate ERISA's provision that employers are free to make their benefits plans as rich or as lean as they wish.[50]

B. QUALITY–QUANTITY: A FLAWED DISTINCTION

Thus the *Dukes* distinction is, in principle, on the right track. Its "quantity" notion corresponds directly with "resources," while "quality" often, though not always, matches "expertise." However, the "quality" notion, as courts use it, has major flaws. Because "quality" is deeply ambiguous, courts tend to make three important mistakes when applying the concept. First, courts tend to be confused about which factual scenarios present genuine issues of quality (expertise) and which are actually problems of quantity (resources). Too often they cite quality when they should cite quantity. Second, probably due to the difficulty of applying the ambiguous notion of quality, courts sometimes resort to a surrogate distinction: if a decision was made by a health plan administrator, it must be a quantity issue, while if it was made by a physician, it must be a quality issue. Chapter 6 has already shown the basic flaw in this thinking. Health plans and their administrators can make errors of expertise as well as of resources; and, reciprocally, physicians can make errors of resources as well as of expertise. Third, courts are also confused about what actually constitutes a denial of benefits. Each of these mistakes needs to be explored.

1. Confusion Number One: Which Cases Present Which Issues

Probably the most persistent problem as courts apply the *Dukes* distinction is that "quality" is a vague, poorly defined notion. Although the paradigm cases presented above implicitly define quality very much as this book defines expertise—namely, in terms of errors of the mind such as inadequate judgement or skill—in fact, many of the actual cases in which courts declare a quality problem have predominantly featured resource issues.

Perhaps courts' penchant to combine expertise and resources under the lone umbrella of quality should not be too surprising. After all, it reflects the same tendency in malpractice law, discussed in Chapter 2, to identify the malpractice standard of care not just in terms of physicians' knowledge and skills, but also in terms of technological resources doctors are expected to provide for their patients regardless of cost. Moreover, in ordinary language the concept of quality is often used to encompass all aspects of a patient's care, including how much care he received, how skillfully it was delivered, and the like.

Examples of how this fuzziness emerges in case law are not difficult to find. One case comes from Chapter 8. *Ouellette v. Christ Hospital*[51] featured a woman who was allegedly discharged prematurely from the hospital after removal of her ovaries. The court decided that the issue concerned quality and was not preempted by ERISA. However, it takes little imagination to see that the core issue was actually resources, not expertise. Ms. Ouellette did not claim that the quality of her treatment while in the hospital was poor. She claimed that she had too few days in the hospital, clearly a resource denial. If state courts find that the plan should have provided a longer hospital stay, then by implication such a decision may well require that plan generally to provide longer hospital stays for surgeries such as Mrs. Ouellette's. In so doing, courts will have effectively mandated a richer benefit package than the employer or its plan intended.

In *In Re. U.S. Healthcare, Inc.,*[52] a newborn was discharged twenty-four hours after delivery and did not thereafter receive the home visit promised by the health plan. The child developed meningitis and died the next day. The plaintiffs argued that the denial of a longer hospital stay was a quality problem, not a benefits denial. The court agreed and remanded the case to state court. On closer analysis, however, it is implausible to believe that the denial of extra time in the hospital does not constitute a denial of resources. As in *Ouellette,* the plaintiffs did not say that the care while in the hospital was of poor quality; they claimed that the baby had too few days of it.[53] And as with *Ouelette,* once a court decides that denial of longer hospitalization is a "quality" problem, it effectively requires the health plan to provide a richer set of benefits than it had intended. To be sure, researchers dispute whether twenty-four-hour discharge policies adversely affect neonatal mortality and morbidity.[54] But equally surely, courts that indirectly mandate longer stays by declaring shorter stays to be a "quality" problem have directly thwarted ERISA's provision that no one can dictate to employers what sort of benefit package they offer.[55]

Other cases manifest the same problem. In *Kampmeier v. Sacred Heart Hospital*[56] the plaintiff was scheduled to undergo ultrasound for her pregnancy. The HMO approved and scheduled the test but, because of administrative procedures, the appointment date was three days after the physician had ordered it. The ultrasound was never performed because the patient went into labor before the three-day period had expired. Had the test been completed, it would have revealed the very large size of the fetus in time to have prompted the physician to perform a cesarean instead of a vaginal delivery. Unfortunately, because this information was not known, the fetus suffered severe shoulder dystocia and other problems during vaginal delivery. The court, noting that the lack of timely ultrasound was not actually the product of an explicit utilization review decision to deny benefits, ruled that the case was a quality problem and could be remanded to state courts.[57] And yet on the face of it, the obvious problem was that the health plan's system for providing benefits was too slow, so that the patient did not actually receive the benefit promised.

Plocica v. NYLCare of Texas, Inc.[58] featured an allegedly premature discharge from a psychiatric hospital, after which the patient ingested antifreeze and died. Again, the case obviously involved denial of a resource—inpatient psychiatric care. And yet because the plaintiff claimed and the court was willing to agree that the complaint concerned only quality of care, the case bypassed ERISA and was remanded to state courts. Once again, by implication of simply declaring a quality problem, courts are potentially requiring employers to provide a richer benefit plan than they had intended.

To be sure, the bare fact that an important resource was denied does not entail that the only or most important problem concerned resources rather than expertise. If errors of expertise were the root cause of the resource denials, then clearly both kinds of problem should be acknowledged, not just the resource denial. In *Moscovitch v. Danbury Hosp.*,[59] for instance, an adolescent psychiatric patient allegedly was transferred prematurely from an inpatient psychiatric facility to a less intensive setting that treated only substance abuse problems. On the day of his arrival there the patient committed suicide. Arguably, the boy did not receive as many days as he needed in the hospital—a resource problem. Yet closer investigation of the facts might reveal important deficiencies of expertise. Perhaps the health plan did not seek the advice of people with adequate training in mental illness when it made its decision that further hospital care was not necessary. Or perhaps it did not select the second facility with adequate care. Alternatively, it is possible that the plan did everything that it reasonably could have: it may have implemented good credentialing and review procedures to select qualified facilities and advisers, so that this unfortunate outcome may simply have happened beyond the health plan's reasonable control. As argued previously, health plans cannot dictate every individual act of care nor should they try, lest the administration of health plans become hopelessly intrusive into the delivery of care. Whatever the actual facts were in this case, the upshot is clear: it was inadequate for the court simply to declare, virtually by fiat, that the problem strictly concerned quality of care.

Although part of the problem, as noted, stems from the conceptual vagueness of "quality," another part of the problem is courts' willingness to let this vagueness be used to plaintiffs' advantage. In some cases the plaintiff needs only to state his claims in the language of quality, and the court seems to be satisfied. Thus, in *Plocica,* cited above, the court noted that the plaintiffs "insist that their claims do not seek reimbursement for past or future medical procedures, hospitalization, or recovery for denial of any benefits."[60] Plaintiffs merely challenged the quality of the medical decision making, including the influence and control exercised by the health plan, and the plan's allegedly negligent acts in its medical decisions, diagnosis, and treatment of Mr. Plocica.[61] The court seemed not to notice that the entire problem and the consequences suffered by the patient and his family stemmed from the denial of a resource, inpatient psychiatric care.[62]

Admittedly, long-standing doctrine holds that "[t]he plaintiff is the master of her complaint, not the defendant."[63] And so long as that is true, " 'the plaintiff may, by eschewing claims based on federal law, choose to have the cause heard in state court.' "[64] However, it is one thing to agree that plaintiffs are entitled to decide to pursue only the claims that belong in state courts. It is another thing for courts to acquiesce to whatever description a plaintiff chooses to put on his complaint—in these cases, to stamp the label "quality" on a complaint—simply to be able to send the case to state courts.

Not all courts have permitted plaintiffs to manipulate the substance of complaints by choice of terminology. In *Jass v. Prudential Health Care Plan, Inc.*,[65] the plaintiff insisted that the denial of extensive physical therapy after her knee surgery constituted a problem of quality, not a deprivation of benefits. In response, the Seventh Circuit explicitly pointed out the plaintiff's ulterior agenda. She had framed her case as a so-called quality issue in order to have it heard in state courts, with their broader causes of action and more generous damage awards, rather than in federal courts. The court was not persuaded and held that her claim concerned benefits denial, regardless how it was framed.

> The question, then, is whether Jass' claim against Margulis is 'really' based on ERISA, . . . or in other words whether the claim is best recharacterised as a Section 502(a)(1)(B) claim to recover benefits due under the terms of the plan. . . . [W]e are not limited by the complaint, but may look beyond it to assure ourselves 'that the plaintiff has not by "artful pleading" sought to defeat the defendant's right to a federal forum.'[66]

In the same vein, the District of Delaware court reminded litigants:

> The Eighth Circuit Court of Appeals held that artful characterization of the action as malpractice did not change the fact that plaintiffs' claims were based on the organization's delay in recertifying payment for surgery. . . . Such a failure constituted an improper processing of a claim for benefits and was, therefore, preempted. . . . Despite plaintiff's attempts to craft defendants' actions as medical malpractice, the wrong committed in this case relates to the administration of the plan, not to the provision or supervision of medical services. In fact, the overarching problem was that no medical treatment was ever initiated let alone provided.[67]

Thus, notwithstanding plaintiffs' rights to decide which complaints to pursue, courts have an important responsibility to clarify causes of action sufficiently that they can be applied with reasonable consistency and predictability. This is partly so that citizens can understand and plan their conduct around the laws that govern them and partly so that legal liabilities and penalties can be assigned fairly. In this instance the *Dukes* distinction needs to be clarified because "quality," at least as courts actually use the term in practice, is too vague and tends too often to encompass resources. At the arbitrary discretion of a plaintiff or a sympathetic judge, issues that from a conceptual standpoint are clearly resource problems have simply been declared to be quality problems so that plaintiffs can find richer damage awards in state courts.[68]

In some cases courts seem openly to ignore ERISA's restrictions in order to achieve what the court deems a more just outcome. In *Pappas v. Asbel,*[69] a factually complex case involving delays in referring an emergency patient to a hospital that was medically adequate and HMO-approved, Pennsylvania courts spent little effort trying to sort out the factual details of a complex case. Instead, they opined that surely Congress could not have intended, back in the 1970s, for ERISA to apply to health care cases in the way it has.[70]

The remedy to the problem, obviously enough in the context of this book, will be to replace the concepts of "quality" and "quantity" with "expertise" and "resources." The latter concepts are considerably clearer because "expertise," unlike "quality," carries no historical or linguistic predisposition to include physical and fiscal resources under the same umbrella as mental and personal faculties like knowledge and skill, judgment and effort. This linguistic shift would help courts to identify, much more clearly than they do at present, which features of a case are rightly preempted to federal courts and which aspects belong in state courts. Admittedly, this improvement in conceptual clarity will not eliminate the need to sort out difficult factual questions. But those, as explored in Chapter 10, are familiar challenges that courts must routinely take up.

2. Confusion Number Two: A Poorly-Chosen Surrogate Distinction

The second confusion is found in some courts' assumption that a neat divide exists between what physicians do and what health plan administrators do, and that this correlates directly with the quality–quantity divide. These courts presume that if a physician made the decision in question the issue must concern quality, while quantity problems can only come from health plan administrators' decisions. *Lancaster v. Kaiser Foundation Health Plan*[71] illustrates the reasoning. An eleven-year-old girl visited her physicians complaining of daily headaches that were frequently accompanied by nausea and vomiting. Although the girl returned many times with the same symptoms, her two physicians, Drs. Campbell and Pauls, prescribed pain medication but offered no further diagnostic workup. Nearly five years later a school psychologist, concerned about the girl's continuing discomfort and her deteriorating academic performance, wrote to the physicians and urged them to evaluate her ongoing headaches more thoroughly. By the time the girl's brain tumor was finally diagnosed, it was very large and required numerous surgeries, none of which were entirely successful.

As with many of the cases discussed above, this case clearly involved resource inadequacies. The physicians failed to undertake important diagnostic testing and failed to refer the girl for specialized consultation. Yet in ruling that Lancaster's injuries should be treated as a deficiency of quality, not of the quantity of benefits provided, the court distinguished between a *"physician's* medical determination concerning appropriate treatment and medication . . . [and] an *administrator's* decision to deny benefits as a matter of coverage or discretion."[72] The court noted that it was physicians who made the decision not to pursue further diagnostic workup and even though they were under financial incentives whose conceded purpose was to reduce the amount of care, "this does not convert these medical malpractice claims into claims for *administrative* denial of benefits."[73] In this way the court set up a surrogate for the *Dukes* distinction: it presumed that physicians' conduct can only concern quality of care, while benefits determinations can only come from administrators.[74]

Superficially, this physician–administrator distinction, functioning as a surrogate for quality–quantity, seems attractive. Rather than applying a fuzzy term like quality, it would be far easier simply to determine whether a physician or an administrator made the error in question and instantly answer the preemption question on that basis. Modern medicine cannot be practiced without considerable use of sometimes costly resources, and the distinction between how well the patient was cared for versus how much care the patient received can blur rather easily.

Unfortunately, the convenience of this surrogate distinction does not excuse the conceptual confusion on which it relies. It is simply erroneous to presume that health plan administrators make all the resource/quantity decisions and that physicians cannot make them. In describing physician errors simply as deviations below the tort standard of care and thereby characterizing these as strictly quality issues,[75] the *Lancaster* court falls into a now-familiar error: it fails to recognize that the traditional standard of care has come to consist of both expertise elements and resource elements—improperly so, as argued in Chapter 2. As this book has made clear, physicians who gain resource control by accepting financial risk can, under some arrangements, have the same authority over resources as any administrator. Reciprocally, health plans can make expertise errors that, like physicians' bad medical judgments, should properly be remanded to state courts. If courts' reasoning more closely followed the expertise–resource distinction proposed in this book, their adjudications in these difficult ERISA cases could be considerably clearer, more cogent, and more consistent.

In an interesting parallel error that relies on the same surrogate distinction, some courts have assumed that, just as physicians cannot commit "quantity" errors, health plans are incapable of making quality–expertise errors. For instance, a number of courts have preempted direct liability claims against health plans, particularly in the context of suits for negligent selection and supervision of providers. The reasoning seems to go this way: since direct duties such as credentialing are undertaken by administrators, and since administrators are the ones who make (ERISA-shielded) benefits decisions, then credentialing activities must likewise be preempted. Thus, for instance, a federal district court in Oklahoma found that "cases involving direct negligence claims against the health maintenance organization arose because of the way the health maintenance organization administered plan benefits."[76]

This reasoning is clearly mistaken. These courts should recall that ERISA's complete preemption[77] applies only to disputes regarding whether the plan has provided the benefits it has promised.[78] The preemption does not aim to shield health plan administrators from liability per se, but rather to ensure that no one dictates to employers the kinds or amounts of benefits they must provide.[79] Therefore, unless the contract expressly promises a certain quality of credentialing as a "benefit due," then plans' credentialing activities do not constitute the resource decisions ERISA aims to shield.[80] As noted in this book, health plans are just as capable of making expertise errors as are physicians, and when they do the case is a tort belonging in state court.[81]

3. Confusion Number Three: What Counts as a Denial of Benefits

In yet another oddity, some courts have construed the concept of benefits–quantity decisions so narrowly that they will only find a denial of benefits where a health plan explicitly refuses to reimburse a claim for payment or to approve a specific request for treatment authorization. In *In re U.S. Healthcare,*[82] an infant was discharged twenty-four hours after birth in accordance with her HMO's general policy. The next day when the child seemed ill, the parents' repeated phone calls to their physician and to the health plan did not result in readmission to the hospital, or even in the in–home nursing visit promised by the HMO. The infant died shortly thereafter from an undiagnosed, untreated meningitis. Although the underlying allegation was that the baby did not receive sufficiently long hospitalization or a home nursing visit—ostensibly a denial of benefits—the Third Circuit was willing to agree with plaintiff that the problem in this case was one of quality, not quantity, of care. As the court reasoned, "[t]he allegations . . . do not raise the failure of U.S.Healthcare to *pay for a benefit or process a claim for benefits* as the basis for the injury suffered."[83]

The First Circuit commits the same error. In a footnote in *Danca v. Private Health Care Sys., Inc.,*[84] that court defines "benefits" as "the monetary payments for medical services, not the services themselves." The court observes:

> ERISA contains no definition of the term 'benefits, nor has any circuit court, to our knowledge, attempted to define the term. . . . Nevertheless, the definition of an ERISA 'plan' suggests that the term 'benefits' is distinct from the care given. . . . Furthermore, Justice Breyer has distinguished between the payment of money, which he characterizes as 'benefits,' *see Boggs v. Boggs,* 520 U.S. 833, 860 (1997) (Breyer, J., dissenting) (characterizing the payment of benefits as 'the writing of checks from [pension and welfare benefit] funds'), and the goods and services that the money purchases, which are not benefits . . . We therefore conclude that 'benefits' in this context, as in the pension context, are the monetary payments for medical services, not the services themselves.[85]

Other courts share the same misconception.[86]

This narrow construction of benefits denials seems to imply that the only way a health plan can make a bona fide benefits decision, preemptable by ERISA, is to be presented with a claim for cash reimbursement or a direct request to authorize (payment for) some specific procedure. While this analysis works well enough in fee-for-service (FFS) plans, it makes no sense in a capitated plan where FFS-style payments are almost never made.[87] After all, capitated plans do not receive, process, or reimburse claims. They simply pay their providers (whether as physician groups or as individual physicians) a fixed sum to deliver a specified array of services. Capitated plans' decisions about benefits are then embedded in general guidelines about appropriate care, in structures for monitoring and encouraging certain approaches to care, and in clinicians' day-to-day decisions and interpretations of those guidelines. The patient may never know that a useful lab test or consult has been denied, because he may never realise that it would have been an appropriate intervention. But the denial is no less real than if a formal claim had been processed and rejected.

Hence we find an odd implication: if these courts' stubbornly FFS-based perspective prevails, ERISA will provide little or no preemption protection for plans that use capitation, while continuing to provide broad protection for FFS plans—even under otherwise identical circumstances. On this view, when a patient in a capitated plan does not receive a treatment out of cost considerations, courts will find that he has not been denied a benefit. At the same time, those courts will declare that an identical patient under medically identical circumstances has indeed been denied a benefit if his not-receiving that treatment happened to emanate from a formal claims process. The result cannot withstand rational scrutiny, yet it is inevitable so long as courts cling to the outdated notion that only health plans and their white-collar administrators can control health care resources. Clearly, this is not the intent of ERISA.[88]

4. Factual Challenges

Once courts are straight about these basic conceptual issues, important factual challenges will arise in litigating such cases. Expertise issues pose fairly routine questions. In the *Lancaster* case, for instance, if plaintiffs want to argue that the health plan failed in a duty of expertise, such as to credential and supervise its physicians properly, factual issues will turn on whether Drs. Campbell and Pauls were generally good physicians who usually provided good care, or whether they exhibited a pattern of problems. If the latter, plaintiffs should have an opportunity to take the health plan into state courts. On the other hand, if this patient's poor care was an aberration in otherwise flawless medical careers for these two physicians, then plaintiffs have little tort case against the health plan. Challenges to the physicians' expertise will raise familiar malpractice factual questions, such as whether these physicians knew what signs and symptoms indicate brain tumors; how carefully they examined this patient and with what frequency; what sorts of diagnostic evaluations are appropriate, and in what sequence, for the work-up of chronic severe headache; and the like.

Since ERISA preemption is the prize for plans and sometimes for providers, and since preemption is only awarded when resource denials are at stake, the more interesting factual questions will focus on whether a resource was in fact denied and, if so, who issued the denial.[89] Those questions, in turn, can only be answered by examining the specific financial structures of the plan to discern who controlled what and who owed which resource duties to the patient.[90]

As noted, courts have little trouble preempting health plans' overt, FFS-style resource denials. Their confusions mainly arise when physicians are the ones making the resource decisions. Hence, some of the most challenging factual questions in this realm will focus on whether the physician actually controlled resources or merely implemented plans' decisions. As outlined in Chapter 6, in some instances physicians have virtually no control while in other situations they have complete personal authority to decide which patients will receive which tests and treatments. Physician–level capitation is usually a paradigm example of the latter, as the physician receives a fixed monthly sum that he can use as he sees fit to provide an array of designated services to his own panel of patients.[91] Depending on the exact financial arrangements, the physician can potentially serve as an ERISA fiduciary, that is, as the one who has the authority and discretion to make the particular resource decision in question. More will be said below regarding fiduciaries.[92]

In *Lancaster,* the court provides insufficient information to determine whether Drs. Campbell and Pauls actually had control over the testing and consulting resources they failed to order for the patient. We do know that the two physicians were under financial incentives, but it is not clear whether they were the kind that convey real control, or whether the incentives were merely rewards to encourage physicians to follow the plan's utilization rules and refrain from "gaming the system."

Even when it is established that a physician is fully authorized to control certain resources, it does not follow from this that every decision that physician makes is a resource decision. Most medical care is simply a matter of seeing that the patient needs (or doesn't need) certain interventions and then providing them (or not). In many of the instances where a physician failed to use a test or treatment he should have used, the failure is simply an expertise problem. He did not know that he should use it, or did not realize that it should be used now rather than later, or was unaware that it is highly beneficial and carries low risk.

Other cases, however, involve resource decisions. The physician knows quite well that a given intervention might be of some medical value but consciously refrains from using it because it is expensive; or he decides that the intervention is "experimental" and thus not covered by the patient's plan or his own provider–contract with the plan; or he decides that another intervention is almost as good and much cheaper; or he believes that the benefit of the test or treatment is too small or unlikely to justify its cost. These are resource decisions.

Although the expertise cases can be distinguished in theory from resource cases, a formidable practical issue looms. The court must be able to determine, in any given case, whether the physician was actually moved by resource concerns or only by medical considerations. The difference is important because, once again, in ERISA cases the ordinary malpractice of medical oversights belongs in state courts while resource denials are preempted to federal courts. If the two kinds of cases must be addressed so differently, then we need a workable way to distinguish between them. The problem is, physicians' reasoning and inner thought processes are open only to themselves. Note, although this discussion focuses on physicians, similar questions—and similar answers—also apply to health plans, since they too make expertise as well as resource decisions.

The first, most obvious answer is to recognise that juries routinely address difficult factual questions like this. Actors' intentions are important at a number of junctures throughout criminal and civil law. While in any given case there can always be lingering doubts, nevertheless certain sorts of evidence would obviously be relevant in cases like these. Some situations are clearly a straightforward malpractice problem, as when a surgeon reads an X-ray backwards and removes the wrong kidney, or where a nurse practitioner punctures a tympanic membrane. These cannot possibly be explained as a resource decision. In other cases certain kinds of evidence can settle the question fairly readily. If the physician has actually written a note in the chart explaining his resource concerns or if witnesses heard him speak about resource reasons for denying this particular test or treatment, such evidence could reasonably lead a jury to believe that the decision was substantially based on resource considerations. If it is also established that this physician was functioning as a bona fide ERISA fiduciary with respect to this particular decision, then one can plausibly conclude that the physician's decision was in fact a benefit decision governed by ERISA.

Shy of such concrete evidence, however, one is asking jurors to read the physician's mind, to determine what he knew and what he thought. With so much at stake for the plaintiff—a broad array of state-based claims and remedies versus a minimal set of federal remedies—one might like to have greater clarity. Accordingly, a preferable approach would be to create a default. When a physician controls resources as an ERISA fiduciary, his failure to use a test or treatment that might have been helpful to a patient should be regarded as potential malpractice issue in the absence of explicit evidence to the contrary. Otherwise stated, only if the physician has specifically and concretely indicated that he considered using that test or treatment, and then relied on a resource rationale for declining to use it, would the court regard the decision as an ERISA fiduciary's resource decision. Such evidence might be a note in the chart, a witnessed statement, or some other clearly documented indication. Absent such clarity, the case would be addressed under ordinary state malpractice law.

Some doubts might be raised about this default approach. For instance, it might be supposed that physicians will be unlikely to admit openly that they are denying resources for financial reasons, even for the ostensibly meritorious purpose of shepherding resources for the benefit of all the patients in their panel. Despite widespread agreement about the need to contain health care costs, it is still rare to hear health plans or providers say they denied an intervention to save money. They are far more likely to support their policies and decisions with ostensibly medical reasoning, such as the treatment's lack of scientific evidence or its potential harms.[93]

In fact, however, physicians who act as ERISA fiduciaries would have a powerful incentive to be up-front any time they make a resource–based denial of care. After all, resource denials are preempted to federal courts with their milder federal sanctions, and the physician–fiduciary who has been forthright about resource rationales is spared the travails of tort litigation. To be sure, even federal courts will scrutinize whatever medical judgments went into the resource decision. But there the standard is much different. As discussed in the next section,[94] courts tend to be very deferential to fiduciaries' decisions.[95] Only if a denial of benefits is arbitrary and capricious or an abuse of discretion are courts likely to overturn the fiduciary's decision.[96] And if they do, the consequence is merely that the treatment or its financial equivalent must be provided. Accordingly, the physician who controls resources has a strong incentive to write an honest note in the chart when he relies on resource considerations to make his decision.

Yet another factor encourages caution in this setting. The very same financial risk that gives these physicians resource control tends to place them in conflicts of interest.[97] When ERISA fiduciaries are in conflicts of interest, courts are less deferential to their decisions. That is, they are more likely to award the treatment or payment the plaintiff requests, making it more difficult for the physician to curb the costs of providing care by denying interventions he deems inappropriate or unnecessary. Conflicted fiduciaries can prevail, but they must be able to justify their resource decisions in terms of overall benefits to the members of the plan. Accordingly, these physician–fiduciaries would have a strong incentive to ensure that their documented resource rationale in any given case reflects careful thought about the broader needs of the other patients in the plan.

C. FIXING THE PROBLEMS: ERISA AND RESOURCE ISSUES

It should be obvious from the foregoing that courts could make an enormous improvement in the currently confused body of ERISA case law by replacing the *Dukes* quality–quantity distinction with the expertise–resources distinction. To begin with, the concepts of expertise and resources are considerably clearer and more straightforwardly, consistently applicable than fuzzy notions like quality. Second, the expertise–resources approach preserves the statute's objective of shielding employers from extraneous requirements to provide or expand their level of benefits. That protection disappears when courts mistakenly place resource issues under the rubric of "quality" and remand them to state courts, thereby potentially forcing employers to augment their benefit plans in ways they had not intended. This result, as noted, is expressly contrary to ERISA. Third, the improved distinction still permits a wide range of claims to proceed to state courts. By acknowledging that health plans as well as physicians can commit errors of expertise, this distinction may in some instances grant plaintiffs greater access to state-based remedies than does the *Dukes* distinction.

The problems of ERISA are not resolved yet, however, because ERISA still manages breaches of resource duty in federal courts. This poses two major differences from non-ERISA health plans, both of which often work to employees' disadvantage and thereby require further scrutiny.

First, ERISA beneficiaries have a narrow legal standard by which to challenge a denial of resources to which they believe they are entitled. By federal statute and by case law, the standard of review in ERISA cases is highly deferential to health plan administrators. ERISA provides that so long as an ERISA fiduciary's benefits decisions are not arbitrary and capricious or an abuse of discretion, they should generally be enforced even when the decision may not be the most reasonable interpretation of the plan.[98] This principle limits a court's ability to issue an injunction mandating coverage or to require the plan to pay for benefits already received.[99]

Second, when it is determined that a denial of benefits was wrong, even injuriously wrong, as when delay or denial of benefits causes significant harm, ERISA offers fewer causes of action and much smaller damages than state-based laws. As noted above, ERISA permits a cause of action only "to recover benefits due . . . under the terms of [the] plan, to enforce . . . rights under the terms of the plan, or to clarify . . . rights to future benefits under the terms of the plan."[100] In contrast, states' tort laws permit wide causes of action and generous damages. Even states' contract laws afford more generous remedies than does ERISA, because state-based breach of contract claims typically permit expectation damages and fairly generous consequential damages for further harms caused by the breach of contract. ERISA has been criticized on both these dimensions.

1. ERISA and the Standard of Review

ERISA plans are typically administered by a fiduciary who, by statutory definition, has discretion in making claims decisions, determining eligibility, and the like. These fiduciaries, like traditional trustees,[101] are responsible to administer the plan "solely in the interest of the participants and beneficiaries"[102] and can be personally liable to make up losses from any breach of this duty.[103] Therefore, courts grant fiduciaries considerable deference[104] and overturn their decisions only if the fiduciary has been arbitrary and capricious.[105]

Two developments have loosened this deference, increasing courts' willingness to overturn ERISA plans' denials of benefits. The first resembles the "judge-made insurance" discussed in Chapter 4. When faced with a desperate patient pleading for a treatment that may represent his or her only hope, courts have sometimes been quick to award benefits by declaring a denial of such a treatment to be arbitrary and capricious—sometimes even when the plan's contract language seems quite clearly to deny those benefits. In *Bailey v. Blue Cross/Blue Shield,*[106] for instance, a woman with advanced breast cancer sought high-dose chemotherapy with peripheral stem cell rescue (a form of bone marrow transplant). The insurer's policy language stated: "Autologous bone marrow transplants and other forms of stem cell rescue . . . with high dose chemotherapy and/or radiation . . . are not covered."[107] Although the policy listed some exceptions to this exclusion, it explicitly stated that breast cancer was not such an exception. Nevertheless, the court found this clause ambiguous.[108] A number of other courts have likewise been willing to overturn denials of benefits on grounds that they were arbitrary and capricious or an abuse of discretion.[109]

The second source of ERISA's loosening concerns fiduciaries with conflicts of interest. Technically, courts must still be deferential to ERISA fiduciaries even when they are in a conflict of interest, as, for instance, when the fiduciary is under financial incentives to save costs by limiting benefits. However, that deference is reduced in proportion to the seriousness of the conflict, thus opening a significant avenue for awarding benefits to patients. In *Brown v. Blue Cross & Blue Shield of Alabama* a patient who failed to obtain precertification was denied benefits. The Eleventh Circuit noted that "[b]ecause an insurance company pays out to beneficiaries from its own assets rather than the assets of a trust, its fiduciary role lies in perpetual conflict with its profit-making role as a business. . . . The inherent conflict between the fiduciary role and the profit-making objective of an insurance company makes a highly deferential standard of review inappropriate."[110] Here, too, a number of courts have happily embraced this leeway for awarding benefits to patients.[111]

Notwithstanding the need for latitude, courts must seek a delicate balance. Patients, who depend on their health plan, must have adequate avenues to challenge improper refusals of care. As pointed out in Chapter 9, health plans should be far clearer and more detailed about what they do and do not cover. And people should have considerably greater opportunity to choose among plans to achieve a personally satisfactory balance of benefits and costs. In the ERISA setting this is difficult to achieve, particularly in a self-funded plan in which the employer simply decides, unilaterally, what benefits workers will receive.

At the same time, health plans must be able to enforce legitimate limits for all the reasons discussed in Chapters 4 and 9. When courts award benefits that clearly go beyond a health plan's limits, they commit either of two kinds of error. Either they unfairly grant special favors to a select few individuals who thereby enjoy advantages not available to others in the plan;[112] or else, if such an individual award becomes generalized into a higher level of benefits for everyone, they raise the costs of that health plan in the future, thereby jeopardizing affordability and ultimately also access to care.[113] In so doing, courts also violate ERISA's express provision that no one may dictate the kinds or amounts of benefits that employers provide.

2. ERISA and Damage Awards

Probably the most controversial feature of ERISA is its refusal, even in cases when wrongful denials of resources have caused terrible harms, to award damages commensurate with the degree of harm or the degree of the health plan's culpability. A number of courts have expressed distress about leaving people with little or no remedy. "The Court is not unmindful this holding leaves plaintiff with no remedy under ERISA for the needless and tragic loss she has suffered. . . . Nevertheless, the Court must respect Congress' intent to have the civil enforcement mechanism of ERISA be the exclusive remedy for such claims."[114]

Nevertheless, the mainstream of U.S. Supreme Court and Circuit Court reasoning upholds ERISA's limits on damages. As the Supreme Court observed in *Massachusetts Mutual Life Ins. Co. v. Russell,* "The six carefully integrated civil enforcement provisions found in §502(a) of the statute as finally enacted . . . provide strong evidence that Congress did not intend to authorize other remedies that it simply forgot to incorporate expressly."[115] In *Mertens v. Hewitt Associates* the Court ruled that the "other appropriate equitable relief" afforded by ERISA does not authorize suits for money damages to compensate prevailing plaintiffs for money damages beyond the actual contractual benefits the defendant owed.[116]

However, several factors are currently at work to mitigate this apparent harshness. First, the *Dukes* line of cases is rapidly opening state-based tort causes of action, with their opportunities for collecting generous damages for "quality"-oriented claims against ERISA plans. As noted above, this book agrees with the basic move, although the appropriate distinction on which to base it is not quality–quantity, but rather expertise–resources.

Second, traditional damage limits are now being questioned even within ERISA-governed cases. In *Haywood v. Russell Corp.* the Alabama Supreme Court argued that federal courts can authorize damages beyond those expressly included in the ERISA statute. According to the *Haywood* court, "Congress intended for the courts to develop a federal common law with respect to employee benefit plans, including the development of appropriate remedies, even if they are not specifically enumerated in Section 502 of ERISA."[117] Those remedies could include "(but certainly [are] not limited to) the imposition of punitive damages on the person responsible for the failure to pay claims in a timely manner."[118]

The Supreme Court may have left the door ajar for expanding damages. The

Mertens case cited above was voted 5–4, and two of the majority justices are no longer on the Court. In a vigorous dissent, Justices White, Rhenquist, Stevens, and O'Conner argued that ERISA can indeed be construed to permit compensatory monetary awards.[119] These dissenters hinted that, given the historical blending of courts of law with courts of equity, even punitive damages and other significant extra-contractual awards might not be beyond the pale.[120]

By the same token, in *Reid v. Gruntal & Co., Inc.,*[121] a federal district court opined that ERISA could award both expectation damages and reliance damages. As the court figured it, Congress based ERISA largely on the common law of trusts as it defined the scope of fiduciaries' duties. Trust law, in turn, permits claims of promissory estoppel that, in turn, permit such a broader range of damages. As the court argued, "[t]he Restatement (Second) of Trusts defines the remedies available under trust law as follows: 'If the trustee commits a breach of trust, the beneficiary may have the option of pursuing a remedy which will put him in the position in which he was before the trustee committed the breach of trust. . . .' "[122]

Somewhat analogously, in *Russell v. Northrop Grumman Corp.*[123] the Eastern District of New York held that equitable relief can include monetary damages so long as they are designed to restore the plaintiff to have " 'the very thing that [he or she] would have received but-for the defendant's illegal action'. . . ."[124] Likewise, in *Weems v. Jefferson-Pilot Life Ins. Co., Inc.,*[125] the Alabama Supreme Court was willing to conclude, on the basis of the U.S. Supreme Court's decision in *Ingersoll-Rand,*[126] that ERISA can permit compensatory and punitive damages. Nevertheless, the prevailing doctrine still precludes broader damages and the future of this issue remains to be seen.[127]

D. ERISA'S FUTURE

Because ERISA treats health plan beneficiaries less generously and sometimes also less fairly than subscribers of private plans, critics of ERISA promote either a legislative elimination of the statute or a major change in it. This book is not the place for extended discussion of such a complex topic, but a few observations are in order.

First, significant changes are already under way, even within ERISA. The *Dukes* avenue into tort claims is already broadening causes of action and thereby available damages, as noted above.

Second, it would not be surprising to find more courts exploring the currently tentative steps toward broader damage allowance, as introduced in *Haywood, Russell,* and *Weems.*

Third, aside from this common law evolution, Congress will probably continue to consider various proposals for legislative change. Some legislators would like to open ERISA health plans to the full panoply of state-based tort and contract litigation; others would like to introduce only limited expansion of remedies, such as to include specified extracontractual but not punitive damages; and others prefer to leave things as they are. Some states, in opening health plans to malpractice liability, have restricted cases to those in which the plaintiff has suffered substantial harm.[128] As this book goes to press, Congress has taken no action. Though the din of criticism grows increasingly harsh, it is interesting to note that Congress has not chosen to modify ERISA despite ample opportunity to do so over the years and despite ample case law evidencing the sometimes unfortunate outcomes for injured ERISA health care beneficiaries.

The reasons can only be speculated upon. An amendment that exposed health plans to malpractice litigation with huge punitive damage awards could potentially raise premium prices and subsequently reduce access to health care, to a point that would leave far more people uninsured than the current number of over forty million. Such a situation could spur a strong demand for some sort of national health care system, a scenario unlikely to be courted by a Congress that has declined, time after time, to institute universal access.

On a more philosophical note, it is, of course, debatable just what sort of changes, either in the statute itself or in its judicial interpretation, would be desirable. On one hand, a number of thoughtful scholars argue that the common law loosening of ERISA preemption is not only desirable, but a sound interpretation of the existing statute. Jacobson and Pomfret, for instance, doubt that Congress, in the process of enacting legislation designed to protect beneficiaries, actually intended to insulate those benefit plans from accountability. They propose that the only real criterion meriting preemption to federal courts is the question whether preemption in a given case "would result in a lack of uniformity that would prevent an employer from offering a chosen plan nationwide."[129] They thus promote a functional approach that would have courts look not just at statutory language, but also at the fairness of the results produced by preemption.[130]

It is not difficult to find case law that appears to share this general orientation. After years of broadly interpreting ERISA, the U.S. Supreme Court narrowed the ambit of preemption in *New York Conference of Blue Cross & Blue Shield Plans v. Travelers Insurance Co.*[131] In its attempt to find funding for the medically uninsured, the state of New York imposed surcharges on commercial health plans, but not on Blue Cross not-for-profit plans. Holding that the statute did not violate ERISA even though it did indirectly raise the costs of ERISA plans and indirectly make Blue Cross plans more attractive, the Court pointed out that "the New York law neither (1) 'mandated employee benefit structures or their administration,' nor (2) provided 'alternative enforcement mechanisms' for ERISA remedies, nor (3) produced such acute, albeit indirect, economic effects . . . as to force an ERISA plan to adopt a certain scheme of substantive coverage or effectively restrict its choice of insurers.' "[132] As the Court noted, Congress meant to insulate ERISA plans from conflicting directives, not to preclude every possible event that might raise the cost of an ERISA plan or pose an economic influence to administrative decisions.[133] "The basic thrust of the pre-emption clause was to avoid a multiplicity of regulation in order to permit the nationally uniform administration of employee benefit plans. Thus, ERISA pre-empts state laws that mandate employee benefit structures or their administration as well as those that provide alternate enforcement mechanisms."[134]

In the same spirit, the Ninth Circuit emphasized in *Parrino v. FHP, Inc.*[135] that the key purpose of ERISA is to establish a uniform body of federal law to govern benefit plans. Similarly, a Michigan court pointed out that the "[p]urpose of ERISA is to ensure that plans and plan sponsors are subject to a uniform body of benefits law, to minimize administrative and financial burden of complying with conflicting directives among states or between states and federal government, and to prevent potential for conflict in substantive law requiring tailoring of plans and employer conduct to peculiarities of each jurisdiction."[136]

On the other side, however, it can be argued that such uniformity has a crucial further purpose. ERISA was not enacted simply to promote uniformity—tidiness—for its own sake. Rather, that uniformity is instrumental toward more important goals. ERISA's provisions for gathering all benefit plans under a single set of federal laws aims to ensure not just that benefit plans like pensions and health care can be administered with relative ease, but also that they remain reasonably affordable, so that employers will choose to offer them in the first place and to continue them over time.[137] *Holmes v. Pacific Mut. Life Ins. Co.*[138] points out that at the time it enacted ERISA, "Congress was concerned that the Social Security system, itself strained by the increasing demands made on it by retired workers, could not be relied upon to provide adequate retirement benefits for the vast majority of covered workers.[139] Congress thus wanted to make sure that employers, rather than the federal government, would predominantly provide for workers' retirement. The court continues: "By 'taking] into account additional costs from the standpoint of the employer', Congress indicated that one of the prime purposes of ERISA was to encourage the private sector to bear a larger share of the responsibility for establishing and maintaining a consistent employee benefit structure. . . . To maintain the desired degree of certainty in payment of plan benefits, it is critical that the actuarial assumptions, upon which the minimum funding calculations are based, be preserved through time. It is for this reason that ERISA preemption, which shields ERISA employee benefit plans from unforeseen liabilities, *including liability arising from the acts of the plan administrators,* is critical to the entire statutory scheme."[140]

More importantly, the Supreme Court held in the seminal case of *Pilot Life Ins. Co v. Dedeaux*[141] that

> the detailed provisions of §502(a) set forth a comprehensive civil enforcement scheme that represents a careful balancing of the need for prompt and fair claims settlement procedures against the public interest in *encouraging the formation of employee benefit plans.* The policy choices reflected in the inclusion of certain remedies and the exclusion of others under the federal scheme would be completely undermined if ERISA-plan participants and beneficiaries were free to obtain remedies under state law that Congress rejected in ERISA. 'The six carefully integrated civil enforcement provisions found in §502(a) of the statute as finally enacted . . . provide strong evidence that Congress did not intend to authorize other remedies that it simply forgot to incorporate expressly.'[142]

The Court enhanced the message in *Varity v. Howe,* by noting "competing congressional purposes, such as Congress' desire to offer employees enhanced protection for their benefits, on the one hand, and, on the other, its desire not to create a system that is so complex that administrative costs, *or litigation expenses,* unduly discourage employers from offering welfare benefit plans in the first place."[143]

The Seventh Circuit echoed the theme. "When setting and changing the terms of a plan, the employer may act to promote its own interests, just as it may do when setting wages. In the short run use of this power may injure retirees; but in the longer run, knowledge that plans may be changed encourages employers to make better offers to their labor force. If employers knew that they were locked in, they would be more conservative in making promises, to the potential detriment of the workers."[144]

In like manner, in *Gable v. Sweetheart Cup Co.* the Fourth Circuit emphasized that Congress meant to preserve the affordability, and thereby protect the availability, of benefits plans. Emphasizing that an employer has a statutory right to terminate or modify its unvested benefits, the court went on:

> We recognize the real hardship that changes in employee benefit plans can visit upon individuals who have worked many years for a company. The enactment of ERISA, however, required Congress to strike a difficult balance between employee rights and available employer resources. In passing ERISA, Congress determined that requiring employers to provide vested employee welfare benefits 'would seriously complicate the administration and increase the cost of plans whose primary function is to provide retirement income.' . . . Were we to hold that the company was nonetheless bound by the original terms of the plan and prohibited from making any amendments, we would strip employers of the protection that Congress intended to provide them and accordingly 'discourage employers from offering any insurance at all.'[145]

Clearly, employers' statutory right to change benefits at any time[146] is not an attempt to promote uniformity. It is an attempt to encourage employers to provide benefits as best they can, even to change or reduce them, if that means they can thereby continue to offer them. A unanimous Supreme Court emphasized this point in *Inter-modal Rail v. Atchison, Topeka & Santa Fe Ry.*

> The flexibility an employer enjoys to amend or eliminate its welfare plan is not an accident; Congress recognized that 'requir[ing] the vesting of these ancillary benefits would seriously complicate the administration and increase the cost of plans.' . . . *Giving employers this flexibility also encourages them to offer more generous benefits at the outset, since they are free to reduce benefits should economic conditions sour. If employers were locked into the plans they initially offered, 'they would err initially on the side of omission.'*[147]

Interestingly, the 1997 *Inter-modal Rail* decision and the 1996 *Varity* decision were issued after, not before, *Travelers* was issued in 1995. Thus, if *Travelers* aimed to loosen the preemption in the name of uniformity, *Inter-modal Rail* reminds us that ERISA's interest in uniformity is not to promote tidiness for tidiness' sake. Its ultimate purpose is affordability of benefits plans alongside fairness and reliability in their implementation. Indeed, even *Travelers* carried a caveat on its permission to raise indirect costs for ERISA plans: indirect economic effects must not be so great that they "force an ERISA plan to adopt a certain scheme of substantive coverage or effectively restrict its choice of insurers."[148]

In the final analysis, some sort of compromise seems appropriate. On the one hand, patients who are grievously harmed when their MCO wrongly fails to provide resources surely need better compensation than the bare cost of the denied treatments. The injustices have become too enormous and too obvious to ignore. On the other hand, it would be seriously harmful, from a broader social standpoint, to take actions that could expose health plans to the sometimes exorbitant, often arbitrary damage awards that have plagued physicians in the malpractice arena for many years.

A middle ground might best be found in two moves, one of which is already under way. First, as argued above, the separation of expertise from resource issues provides a legitimate avenue into state-based tort litigation, albeit only for breaches of expertise duties. Second, if ERISA's federal remedies were broadened to cover the full panoply of expectation damages, like state-based contract remedies,[149] then even in cases involving no torts, injured patients would not be left to bear the financial burdens of their MCOs' mistakes. Health plans would potentially face larger damage payouts, but not the enormity and unpredictability of punitive damages.

12

REFLECTIONS

I am a member of the Baby Boom generation. We came of age in the '60s and '70s, and it was an extraordinary time to grow up. Virtually everyone our age or older remembers precisely what we were doing on November 22, 1963, at about one o'clock in the afternoon Central Standard Time. From that moment, the assassination of the nation's thirty-fifth President, and continuing for barely more than a decade, the country went through a period of social turbulence whose equal would be hard to find:

- the civil rights struggle, with its sit-ins, boycotts, marches, burnings, attack dogs, church bombings, murders, lynchings, Black Panthers, and inner-city riots;
- two more assassinations, from a beloved civil rights leader to the brother of the fallen President, and an attempt to slay a Southern governor whose old-time segregationist message made him, even then, an odd sort to be running for President;[1]
- the Vietnam War, with its own brand of sit-ins, boycotts, marches, draft card burning, draft-dodging, and violence, including the killing of four students at Kent State University;
- women's liberation and the quest for gender equality alongside the quest for racial equality;
- free love, drugs, and rock'n'roll, from hippies to Woodstock;

- the Watergate scandal, from dirty tricks, buggings, and break-ins, to coverups and Congressional hearings, culminating in the resignation of Richard Nixon in August of 1974.

During that brief decade, from the assassination of one President to the abdication of another, the nation rewrote many of its social rules. Those who presumed themselves ordained to rule, whether by gender or by race or by nationality, suddenly found their world far more complex than they ever envisioned it could be. The changes have been profound and pervasive, and we still have not quite sorted everything out.

In its own way, the world of health care is amidst a transition nearly as profound, even if less dramatic and, on the whole, less deadly. Here, too, values at the very core of our beliefs—values about what health care ought to do, and how, and for whom—are being upended. We have gone from a time in which costs were essentially irrelevant, to a time in which virtually everything must pass some test of cost-worthiness.[2]

The transition is painful because we are looking back on an era—an era lasting only a few decades, really—in which resources were virtually limitless, and resource ethics were easy. With a few exceptions for burdensome excesses at the end of life and for vulgar exploitation promoting pointless invasions to enrich providers, it was an open-handed ethic that said we can always do more, we can always try harder, and if our efforts (and our expenditures) come to naught, at least we gave it our best shot.[3] Nearly all our medical research was devoted to developing spectacular new drugs, devices, and procedures. Anything dubbed "safe and effective" became ipso facto "necessary" and assured of third-party payment, thereby further fueling the furnaces of research and the coffers of providers everywhere.

To have gone on for so long as we did, believing that there never would be or should be any need to draw limits, will undoubtedly mystify and probably amuse future observers. But as for us, here and now, we need to acknowledge that those days are gone. We need to find new ways to define health and health care, and to decide what our health plans and providers owe to us and what we owe to each other as citizens helping one another to meet basic needs.

On a radically different and constantly evolving economic infrastructure, we are rewriting virtually all of health care from the ground up, largely without a road map. Whereas research focused for so long on wondrous new toys and dramatic saves, suddenly providers are expected to prove the worth of their most routine care. The expectation is probably a good idea, at least up to a point, because so much of ordinary medicine has been founded on clinical anecdotes and local habits, not on science. But that expectation is also nearly impossible to meet, at least for the present. The right kind of research doesn't exist. Not yet, anyway. Not enough of it. Still, we are learning, in bits and pieces, that medical routines previously considered mandatory are not so sacred after all. What was once minimal may now seem excessive. What was once considered outrageous, like sending patients home with indwelling intravenous lines, is now routine. "Standard of care" has become a fast-moving, multidirectional mythical target.

We are also reorganizing very basic relationships and power structures. Physicians can no longer order whatever tests and treatments they want, simply on the basis of their clinical judgment; patients can no longer demand whatever care they want; and payers will no longer write a check just because someone asks them to.

In the process, we are rewriting our moral road map, at least as it concerns health care. As the eighteenth century philosopher David Hume pointed out, it is not until we meet scarcity that we find a need for justice.[4] As we are painfully discovering, the values that were so obviously right in a period of limitless resources simply do not fit the realities of our emerging scarcity. When money flowed from an artesian well there were no opportunity costs to pay after a choice to do this for one person and that for another, because no matter how much money we spent, there was always more. But now there is a cap on the well with a meter attached to it. We still draw plenty from that well, and our allotment still has a fair amount of flexibility, but we must justify how much we use, and we must explain why we used our resources this way rather than that.

It is no wonder, then, that we also need to rewrite our legal road map. The law, after all, embodies our deepest, most important shared social values. As a body of doctrine that emerges partly from politically charged processes of legislation, but especially from the evolution of jurists' thinking in the common law, medical law has been, so to speak, "marching with medicine, but in the rear and limping a little."[5] For the most part, it is probably just as well that law does not change as fast as medical science. Medicine looks to what is promising, while law must focus on what is abiding. And yet our legal doctrines must stay reasonably in step with the world around them lest they become irrelevant, or worse, detrimental to justice as it resolves the difficult conflicts among human beings, their aims and actions, and the scarcities within which we must try to find a harmony. This book has proposed one way in which that task might be accomplished.

NOTES

CHAPTER 1

1. "The frequency of claims filed against physicians between 1970 and 1975 increased 42%, and the average damage award increased from $12,993 in 1970 to $34,297 in 1975, with medical malpractice insurance premiums for physicians rising 410% during the same period." Kinney, Gronfein 1991, at 171 n. 16. "The key characteristics of claims affecting the availability and affordability of medical malpractice insurance are their frequency and their severity (that is, their size in dollar terms). Increases in claim frequency and severity helped trigger the two malpractice crises of the 1970s and 1980s." *Id.*, at 176.

See also Danzon, 1985; Bovbjerg, 1989; Wadlington, 1991; Gronfein, Kinney, 1991; Horwitz, Brennan, 1995; Reynolds, Rizzo, Gonzalez, 1987; Robinson, 1986(b); Morlock, Malitz, 1991, at 4; Posner, 1986, at 37–38; Bovbjerg, Schumm, 1998, at 1052–58.

2. "On an aggregate basis, there was one malpractice tort claim filed by patients for every 7.5 negligently inflicted injuries. Because about one in two patient claims is ultimately paid, this means that the tort litigation/insurance system paid one claim for every 15 tort incidents." Weiler, Newhouse, Hiatt, 1992, at 2355.

"Many more incidents of malpractice occur . . . than result in a claim for damages. Records of patients discharged from two hospitals during 1972 revealed a large number of severe injuries resulting from malpractice; of these, only one in every 15 led to malpractice claims." Schwartz, Komesar, 1978, at 1286.

In commenting on a new study, Orentlicher notes: "Eighteen years after landmark California data and 8 years after equally important New York data, malpractice occurrence and malpractice claims data from Colorado and Utah in 1992 paint essentially the same picture as the earlier results: a small percentage of injured patients actually sue, and when claims are brought, a high percentage of them do not involve malpractice. In other words, the tort system includes many false-positives (patients who sue in the absence of negligence) and even more false-negatives (patients who do not sue despite having been harmed by negligence). As a result, the law often subjects the wrong physicians to legal process, it generally does not hold physicians accountable for their negligence, and it fails to ensure adequate compensation for injured patients." Orentlicher, 2000, at 247 (citing Studdert, Thomas, Burstin, et al. 2000).

See also Localio, Lawthers, Brennan TA, et al., 1991; Brennan, Colin, Burstin, 1996; Brennan, Leape, Laird, et al., 1991; Leape, Brennan, Laird, et al., 1991; Danzon, 1985, at 23–25.

3. For further discussion, see Morreim, 1991(a).

4. Blumenthal, 1999, at 1916.

5. Blumenthal, 1999, at 1917.

6. Morreim, 1994(a).

7. Butler, Haislmaier, 1989.

8. Morreim, 1994(a), at 80.

9. Morreim, 1994(a), at 81–82.

As Havighurst observes: "Although the medical profession's advocacy of quality in medical care without regard to cost appeared to reflect a sincere concern for patient welfare, it also served providers' economic interests. Not only did the suppression of normal economizing impulses pave the way for expansive and demand-increasing definitions of the need for providers' own services, but it also allowed providers to set their fees and charges on a noncompetitive and therefore highly lucrative basis." Havighurst 1986(a), at 151.

10. Axelroth v. Health Partners of Alabama, 720 So.2d 880 (Ala. 1998).

11. Hardwig, 1987.

12. As an example, even the best screening protocols for preventive interventions such as mammography, will inevitably produce at least a few instances in which someone's latent illness is not detected and which might have been detected if the screening protocol had spent more money to be more thorough. When courts face the lone individual whose cancer was not detected, however, they have a tendency to focus on that individual to the neglect of health plans' need (and the need of all the other members in that plan) to enforce reasonable resource policies. See Leahy, 1989, at 1520–21; Eddy, 1993(a).

13. Employee Retirement Income Security Act, 29 U.S.C. §§ 1001–1461. For a more detailed discussion of ERISA, see Chapter 11.

14. Corcoran v. United Healthcare, Inc., 965 F2d 1321 (5th Cir 1992), cert denied 113 S.Ct. 812 (1992).

15. Furrow, Johnson, Jost, Schwartz, 1997, at 92–110; Baker, 1992.

16. Ginzberg, 1987, at 1152; Furrow, 1994, at 407.

CHAPTER 2

1. Keeton, Dobbs, Keeton, et al. 1984.

2. See Morreim, 1987; Morreim, 1992(a); Morreim, 1989; Morreim, 1985–86; see also Havighurst, 1995, at 268–70.

3. "Generally, the standard of care for a physician is one established by the profession itself." Spensieri v. Lasky, 723 N.E.2d 544, 548 (N.Y. 1999) (citing: Toth v. Community Hosp, 239 N.E.368 (N.Y. 1968)).

4. The physician must "have and use the knowledge, skill and care ordinarily possessed and employed by members of the profession in good standing." Keeton, Dobbs, Keeton, et al. 1984, at 187. See also Holder, 1978, at 43–45; Marsh, 1985, at 160, 172; McCoid, 1959, at 558–59, 605–14; Pearson, 1976, at 528; Robinson, 1986(a), at 173; Siciliano, 1991, at 447; Note, 1985, at 1008; Johnson, 1970, at 741–42; Henderson, Siliciano, 1994, at 1384–89; Frankel, 1994, at 1315; King, 1975, at 1234–36; Havighurst 1986(b), at 266–67.

See also Clark v. United States, 402 F.2d 950, 952 (4th Cir. 1968); Kingston v. McGrath, 232 F.2d 495, 498 (9th. Cir. 1956); Becker v. Janinski, 15 N.Y.S. 675, 676 (1891); Pike v. Honsinger, 155 N.Y. 201, 49 N.E. 760 (1898).

5. Wilkinson v. Vesey, 295 A.2d 676 (R.I. 1972); Clark v. United States, 402 F.2d 950 (1968); Kingston v. McGrath, 232 F.2d 495 (Idaho 1956); Peterson v. Hunt, 84 P.2d 999 (Wash. 1938); Price v. Neyland, 320 F.2d 674 (D.C. 1963); Smith v. Yohe, 194 A.2d 167 (Pa. 1963); Coleman v. Wilson, 85 N.J.L. 383 (N.J. 1913); Ramberg v. Morgan, 218 N.W. 492 (Iowa 1928); Hicks v. United States, 368 F.2d 626 (1966); McCoid, 1959, at 575–577; Mehlman, 1985, at 287 (discussing Blake v. District of Columbia).

6. Siciliano, 1991, at 463. See also Henderson, Silician, 1994, at 1396–97.

7. "Malpractice doctrine's focus on usual and customary practice reflects the belief that there is a 'best way' to practice medicine, one that is supported by a professional and scientific consensus. Courts allow few exceptions to this unitary standard of care. . . . Although the courts never say so directly, this duty of care embodied in malpractice doctrine seems to obligate physicians to make

their medical decisions without regard to the cost (or cost-effectiveness) of the treatments or tests they are prescribing. Once a physician accepts a patient for treatment . . . she becomes the patient's fiduciary. She may not vary the kind or degree of care she provides because of her patient's financial status." Frankel, 1994, at 1315–16.

See also Havighurst, 1986: 49: 143–72, at 143, 149; Hershey, 1986, at 61–62; King, 1975, at 1234; Stone, 1985, at 310; Note, 1985, at 1010.

8. Buttersworth v. Swint, 186 S.E. 770 (1936); Childers v. Frye, 158 S.E. 744 (N.C. 1931); Becker v. Janinski, 15 N.Y.S. 675 (1891); Holder, at 1–3, 372; Curran, Moseley, 1975, at 78.

9. Becker v. Janinski, 15 N.Y.S. 675, 677 (1891); see also Tunkl v. Regents of Univ. Of Calif., 60 Cal. 2D 92, 103, 383 P.2d 441, 448 32 Cal. Rptr. 33, 40, (1963).

10. Tunkl v. Regents of Univ. of Cal., 383 P.2d 411, 448 (Cal. 1963).

11. Marsh, 1985, at 170. See also Clark v. United States, 402 F.2d 950, 953 (4th Cir. 1968); Kingston v. McGrath, 232 F.2d 495, 499 (9th. Cir. 1956); Smith v. Yohe, 412 Pa. 94, 105, 194 A.2d 167, 173 (1963); Wilkinson v. Vesey, 110 R.I. 606, 615–16, 295 A.2d 676, 683 (1972); Holder, 1978, at 77; Furrow, 1982, at 12.

12. Becker v. Janinski, 15 N.Y.S. 675, 677 (1891); Ricks v. Budge, 91 Utah 307, 314–16, 64 P.2d 208, 211–13 (1937); Meiselman v. Crown Heights Hospital, 34 N.E.2d 367 (N.Y. 1941) (the patient's refusal to pay is not a defense to abandonment). See also Holder, 1978, at 126, 373; Wadlington, Waltz, Dworkin, 1980, at 470–73; Marsh, 1985, at 165, 178–85; Crothers, 1974, at 938.

13. A case of this sort, Black v. District of Columbia, No. 2623–80 (D.C. Super. Ct. June 30, 1981), is discussed in Mehlman, 1985, at 287.

On some views, any form of nontreatment or inadequate treatment based on nonmedical considerations such as cost could constitute a form of abandonment. See Becker v. Janinski, 15 N.Y.S. 675 (1891); Ricks v. Budge, 91 Utah 307, 64 P.2d 208 (1937); Holder, 1978, at 378; Marsh, 1985, at 179; Crothers, 1974, at 938.

14. Small v. Howard, 128 Mass. 131, 135 (1880); Pike v. Honsinger, 155 N;.Y. 201, 209–10, 49 N.E. 760, 762 (1898); Becker v. Janinski, 15 N.Y.S. 675, 676 (1891).

15. Siliciano, 1991, at 441. Siliciano goes on to note: "The vast burgeoning of medical technology, the rapid inflation of medical costs, and the rise of defensive medicine during the last quarter century have greatly increased the costs of what is considered to be legally adequate care" (at 456).

Similarly, Frankel notes that "[t]ort doctrine holds medical providers to a certain standard of care, and the actions and interventions that the law requires are set without regard to cost. . . . Efforts to contain medical costs by forcing physicians to alter their practices to take account of economic concerns cut directly across the grain of this ideal. Plans for cost containment thus risk direct collision with the tort system." Frankel, 1994, at 1302. See also Morreim, 1989, at 358 (discussing abandonment doctrine and the pressures to ignore costs).

16. Muse v. Charter Hospital, Inc., 452 S.E.2d 589 (N.C. Ct. App.), aff'd, 464 S.E.2d 44 (N.C. 1995).

17. Muse v. Charter Hospital, Inc., 452 S.E.2d 589, 594 (N.C. Ct. App.), aff'd, 464 S.E.2d 44 (N.C. 1995).

18. In a lone dissent, Judge Orr acknowledged that:

> [there was] evidence that defendant hospital had a policy or practice of discharging patients when their insurance ran out. This practice was obviously done for a business purpose; however, the evidence reveals that the policy was subject to being overridden on occasion by request of the treating physician or other financial consideration. . . .
>
> Dr. Barnhill testified that the policy did not influence his decision, and more importantly, that a range of treatment options including a state psychiatric hospital were available for the patient. No evidence was presented that could lead a jury to conclude that the policy in question involved a deliberate purpose not to discharge some duty necessary to the safety of the person in question. While it can be said that the policy to discharge was deliberate, there is no evidence that the hospital expected, anticipated or intended for the patient to be released in circumstances that put the person's safety in jeopardy.

Muse, 452 S.E.2d at 600 (Orr, J., dissenting).

19. Wickline v. State of California, 192 Cal. App. 3d 1630, 1645 (1987) (dicta).

20. "We must remember that doctors, not insurance executives, are qualified experts in determining what is the best course of treatment and therapy for their patients. Trained physicians, and them [sic] alone, should be allowed to make care-related decisions (with, of course, input from the patient). Medical care should not be subject to the whim of the new layer of insurance bureaucracy

now dictating the most basic, as well as the important, medical policies and procedures from the boardroom." Herdrich v. Pegram, 154 F.3d 362, 377 (7th Cir. 1998), rev'd, 120 U.S. 2143 (2000).

See also Pappas v. Asbel, 675 A.2d 711, 716 (Pa.Super. 1996): "Considerations of cost containment of the type which drive the decision making process in HMO's did not exist for employee welfare plans when ERISA was enacted. It cannot therefore be argued that the type of recovery sought here was deliberately excluded from the Congressional schema in order to protect ERISA plans from conflicting directives which would, in attempting to control expenses, affect medical judgments." In other words, medical judgments ought to prevail over health plans' cost concerns. Aff'd, Pappas v. Asbel, 724 A.2d 889 (Pa. 1998), vacated, 120 S.Ct. 2686.

See also Mt. Sinai Hospital v. Zorek, 271 NYS2d 1012, 1016 (NY Civ Ct 1966): "Only the treating physician can determine what the appropriate treatment should be for any given condition. Any other standard would involve intolerable second-guessing, with every case calling for a crotchety Doctor Gillespie to peer over the shoulders of a supposedly unseasoned Doctor Kildare. The diagnosis and treatment of a patient are matters peculiarly within the competence of the treating physician. The diagnosis may be insightful and brilliant, or it may be wide of the mark, but right or wrong, the patient under his doctor's guidance proceeds upon his theories and sustains expenses therefor. . . . The doctor who orders hospital confinement for the removal of a simple splinter or the lancing of a boil has almost certainly exceeded the bounds of proper medical judgment in providing for his patient. . . . Once the treating doctor has decided on a course of treatment for which hospitalization is necessary, his judgment cannot be retrospectively challenged."

Finally, a classic statement comes from Clark v. United States: "If a physician, as an aid to diagnosis, . . . does not avail himself of the scientific means and facilities open to him for the collection of the *best* factual data upon which to arrive at his diagnosis, the result is not an error of judgment but negligence in failing to secure an adequate factual basis upon which to support his diagnosis or judgment." Clark v. United States, 402 F.2d 950, 953 (quoting Smith v. Yohe, 194 A.2d 167, 173 (Pa. 1963)).

21. Fuchs, 1984, at 1575; Thurow, 1985, at 611–12.

22. Kuttner, 1999, at 248.

23. See Morreim, 1987, at 1722; Morreim, 1992(a), at 161; Morreim, 1989, at 360; Morreim, 1985–86, at 1036; Morreim, 1991(c), at 288.

24. Personal communication, Dr. James Brown, medical director, The Regional Medical Center at Memphis (20, Jan. 1987).

25. See Morreim, 1987; Morreim, 1992(a); Morreim, 1989; Morreim, 1985–86.

26. Portions of the analysis in this section can be found in Morreim, 1997(a).

27. Miller, 1996; Lipson, De Sa, 1996, at 75.

28. See Morreim, 1994(a), at 80–81.

29. As of 1989, utilization review panels refused to authorize payment for proposed medical interventions only one to two percent of the time. See Institute of Medicine, 1989, at 77.

By 1999, one large FFS-based HMO, United Healthcare, announced that it would forego its more traditional utilization review in favor of a broad profiling of its physicians' practice habits, in large part because it denied so few requests that the system was not cost-effective. See Burton, 1999. Shortly thereafter, Aetna, the nation's largest health insurer, announced plans to move in the same direction. See Gentry, 1999.

Various commentators foreshadowed United's move. "Evidence suggests that the principal process of review, the case-by-case review, may not be cost-effective and may not be conducive to improving quality. . . . [T]he American College of Physicians recommends that routine case-by-case reviews be abandoned and replaced by profiling of patterns of care." American College of Physicians, 1994, at 423, 426. See also Kassirer, 1994. The question of whether this approach will successfuly contain costs remains to be answered, but it does represent an interesting shift from external management toward an essentially incentive-based approach—here not as direct cash incentives, but rather via the prospect that a high-cost physician might be deselected from the plan.

30. See Hall, 1994, at 34.

31. See Burnum, 1987, at 1221; Hardison, 1979, at 193; Reuben, 1984, at 592.

32. For further discussion of judge-made insurance, see Abraham, 1981, at 1155; Anderson, Hall, Steinberg, 1993, at 1636; Ferguson, Dubinsky, Kirsch, 1993, at 2116; Hall, Anderson, 1992, at 1655; Kalb, 1990, at 1118; Morreim, 1995(a), at 251.

33. See generally Brennan, 1991, at 67, 78.

34. See Farmer, 1993, at 316.

35. See Eichhorn, 1989, at 575–76; Eichhorn, Cooper, Cullen, et al., 1986; Goldsmith, 1992. For further discussion, see Allred, Tottenham, 1996, at 537.

36. See Ayres, 1994, at 154; Hafferty, Light, 1995, at 136; White, 1994, at 899; Woolf, 1993(a), at 2647; Stevens, 1993, at 73.

37. See Havighurst, 1995, at 117.

38. Direct limits are usually enforced through utilization management, while indirect limits are achieved by shifting financial risk to providers who, in turn, limit the care. "Managed care" can refer to widely varying arrangements in the financing and delivery of health care. However, a common description, articulated by Marc Rodwin, will be used here.

> Managed care refers to health insurance combined with . . . controls over the delivery of health services. Managed care organizations (MCOs) exercise control over the kind, volume, and manner in which services are provided by choosing providers, or by controlling their behavior through financial incentives, rules, and organizational controls. Under traditional indemnity insurance and fee-for-service medical practices, the insurers enter into a contract with the insured party and reimburse the individual for certain medical expenses that are incurred. The individual receives medical services from any provider he or she chooses and usually pays a fee for each service rendered, with the insurer having no control over the choice of provider or provision of services. Managed care changes this relationship either (1) by directly providing the contracted-for services; or (2) by exercising control over the services provided. . . . Many indemnity insurers now provide managed care in that they exercise control over their beneficiaries' use of medical services. They require pre-authorization for . . . expensive referrals or procedures. They do not reimburse claims from medical providers for services rendered if the organization decides they were not necessary.

Rodwin, 1996, at 1009.

The Texas Civil Practices and Remedies code defines a managed care entity as "any entity which delivers, administers, or assumes risk for health care services with systems or techniques to control or influence the quality, accessibility, utilization, or cost and prices of such services to a defined enrollee population" (TEXAS Civ. Prac & Rem. Code §§88.001(8)).

In this book, then, "managed care" will refer to any health plan that serves, not only to finance patients' access to health care, but to "manage" the care by determining, at least in some instances, that certain sorts of care will be preferred over others on medical or economic grounds or both. MCOs thus range from the most traditional kinds of health maintenance organizations (HMOs) that have their own medical staffs, clinics, and hospital facilities, to managed indemnity insurers that scrutinize care prospectively and concurrently, even as they reimburse on a (usually discounted) fee-for-service basis. In this sense the managed health plan is involved in providing as well as financing the care. It is in the context of "providing" care that allegations about corporate practice of medicine arise.

39. Although historically indemnity insurers provided retrospective reimbursement for services rendered, much like any other insurer, in recent years most insurers have initiated other kinds of review. In prospective review the insurer requires providers and/or patients to secure advance agreement that the proposed intervention will be covered, while under concurrent review the health plan reviews with providers, sometimes on a daily basis, the appropriate management, for instance, of patients who are hospitalized. See Andreson, 1998, at 433–35. Whereas retrospective review focuses only on who pays for what, prospective and concurrent review can influence decisions about care. Medical interventions are costly, and without some assurance of payment, patients and providers are more likely to defer it.

"Utilization review" (UR) and "utilization management" (UM) are nearly, though not precisely, interchangeable terms. UR is the narrower concept, usually applied to a health plan's decisions about which interventions it will cover for which patients. Such review can be retrospective, prospective, or concurrent. UM is a broader concept, encompassing UR and additionally some other tactics by which an MCO might try to limit or guide utilization. Disease management programs, for instance, typically focus on chronic ailments such as asthma, diabetes, and congestive heart failure and attempt to help patients to maximize their control over their disease through careful adherence to medication and lifestyle regimens. See Harris, 1996; Epstein, 1996; Henning, 1998; Bodenheimer, 1999. Demand management programs, as another example, might feature a twenty-four-hour telephone information service staffed by nurses or other trained personnel to help patients determine whether they need to seek medical care. See Demand management: The new way to cost containment: when managed care is not enough. Health Care Business Digest 1996; 1(2): 36–37.

40. "Today, seventy-five national organizations have developed some 1,800 sets of guidelines, while individual hospitals, managed care organizations, private researchers, and pharmaceutical manufacturers have developed thousands of others." Gabel, 1997, at 142.

For a useful overview of various managed care structures, see Weiner, deLissovoy, 1993. For a good discussion of the increasing diversity of ways in which to compensate providers, see Robinson, 1999.

41. See, e.g., Milliman & Robertson, 1994 (cited in Hirshfeld, 1996, at 35); also cited in Rosenbaum, Frankford, Moore, et al., 1999, at 231.

Companies to which Milliman & Robertson (M&R) sells its guidelines include Cigna, Prudential, United Healthcare Corp, and U.S. Healthcare, Inc., among others. See Anders, 1994; Zoloth-Dorfman, Rubin, 1995, at 350.

42. See Farmer, 1993, at 315–16; Perry, 1994, at 65, 70; Terry, 1994, at 26B.

43. See Frankel, 1994, at 1320. See also Azavedo, 1996, at 156; Lipson, De Sa, 1996, at 62, 70; Slomski, 1994, at 87; Wetzell, 1996, at 15.

44. The Office of Technology Assessment was involved in such activities at certain points. And the Agency for Health Care Policy and Research (AHCPR) was instructed to create guidelines for conditions such as cataracts, depression, and pain management through its Forum for Quality and Effectiveness in Health Care. See 42 U.S.C. §§299, 299b-1 to -3 (1994 & Supp. 1995). See also Grimes, 1993, at 3032; Hall, Anderson, 1992, at 1664; Rosoff, 1995, at 373; Sox, Woolf,1993; Woolf, 1992, at 947–8; Stevens, 1993, at 67; Wennberg, 1992, at 67–68.

However, political pressures closed the government's Office of Technology Assessment and precipitated major cutbacks in the scope of the AHCPR. Deyo, Psaty, Simon, et al., 1997; Kahn, 1998. See also Sofamor Danek v. Gaus, 61 F.3d 929 (D.C. Cir. 1995).

45. See See Leape, 1995, at 1536; Woolf, 1992, at 947; Stevens, 1993, at 67; Morreim, 1991(b).

46. Woolf notes that "[g]uidelines can rarely define optimal care with certainty, due to poor science, imperfect analytic processes, and differences in patients. Recommendations are often worded in highly specific language that achieves clarity at the expense of scientific validity." Woolf 1993(a), at 2646.

Elaine Power points out the wide variations among clinical practice guidelines and observes that "[t]hese guidelines activities are uncoordinated, however, and different agencies sometimes issue different guidelines on the same topic. Occasionally, their recommendations conflict.

"At least some of these differences are probably attributable to the vastly different methods used to create the guidelines. Methodological differences include the types of people selected to be in the expert group, methods used to collect and synthesize evidence, methods used to structure the group discussion and arrive at consensus, and [sic] degree to which recommendations are linked directly with the evidence behind them." Power, 1995, at 205. See also Hayward, Wilson, Tunis, et al., 1995, at 572.

47. Some insurance companies identify their experts for consensus by asking physician friends of administrators; others ask the insurer's company physician to read textbooks and discuss the relevant issues with other insurance company physicians; others establish more formal technology assessment committees. See Holder, 1994, at 19. See also Ross, 1998; Culpepper, Sisk, 1998.

48. In a study conducted by the General Accounting Office, payment for a chest X-ray was 451 times more likely to be denied in Illinois than in South Carolina, while payment for a physician office visit was almost ten times more likely to be denied in Wisconsin than in California. See Pretzer, 1995, at 92–93. See generally United States General Accounting Office, Mar. 1, 1994; United States General Accounting Office, Dec. 19, 1994.

49. See Kerr, Mittman, Hays, et al., 1995, at 503.

50. Under capitation the health plan pays a fixed monthly sum to providers, whether individually or as a group, to provide specified care for the patient. For a more detailed discussion of capitation arrangements, See Chapter 6 § B-2. See also Berwick, 1996.

51. See Terry, 1994, at 26E.

52. Terry, 1994.

53. See Terry 1994(b), at 124.

54. See Zoloth-Dorfman, 1994, at 26, 31–32.

55. Oberman, 1994, at 1.

Some states are establishing medical standards in hopes of reducing malpractice litigation. See Hyams, Shapiro, Brennan, 1996, at 305–6. Maine undertook a five-year Medical Liability Demonstration Project. Crane, 1994, at 32. In the areas of gynecology, emergency medicine, anesthesiology, and radiology physicians who volunteer for the program and follow established guidelines will be immune from liability. See *id.* at 33–34; Stevens, 1993, at 83.

56. See Stevens, 1993, at 74–75. An obstetrics protocol, for instance, may ask the physician to watch and wait for a certain length of time before attempting a cesarean delivery. See *id.* at 76.

However, if the region's only anesthesiologist is about to go home for the night, it may make considerably more sense to curtail the protocol a bit. See *id.*

A different approach comes from the Colorado Court of Appeals. See *Quigley* v. *Jobe,* 851 P.2d 236 (Colo. Ct. App. 1992). For medically sound reasons, a physician had declined to follow the guidelines of his malpractice insurer, COPIC, in diagnostic evaluation of a breast mass. See *id.* at 237–38. The mass turned out to be malignant, but in subsequent litigation the Colorado court ruled that malpractice insurers' guidelines were not admissible as evidence. The guides were promulgated by a private insurance company and did not reflect any general standard of care. Further, the jury might have been prejudiced by any mention of the guidelines, because that would disclose that the doctor had insurance coverage. *See id.* For further discussion of this case, see Crane, 1994, at 31; Oberman, 1994.

57. So long as informed consent is a significant element of decision making in medicine, "highly complex medical decisions must ultimately pass through the portal of patient ignorance and fear." Henderson, Siliciano, 1994, at 1392.

58. See Havighurst, 1992, at 1785; Reinhardt 1992(a), at 141; Reinhardt 1992(b); Weaver,1992.

59. Localio, Lawthers, Brennan TA, et al., 1991; Brennan, Colin, Burstin, 1996; Brennan, Leape, Laird, et al., 1991; Leape, Brennan, Laird, et al., 1991; Weiler, Newhouse, Hiatt, 1992, at 2355; Schwartz, Komesar, 1978, at 1286; Danzon, 1985, at 23–25.

60. See Entman, Glass, Hickson, et al., 1994, at 1591.

61. See Beckman, Markakis, Suchmen et al., 1994, at 1368–69; Hickson, Clayton, Githens, et al., 1992, at 1362; Hickson, Clayton, Entman, et al., 1994, at 1586; Huycke, Juycke, 1994, at 797; Levinson, 1994, at 1620; Anderson, 1995, at 39, 42; Kam, 1995, at 42, 44.

62. See Levinson, Roter, Mullooly, et al., 1997, at 558.

63. See Gosfield, 1995, at 233; Rosoff, 1995, at 370–71; Stevens, 1993, at 69–73.

64. E.g., Tefft v. Wilcox, 6 Kan. 46 (1870); Small v. Howard, 128 Mass. 131 (1880); see also Holder, 1978, at 58–61; McCoid, 1959, at 569–75; Johnson, 1970, at 730–31.

65. E.g., Shilkret v. Annapolis Emergency Hosp. Ass'n, 276 Md. 187, 349 A.2d 245 (1975); Brune v. Belinkoff, 235 N.E.2d 793 (1968); Naccarato v. Grob, 384 Mich. 248, 180 at 598; McCoid, 1959, at 569–75; Johnson, 1970, at 732–41.

66. Hall v. Hilbun, 466 So. 2d 856, 872–73 (Miss. 1985).

67. Keeton, Dobbs, Keeton, et al. 1984, at 187–88.

68. Schloendorff v. Society of New York Hospital, 105 N.E. 92 (1914); Canterbury v. Spence, 464 F.2d, 772, 781–82 (D.C. Cir.), cert denied, 409 U.S. 1064 (1972); Cobbs v, Grant, 8 Cal. 3d 229, 242–43; 502 P.2d 1, 9–10, 104 Cal. Rptr. 505, 513–14 (1972); Miller v. Kennedy, 11 Wash. App. 272, 522 P.2d 852 (1974), aff'd, 85 Wash. 2d 151, 530 P.2d 334 (1975).

69. Abrams, 1986; Blumstein, 1983, at 389–90; Council on Ethical and Judicial Affairs, 1986; Kapp, 1984, at 251; Marsh, 1985, at 177–78. According to this approach, physicians should inform patients not only about services that are not covered by third-party payors but also about payors' utilization review policies and efforts to curtail ongoing services. See Hershey, 1986, at 61–62.

70. Hall 1997(a); Hall, 1997(b), at 209–227.

71. Morreim, 1991(c); Morreim, 2000(a); Morreim, 1997(b); Morreim, 1998; Morreim 1995(b).

72. According to one recent study, of businesses that provide health plans at all, 84% offered only one plan. Blendon, Brodie, Benson, 1995, at 243; American College of Physicians, 1996, at 845.

Another study concluded that 78% of firms offer just one plan, although often with multiple products, such as a POS version of an HMO. Berenson, 1997, at 173.

From another vantage point, a study looking at workers rather than employers found that 48% of employees have only one health plan available, while 23% have only two plans to choose from, and 12% have three plans to choose from. Etheredge, Jones, Lewin, 1996, at 94.

73. Ash v. New York University Dental Center, 564 N.Y.S.2d 308, 311 (A.D. 1 Dist. 1990). Historically, courts have routinely discarded "exculpatory clauses" in which a patient agrees to forego his right to sue for substandard care. See, e.g., Tunkl v. Regents of University of California, 383 P.2d 411 (Cal. 1963); Olson v. Molzen, 558 S.W. 2d 429 (Tn. 1977); Emory University v. Porubiansky, 282 S.E. 2d 903 (Ga. 1981); Cudnick v. William Beaumont Hospital, 525 N.W.2d 891 (Mich. App. 1994); Meiman v. Rehabilitation Center, Inc., 444 S.W.2d 78, 80 (Ky. 1969); Wheeler v. St. Joseph Hospital, 133 Cal. Rptr. 775 (Cal. App. 1977); DiDomenico v. Employers Co-op. Industry Trust, 676 F.Supp. 903, 907–08 (N.D. Ind. 1987).

For further discussion, see also Robinson, 1986(a); Epstein, 1986; Epstein, 1976; Havighurst, 1986(b).

74. For an excellent discussion of the potential and the drawbacks of using information to address the challenges of managed care, see Sage, 1999.

75. Hall, 1997(b), at 171–182, 198–209; Miller, Sage, 1999.

76. See Hershey, 1986, at 61–62.

77. For further discussion of the nuances of making economic disclosures, see Morreim, 1991(c).

78. Keeton, Dobbs, Keeton, et al. 1984, at 189; Blumstein, 1983, at 391; Bovbjerg, 1975, at 1377, 1384; Havighurst 1986(b), at 265, 266–67; McCoid, 1959, at 605–09; Pearson, 1976, at 528; Knotterus, 1984, at 464; Henderson, Siliciano, 1994, at 1383–89.

79. Schuck, 1983, at 413; Holder AR. Medical Malpractice Law (2d. Ed. 1978). New York: John WIley & Sons, 1978, at 47–48; Blumstein, 1983, at 391; McCoid, 1959, at 565.

80. United States v. Carroll Towing, 159 F.2d 169 (2d Cir. 1947).

81. United States v. Carroll Towing, 159 F.2d 169, 173 (2d Cir. 1947).

82. Hall, 1989, at 348.

83. One estimate pegged the cost of defensive medicine at $13.7 billion per year. Reynolds, Rizzo, Gonzalez, 1987, at 2778; see also Bovbjerg, 1975, at 1397; Zuckerman, 1984, at 128.

The Office of Technology Assessment recently concluded that up to 8% of diagnostic testing is "consciously defensive," while another study proposed that liability reform might save up to $50 billion per year without compromising outcomes. Anderson, 1999, at 2399; citing: Kessler, McClellan, 1996. Anderson, 1999, also argues that, aside from defensive medicine that goes beyond the standard of care, that standard itself is inflated by defensive medicine.

84. Veatch, 1981, 285.

85. See Morreim, 1991(a), at 8–20.

86. Lange, Hillis, 1998, at 1839; Avanian, Landrum, Normand, et al., 1998, at 1901.

87. Burnum, 1987; Wong, Lincoln, 1983; Holoweiko, 1995, at 180–81; Woosley, 1994, at 250; Avorn, Chen, Hartley, 1982.

88. Wennberg JE, 1996; Wennberg, 1997; Wennberg, 1986; Chassin, Brook, Park, et al., 1986; Wennberg, Freeman, Culp, 1987; Chassin, et al., 1987; Wennberg, 1990; Leape, Park, Solomon, et al., 1990; Leape, Park, Solomon, Chassinet al., 1989; Wennberg, 1991; Cleary, Greenfield, Mulley, et al., 1991; Fisher, Welch, Wennberg, 1992; Greenfield, Nelson, Subkoff, et al., 1992; Welch, Miller, Welch, et al., 1993; Miller, Miller, Fireman, et al., 1994; Detsky, 1995; Guadagnoli, Hauptman, Avanian, et al., 1995; Pilote, Califf, Sapp, et al., 1995; Weiner, Parente, Garnick, et al., 1995; MonaneL, Kanter, Glynn, et al., 1996; Ashton, Petersen, Souchek, et al., 1999; O'Connor, Quinton, Traven, et al., 1999; Wennberg, 1999; Wennberg, Freeman, Shelton, et al., 1989; Wennberg, Kellett, Dickens, et al., 1996; Fisher, Wennberg, Stukel, et al., 1994; Wennberg, 1987; Van de Werf, 1995; Welch, Miller, Welch, 1994.

89. Fuchs, 1984, at 1576.

90. Another example comes from as far back as 1975, when it was was noted that if physicians screened for colon cancer with six serial stool guaiac tests, that sixth test would cost $50 million for each new cancer detected. Aside from the dangers of false-positive diagnostic results and unwanted side effects, the marginal benefits simply do not merit their costs. Neuhauser, Lewicki, 1975, at 226.

91. Note, 1985, at 1018.

92. Kapp, 1984, at 249–50.

93. Cases focusing on the "loss of a chance" doctrine include: Waffen v. Departent of Health & Human Servs., 799 F.2d 911 (4th Cir. 1986); DeBurkarte v. Louvar, 393 N.W. 2d 131, 139 (Iowa 1986); Valdez v. Lyman-Roberts Hosp. 638 S.W.2d 111,116 (Tex.Ct. App. 1982); Andersen v. Brighman Young University, 879 F.Supp. 1124 (D.Utah 1995); Boburka v. Adcock, 979 F.2d. 424 (6th Cir. 1992); Bromme v. Pavitt, 7 Cal. Rptr. 2d 608 (Cal. App. 3 Dist. 1992); DeBurkarte v. Louvar, 393 N.W. 2d 131 (Iowa 1986); Delaney v. Cade, 873 P.2d 175 (Kan. 1994); Estep v. Ross E. Pope, D.O., P.C., 842 P.2d 360 (Okl. App. 1992); Falcon v. Memorial Hosp., 462 N.W. 2d 44 (Mich. 1990); Greco v. U.S., 893 P.2d 345 (Nev. 1995); Kilpatrick v. Bryant, 868 S.W.2d 594 (Tenn. 1993); Leubner v. Sterner, 493 N.W. 2d 119 (Minn. 1992); Manning v. Twin Falls Clinic & Hosp., 830 P.2d 1185 (Idaho 1992); Roberts v. Ohio Permanente Med. Group, 668 N.E. 2d 480 (Ohio 1996); Short v. U.S., 908 F. Supp. 227 (D.Vt. 1995); Steineke v. Share Health Plan, 518 N.W. 2d 904 (Nev. 1994); Thompson v. Sun City Community Hospital, Inc., 688 P.2d 605 (Ariz. 1989); Wendland v. Sparks, 574 N.W. 2D 327 (Iowa 1998); Andersen v. Brighman Young University, 879; Baer v. Regents of University of Cal., 972 P.2d 9 (N.M. App. 1998); Borkowski v. Sacheti, 682 A.2d 1095 (Conn. App. 1996); Bromme v. Pavitt, 7 Cal. Rptr. 2d 608 (Cal. App. 3 Dist. 1992); Crawford v. Deets, 828 S.W.2d 795 (Tex. App.—Fort Worth 1992); Smith v. State, 647 So.2d 653 (La.App.2 Cir. 1994); Straughan v. Ahmed, 618 So.2d 1225 (La. App. 5 Cit. 1993); Weatherly v.

Blue Cross Blue Shield Ins., 513 N.W.2d 347 (Neb. App. 1994); Windisch v. Weiman, 555 N.Y.S.2d 731 (A.D. 1 Dept. 1990).

94. Suppose, for example, that a new hospital policy discourages physicians from obtaining the chest X-rays that previously had been routinely obtained for all patients admitted to the hospital. Suppose further that a patient had early lung cancer that would have been detected by this routine test but was not diagnosed until much later due to the cost-oriented elimination of this routine. This patient might argue that her chance of survival was substantially diminished by the curtailment of custom. This argument cannot be made, for example, by the patient who did not receive magnetic resonance imaging as a "routine admission procedure," for this latter test has never been a "routine" of admission. The difference is not so much one of medical substance as of history. One can only claim that duties of custom have been breached when there was a custom in the first place.

95. Peters, Rogers, 1994; Ferguson, Dubinsky, Kirsch, 1993, at 2116 (1993); Grimes, 1993; Garber, 1992; Reiser, 1994. See also Abraham, 1981, at 1155; Anderson, Hall, Steinberg, 1993, at 1636; Hall, Anderson, 1992, at 1655; Kalb, 1990, at 1118; Morreim, 1995(a), at 251.

96. Helling v. Carey, 519 P.2d 981 (Wash, 1974).

97. Helling v. Carey, 83 Wash. 2D 514, 519 P.2d 981 (1974); cf. The T.J. Hooper, 60 F.2d 737 (2d. Cir. 1932) (tugboat held to be unseaworthy because it lacked radio equipment to receive storm warnings, even though use of such equipment was not widespread). See also United Blood Services v. Quintana, 827 P.2d 509, 520 (Colo. 1992) (prevailing practice is not always conclusive proof of due care); Toth v. Commuity Hosp., 22 N.Y.2d 255, 239 N.E. 2D 368, 292 N.Y.S.2d 440 (1968).

98. Peters, 2000.

99. Newborns' and Mothers' Health Protection Act of 1996, Pub. L. No. 104–204, 110 Stat. 2935 (codified as amended scattered sections of 29 U.S.C. and 42 U.S.C. "The law provides that group health insurance plans may not restrict postpartum hospital stays for a mother or a newborn to less than 48 hours in the case of a vaginal delivery and 96 hours in the case of a Ceasarean section delivery. See § 711(a)(1), 110 Stat. at 2936." Korobkin, 1999, at 3.

"Since 1995, 41 states have mandated coverage for extended postpartum hospital stays." Korobkin, at 17, n. 84. "Fourteen states have enacted legislation mandating minimum-stay requirements for mastectomy patients" Korobkin, at 17, n. 85.

See also Hoffman, 1999: "In 1998, Congress enacted the 'Women's Health and Cancer Rights Act of 1998,' amending ERISA. The Act requires all group health plans and health insurance issuers offering coverage for mastectomies to provide reimbursement for reconstructive surgery that is associated with a mastectomy" (citing 29 U.S.C. § 1185(b) (Supp. 1999)) (at 252). See also Theodos, 2000.

Numerous states and the federal government (for federal employees) have mandated coverage for autologous bone marrow transplant (ABMT) for breast cancer. "On September 10, 1994, the United States Office of Personnel Management (OPM) 'mandat[ed] immediate coverage of HDC/ASCR for all diagnoses for which it is considered standard treatment and, in addition, specifically for breast cancer, multiple myeloma, and epithelial ovarian cancer' for the approximately 200 insurers participating in the Federal Health Benefits program, which covers nine million federal employees." ECRI, February 1995, at 10. See also Holoweiko, 1995, at 172; Hoffman, 1999.

Alongside these government initiatives, numerous courts have issued injunctions forcing payors to cover the ABMT for breast cancer. See, e.g., Harris v. Blue Cross Blue Shield of Missouri, 995 F.2d 877 (8th Cir. 1993); Wilson v. Group Hospitalization, 791 F.Supp. 309 (D.D.C. 1992); Pirozzi v. Blue Cross-Blue Shield of Virginia, 741 F.Supp. 586 (E.D. Va. 1990); Calhoun v. Complete Health Care, Inc., 860 F.Supp. 1494 (S.C.Ala. 1994); Henderson v. Bodine Aluminum, Inc. 70 F.3d 958 (8th Cir. 1995); Dahl-Eimers v. Mutual of Omaha Life Ins. Co., 986 F.2d 1379 (11th Cir. 1993); Wilson v. CHAMPUS, 65 F.3d 361 (4th Cir. 1995); Bailey v. Blue Cross/Blue Shield of Va., 67 F.3d 53 (4th Cir. 1995).

100. Beebe, Britton, Britton, et al., 1996; Chin, 1997; Edmonson, Stoddard, Owens, 1997; Liu, Clemens, Shay, et al., 1997; Gazmarian, Koplan, Cogswell, et al., 1997; Lane, Kauls, Ickovics, et al., 1999.

101. See below, § C-1.

102. Bovbjerg, 1975, at 1377; Havighurst, 1986(b), at 269.

103. See, e.g. American College of Physicians, 1994(b); Deyo, 1994; Jensen, Brant-Zawadzki, Obuchowski, et al., 1994; Kleinman, Kosecoff, Dubois, et al., 1994, at 1250–1255; Katzman, Dagher, Patronas, 1999; Berkowitz, 1993; Ewigman, Crane, Frigoletto, et al., 1993; James, 1987; Schwartz, 1984, at 90.

104. The question of whether guidelines help or hurt physicians in court remains a subject of

active discussion. See Garnick, Hendricks, Brennan, 1991; Brennan, 1991; Havighurst, 1990; Leahy, 1989; Crane, 1994; Garnick, Hendricks, Brennan, 1991.

105. For further discussion, see, e.g., Hornbein, 1986; Morreim, 1985–86, at 1037–93; Burstin, Lipsitz, Brennan, 1992; Leape, 1995; Bovbjerg, 1975; Chassin, 1988; Giordani, 1989; Hirshfeld, 1992; Mann, 1975; Siliciano, 1991.

106. There is also a danger that such guidelines could be taken too literally. May, 1985. While every physician knows that good medicine cannot be practiced by strict adherence to "cookbooks," it may nevertheless be tempting to suppose that so long as one does everythng recommended by the protocol, he is legally, even if not medically, secure—even though the patient's condition may require further care. Reciprocally, and just as dangerously, the physician might be tempted to suppose that he must do everything recommended in the guideline, whether or not the patient needs it. The resulting useless interventions could cause needless iatrogenic injuries and also a further escalation, not a diminution, of health care expenditures.

107. For further discussion of the potential role of guidelines in tort malpractice, see Garnick, Hendricks, Brennan, 1991; Brennan, 1991.

108. See McHugh v. Audet, 72 F. Supp. 394, 400 (M.D. Pa. 1947); Jones v. Chidester, 610 A.2d 964, 967–69 (Pa. 1992).

109. Chumber v. McClure, 505 F.2d 489, 492 (6th Cir. 1974); Holder, 1978, at 47–48; Blumstein, 1983, at 391; McCoid, 1959, at 565.

110. Blumstein, 1983, at 392; Schuck, 1983, at 413.

111. King, 1975, at 1236.

112. King, 1975, at 1241–43.

113. King, 1975, at 1252.

114. Peters, 2000.

115. Henderson and Siliciano note that instead of acknowledging the plain truth that "wealth matters[,] . . . tort law has traditionally refused to recognize formally the crucial role of patient resources in determining the kind and degree of medical treatment the patient receives." Henderson, Siliciano, 1994, at 1396–97.

116. Preventive screening provides an example. Relatively little evidence indicates that mammography is of benefit for women under age fifty. Although, of course, the test can detect some breast cancers in this age group, the number is rather small. See Salzmann, Kerlikowske, Phillips, 1997; Woolf, Lawrence, 1997; Taubes, 1997; Ransohoff, Harris, 1997; Davis, Love, 1994; Kerlikowske, Grady, Rubin, et al., 1995; Lindfors, Rosenquist, 1995; Kerlikowske, Salzmann, Phillips, et al., 1999; Gotzsche, Olsen, 2000.

An "artesian" approach will tend to recommend it anyway, with the thought that detecting even a few cancers in these women is still of benefit. A managed care approach, in contrast, is more likely to limit the test to whatever segment of the population will quite clearly benefit, then direct any savings toward alternative care that is more likely to benefit other members of the population the MCO serves. No matter where one sets thresholds for various screening procedures, it is certain that some cases of the illness in question will be detected and some will not. The question of where to set those thresholds is a value judgement that weighs the value of increasing the detection rate for this illness against alternative possible uses of the same resources. Just as there are many different ways of resolving this value question, it is equally clear that people may disrespect those whose values differ significantly. See Leahy, 1989, at 1520; Eddy 1993(a); Eddy, 1994.

See, e.g., Berthelot v. Travelers Ins. Co., 973 F.Supp. 596 (E.D.La. 1997), in which women between the ages of thirty-five and forty undertook class action litigation to require their health plans to disclose state laws regarding the availability of this test (the court held that ERISA does not require such disclosure). See also Berthelot v. Travelers Ins. Co., 2000 WL 222155 (E.D.La. 2000) (federal court finding it did not have jurisdiction).

117. In the effort to discern whether available legal doctrines can resolve the tension between physicians' traditional tort obligations and their newer economic constraints, further questions arise concerning equal protection issues. Interested readers are referred to Morreim, 1987, at 1738–44. See also Henderson, Siliciano, 1994; Siliciano, 1991.

118. These values were cited above to include "more is better," "high-tech is better than low-tech," and the like. See Morreim, 1994(a), at 80–81.

119. Diversity of medical practices is not itself new, though today its breadth and depth is clearly new. An array of studies discussing practice variations is listed above, § B-3, at n. 88.

120. Henderson, Siliciano, 1994.

121. No. 219692, 1993 WL 794305 (Riverside County Super. Ct./Central Cal. Dec. 23, 1993). See also Furrow 1997, at 447; Meyer, Murr, 1994, at 36. Other issues in the case also arose,

including administrators' conflicts of interest and the care with which the HMO reviewed the HDC/ABMT procedure as it made its coverage decision. These controversies, while interesting and important in their own right, are not the topic here and thus will not be pursued.

122. See Hoffman, 1999; Peters, Rogers, 1994, at 476; Morreim, 1995(a), at 251.

123. See ECRI, February 1995.

124. As noted in one commentary,

> problems have arisen in efforts to recruit women for trials designed to assess the benefit of HDC/ABMT in the treatment of metastatic breast cancer. Because of the availability of HDC/ABMT outside of clinical trials, many women with metastatic breast cancer have not been willing to accept the chance of being randomized to a control group in a trial designed to evaluate the effectiveness of HDC/ABMT. As a result, it has taken much longer than expected to obtain an adequate number of participants in these studies to resolve the uncertainty over the value of this technology.

Steinberg, Tunis, Shapiro D, 1995, at 150. See also Kolata, 1995; Kolata, Eichenwald, 1999.

125. Of five studies released in 1999, four indicated that high-dose chemotherapy with bone marrow transplant was no better for breast cancer than conventional chemotherapy. A fifth study, done in South Africa, suggested some benefit. However, several months later, as scientists looked at this study more closely in an effort to replicate its results, the principal investigator admitted to having falsified some of the data "out of a foolish desire to make the presentation more acceptable" to the scientific meeting sponsored by the American Society of Clinical Oncology. Weiss, Rifkin, Stewart, et al., 2000, at 1003. See also Antman, Heitjan, Hortobagyi, 1999; Gradishar, 1999; Rowlings, Williams, Antman, et al., 1999; Horton, 2000; Bergh, 2000.

Another study completed even more recently came to the same conclusion, namely, that bone marrow transplant offers no advantage over conventional chemotherapy. See Stadtmauer, O'Neill, Goldstein, et al., 2000; Lippman, 2000.

126. See Barnett v. Kaiser Found. Health Plan, Inc., 32 F.3d 413 (9th Cir. 1994). In *Barnett,* the Ninth Circuit upheld Kaiser's denial of a liver transplant for a man with hepatitis B. See id. at 417. The man's disease was e-antigen positive, meaning that the virus was replicating rapidly outside the liver and any transplanted liver would very likely soon be infected. See *id.* at 414. Despite the fact that other medical centers are willing to perform transplants on such patients, the court accepted Kaiser's medical criteria, which deemed e-antigen positive status to be an absolute contraindication to liver transplant. See *id.* at 416. For another example of the tension between medical community practices and other kinds of standards, see Weaver v. Reagen, 886 F.2d 194, 196–200 (8th Cir. 1989) (holding that the state's Medicaid program should honor the medical community's general acceptance of using AZT in AIDS patients even when they do not yet meet stringent criteria such as a history of pneumocystis pneumonia or CD4 counts below 200).

127. See McCoid, 1959, at 631–32.

128. See Bovbjerg, 1975, at 1389–90; King, 1975, at 1236–37.

129. Bovbjerg, 1975, at 1377–78; 1394–95; Furrow, 1982, at 14; King, 1975, at 1237.

130. For further discussion, see Chapter 5, Section C-2.

131. See Bovbjerg, 1975, at 1396–97.

132. See Terry 1994, at 26E; Terry 1994(b), at 124; Zoloth-Dorfman, 1994, at 31–32. Also see above, at A-3.

133. See Morreim, 1992(a), at 162; Morreim, 1989, at 358.

134. See Anderson, Hall, Steinberg, 1993, at 1636.

135. See Corcoran v. United Healthcare, Inc., 965 F.2d 1321, 1331–32 (5th Cir. 1992).

136. See Morreim, 1995(a), at 254–55; see also Chapter 9, infra.

137. For further discussion of incentive structures such as capitation, see Chapter 6 § B-2, Berwick, 1996.

138. See Wickline v. State, 192 Cal. App. 3d 1630, 1645 (1987) (stating in dicta that physicians are expected to keep a patient in the hospital if the hospital is where that patient needs to be—regardless of insurer's decisions about payment).

Frankel observes: "By focusing exclusively on the discharge order and relying unthinkingly on who had *customary* authority to make that decision, the court ignored the plaintiff's primary contention: that the old custom had given way to a new medical practice culture." Frankel, 1994, at 1306.

139. "As a result of this current temporal parallax in case law, where precedent does not keep pace with market changes, the treating physician is still, for the most part, legally accountable for decisions or policies including some beyond his control." Gosfield, 1995, at 231.

"Traditionally, physicians have had a monopoly on the power to define appropriate medical outcomes, but as a result of that monopoly, they bore sole liability for negligent medical decisions." Frankel, 1994, at 1318; see also Morreim, 1987, at 1724–25; Morreim, 1992(a), at 161; Morreim, 1989, at 359.

140. Employee Retirement Income Security Act, 29 U.S.C. §§ 1001–1461 (1994). ERISA is a federal law enacted to ensure that employee benefits plans are established on a fiscally sound basis so that employees can be confident of receiving their pensions, health plans, and any other promised benefits when their time of need arises. See *id.* § 1001. In exchange for various funding requirements, the government placed all employee benefits under a uniform set of federal laws. See *id.* § 1001b. For further discussion regarding ERISA, see Morreim 1995(a); 23: 247–265, at 251–52.

141. See 29 U.S.C. § 1144(a) (1994).

142. See Nealy v. U.S. Healthcare HMO, 844 F. Supp. 966, 975 (S.D.N.Y. 1994); Harrell v. Total Health Care, Inc., 781 S.W.2d 58, 62 (Mo. 1989).

143. Payors, as noted, have traditionally written contracts to cover all "medically necessary" care and then permitted the medical profession and its "accepted practice" to determine which care was "necessary" and which was not. See Havighurst, 1995, at 15–17, 110–16.

144. As noted by Bovbjerg:

> [B]y accepting medical custom as the legal standard of care, malpractice law has implicitly left both the assessment of risk and the valuation of cost and results to the judgment of medical practitioners. It should be recognized that the standards thus established can only be as good as the circumstances and incentives which give rise to medical custom. . . .
> Neither the theory nor the law of customary practice standards gives much attention to the possibility that an entire industry may set standards too high, or perhaps too high in some areas and too law in others.

Bovbjerg, 1975, at 1393–4.

145. As noted by Hayward and others, guidelines "reflect value judgments about the relative importance of various health and economic outcomes in specific clinical situations." Hayward, Wilson, Tunis, et al., 1995, at 571.

146. See Bovbjerg, 1975, at 1377. Bovbjerg went on to propose that courts acknowledge an alternate, more cost-conscious standard of care for HMOs. See *id.* at 1408–14. Although the concept was well ahead of its time, it could not be applied to current economic conditions. The diversity among HMOs and other kinds of health plans is too great to permit a single alternative, nor would it be desirable to suppose that "mainstream" medicine can suitably continue to function under a single standard.

147. Similarly, a screening test might be implemented at a higher rather than lower frequency to reduce the risk that an illness might not be detected at an earlier, more curable stage. See Leahy, 1989, at 1520.

148. See GUSTO Investigators, 1993(a); GUSTO Investigators 1993(b); Lee, Califf, Simes, 1994.

149. See Barrett, Parfrey, Vavasour, et al., 1992; Barrett, Parfrey, McDonald, 1992; Hirshfeld, 1992; Powe, 1992; 183:21–22; Steinberg, Moore, Powe, et al., 1992.

150. See Eddy, 1992; 268: 2575–2582, at 2580. As a final example, values issues are particularly highlighted in the so-called futility debate. On the one hand, vitalists maintain that all life is infinitely precious, regardless of its quality, and conclude that no expense should be spared to prolong even the lives of patients who are permanently unconscious. In vigorous opposition, others claim that such costly care at others' expense is utterly unwarranted when there is no hope of returning patients to conscious function. For further discussion of this debate, see Morreim, 1995(c); Morreim, 1993, at 33.

151. See generally Orient, 1994, at 81–82; Frankel, 1994, at 1320.

152. Pegram v. Herdrich, 120 U.S. 2143, 2150 (2000).

153. Corporations have long recognized that whatever they spend on health care is not available for improving employees' salaries or other benefits or enhancing other phases of corporate operations. An executive from Xerox Corporation pointed out in 1994: "Our employees won't get merit raises this year, and we're taking out at least 10,000 jobs worldwide. Meanwhile, medical inflation is still 1 to 2 times the overall CPI." Slomski, 1994, at 88. Governments, likewise, must make trade-offs between health care expenditures and alternate programs, from roads to education to defense.

154. The view that physicians have no special expertise to make the value judgments associated with medical care is particularly articulated by philosophers such as Robert Veatch. See, e.g., Veatch, Spicer, 1992; Veatch, 1994.

155. A California appellate court poignantly noted the implications of such power as it upheld a law prohibiting physicians from owning substantial interests in pharmacies. See Magan Med. Clinic v. California State Bd. of Med. Exam'rs, 57 Cal. Rptr. 256 (Cal. Ct. App. 1967):

> The doctor dictates what brand the patient is to buy [,]. . . . orders the amount of drugs and prescribes the quantity to be consumed. In other words, the patient is a captive consumer. There is no other profession or business where a member thereof can dictate to a consumer what brand he must buy, what amount he must buy, and how fast he must consume it and how much he must pay with the further condition to the consumer that any failure to fully comply must be at the risk of his own health. If the doctor interferes with the patient's free choice as to where he purchases his prescribed medicine, the patient then becomes a totally captive consumer and the doctor has a complete monopoly.

Id. at 263.

CHAPTER 3

1. For further discussion of this historical trend, see Chapter 4; see also Weiner, deLissovoy, 1993, at 76–77; Butler, Haislmaier, 1989; Thurow, 1984; Thurow, 1985.
2. 29 U.S.C. § 1001–1461.
3. "Stagflation" is a term coined in the 1970s, when the economy bore double-digit inflation, yet remained essentially stagnant, showing little real growth.
4. Holmes v. Pacific Mut. Life Ins. Co, 706 F.Supp. 733, 735 (C.D.Cal. 1989).
See also Mertens v. Hewitt Associates: "Concerned that many pension plans were being corruptly or ineptly mismanaged and that American workers were losing their financial security as a result, Congress in 1974 enacted ERISA, 'declar[ing] [it] to be the policy of [the statute] to protect . . . the interest of participants in employee benefit plans and their beneficiaries, by requiring the disclosure and reporting to participants and beneciaries of financial and other information with respect [to the plans], by establishing standards of conduct, responsibility, and obligation for fiduciaries of employee benefit plans, and by providing for appropriate remedies, sanctions, and ready access to the Federal courts' (29 U.S.C. § 1001(b))" Mertens v. Hewitt Associates, 113 S.Ct. 2063, 2072 (1993).
5. ERISA distinguishes in certain ways between pension plans and welfare benefit plans such as health insurance. "Congress has distinguished between 'employee pension plans' and 'employee welfare benefit plans,' exempting the latter from much of ERISA's panoply of requirements including its vesting provisions. 'Welfare benefits such as medical insurance . . . are not subject to the rather strict vesting, accrual, participation, and minimum funding requirements that ERISA imposes on pension plans.'" Pitman v. Blue Cross & Blue Shield, 24 F.3d 118, 121 (10th Cir. 1994). In the context of this book, however, this difference will not play a role.
ERISA does not apply to literally every employment situation. Government workers and employees of churches are not covered by ERISA, for example. More precisely, "ERISA applies only to benefit plans offered by employers engaged in interstate commerce. *See* 29 U.S.C. § 1003(a)(1)." Settles v. Golden Rule Ins. Col, 927 F.2d 505, 507–8 (10th Cir. 1991). Other than these limited exceptions, however, almost all benefit plans that workers receive as part of their employment are governed by ERISA.
6. Mertens v. Hewitt Associates, 113 S.Ct. 2063 (1993); Massachusetts Mutual Life Ins. Co. v. Russell, 473 U.S. 134 (1985); Novak v. Andersen Corp., 962 F.2d 757, 760 (8th Cir. 1992).
Some observers would argue that federal remedies are actually greater than mainstream legal thinkers envision and can encompass compensatory damages, reliance damages, and perhaps even punitive damages under the provisions for equitable relief. See, e.g., Weems v. Jefferson-Pilot Life Ins. Co., Inc., 663 So.2d 905 (Ala. 1995); Reid v. Gruntal & Co., Inc., 763 F.Supp. 672 (D.Me. 1991); Russell v. Northrop Grumman Corp., 921 F.Supp. 143 (E.D.N.Y. 1996).
7. Corcoran v. United Healthcare, Inc., 965 F2d 1321 (5th Cir 1992), cert denied 113 SCt 812 (1992). See also Nealy v. U.S. Healthcare HMO., 844 F.Supp. 966 (S.D.N.Y. 1994); Cannon v. Group Health Service of Oklahoma, Inc., 77 F.3d 1270 (10th Cir. 1996); Turner v. Fallon Community Health Plan Inc., 953 F.Supp 419 (D.Mass 1997); Tolton v. American Biodyne, Inc., 48 F.3d 937 (6th Cir. 1995).
8. The Texas statute permits malpractice-type actions against health insurers, health maintenance organizations, and other managed care entities. See Tex. Civ. Prac. & Rem. Code §§ 88.001-003 (West Supp. 1997). However, potential plaintiffs must first exhaust the internal appeals applicable

under Texas utilization review requirements. See *id.* § 88.003. The Texas law also included a number of other provisions, as it: established an independent appeals process for coverage denials; forbade health plans to remove physicians because they had advocated for patients; and forbade indemnification, or "hold harmless," clauses.

Regarding health plans and malpractice, the act established that a "health insurance carrier, health maintenance organization, or other managed care entity for a health care plan has the duty to exercise ordinary care when making health care treatment decisions and is liable for damages for harm to an insured or enrollee proximately caused by its failure to exercise such ordinary care." §88.002(a). Ordinary care is defined as "that degree of care that a health insurance carrier, health maintenance organization, or managed care entity of ordinary prudence would use under the same or similar circumstances," when making benefits decisions. §§ 88.001–002. An organization can be held liable for damages proximately caused by its failure to exercise ordinary care. See *id.* § 88.002(a). An organization can also be held liable for harm caused by its employees, agents, ostensible agents, or "representatives who are acting on its behalf and over whom it has the right to exercise influence or control or has actually exercised influence or control which result[s] in the failure to exercise ordinary care." *Id.* § 88.002(b).

The act applies only to "a cause of action that accrues on or after the effective date of [the] Act [Sept. 1, 1997]." 1997 Tex. Sess. Law. Serv. Ch. 163, § 9 (West).

9. Corporate Health Ins. Inc. v. Texas Dept. of Ins., 12 F.Supp.2d 597 (S.D.Tex. 1998). Although the federal district court held that several other parts of the statute were preempted by ERISA, the portion permitting lawsuits against MCOs was not preempted: "The Act allows an individual to sue a health insurance carrier, health maintenance organization, or other managed care entity for damages proximately caused by the entity's failure to exerecise ordinary care when making a health care treatment decision. . . . In addition, under the Act, these entities may be held liable for substandard health care treatment decisions made by their employees, agents, or representatives" (at 602).

On appeal, the Fifth Circuit affirmed in part and reversed in part. The court agreed that tort suits against ERISA health plans were not preempted. Indeed, the only portion of the Texas statute that violates ERISA, the court held, is the requirement for independent review of benefits denials. By permitting an outside entity to rule that a plan should have provided a particular intervention, the statute potentially imposes a state administrative regime governing benefit determinations. The other feature struck down by the district court, concerning anti-retaliation and anti-indemnity provisions, was reinstated by the Fifth Circuit. Corporate Health Insurance, Inc. v. Texas Dept. of Insurance, 215 F.3d 526 (5th Cir. 2000).

10. These states include Georgia, Missouri, California, and Washington. See Ga. H.B. 732, 145th Gen. Assembly, Reg. Sess. (Ga. 1999); Ga. S. Res. 210, 145th Gen. Assembly, Reg. Sess. (Ga. 1999); Mo. H.B. 335, § A, 89th Gen. Assembly, 1st Reg. Sess. (Mo. 1997) (codified as amended at Mo. Ann. Stat. § 354.505; Cal. Civ. Code § 3428 (West 1999); 2000 Wash. Legis. Serv. 6199 (West) (Second Substitute Senate Bill 6199, as amended by the House; passed by Senate 3/6/200; passed by House of Representatives 3/3/2000).

Missouri's H.B.335 deleted "subsection (3) from Missouri Revised Statute section 354.505. Prior to H.B. 335, that subsection provided that '[a]ny [HMO] authorized under [s]ections 354.400 to 354.550 shall not be deemed to be practicing medicine and shall be exempt from the provisions of Chapter 334, RSMo.' Concurrent with the elimination of this provision, H.B. 335 adds HMOs to the definition of health care provider under Missouri's medical malpractice statutes. It also includes HMOs in the peer review protections of Chapter 537. The significance of these changes remains to be seen. According to a bulletin issued by the Department of Insurance, the Department interprets the amendment to Missouri Revised Statute section 354.505 as making HMOs subject to medical malpractice claims. There are, however, strong arguments that the amendment should not be interpreted to create a liability that would not otherwise exist." Garrison, 1998, at 782–83.

11. See, e.g., Dukes v. U.S. Health Care, Inc., 57 F.3d 350 (3rd Cir. 1995); Roessert v. Health Net, 929 F.Supp. 343 (N.D.Cal. 1996); Rice v. Panchal, 65 F.3d 637, 644 (7th Cir 1995); *In Re* Estate of Frappier, 678 So.2d 884 (Fla.App. 4 Dist. 1996); Santitoro v. Evans, 935 F.Supp. 733 (E.D.N.C. 1996); Prihoda v. Shpritz, 914 F.Supp. 113 (D.Md. 1966); Kampmeier v. Sacred Heart Hospital, 1996 WL 220979 (E.D. PA); Pappas v. Asbel, 675 A.2d 711 (Pa.Super. 1996), aff'd: Pappas v. Asbel, 724 A.2d 889 (Pa. 1998), vacated, 120 S.Ct. 2686; Haas v. Group Health Plan, Inc., 875 F.Supp. 544 (S.D.Ill. 1994); Kearney v. U.S. Healthcare, Inc., 859 F.Supp. 182 (E.D.Pa. 1994); Jackson v. Roseman, 878 F.Supp 820 (D.Md. 1995); Schachter v. Pacificare of Oklahoma, Inc., 923 F.Supp. 1448 (N.D.Okl. 1995); Lancaster v. Kaiser Foundation Health Plan, 958 F.Supp. 1137 (E.D.Va. 1997); Newton v. Tavani, 962 F.Supp. 45 (D.N.J. 1997); Ouelette v. Christ Hosp. 942

F.Supp. 1060 (S.D.Ohio 1996); Bauman v. U.S. Healthcare, Inc., 1 F.Supp.2d 420 (D.N.J. 1998) (aff'd In re. U.S.Healthcare, Inc., 193 F. 3d 151 (3rd Cir. 1999), cert. denied 120 S.Ct. 2687); Negron v. Patel, 6 F.Supp.2d 366 (E.D.Pa. 1998); Moscovitch v. Danbury Hosp., 25 F.Supp.2d 74 (D.Conn. 1998); Herrera v. Lovelace Health Systems, Inc., 35 F.Supp.2d 1327 (D.N.M . 1999).

For a more detailed discussion, see Morreim, 1997(b).

12. Allred, Tottenham, 1996.

13. Corporate practice of medicine will be discussed further below, and in Chapter 8, § A-4. For now, suffice it to say that the prohibition against corporations' practicing medicine is largely a product of common law developed during the early part of the twentieth century. Courts identified several potential hazards as they pointed to licensure laws and held that only licensed individuals, not corporations, can practice medicine, optometry, dentistry, law, and other professions.

"First, physician employment by corporations controlled by lay persons arguably may reduce physician autonomy over medical judgments. Second, employed physicians may experience a sense of divided loyalty between their profit-seeking employer and their treatment-seeking patients. Finally, public policy arguments have been raised to attack the commercialization of the medical profession. Critics of commercialization within the health care arena are concerned that investors in for-profit medical entities that employ physicians will exert too much pressure on their physician-employees to promote the sale of professional services in order to obtain large profits. This may create pressure on employed physicians to place a greater emphasis on profitability over quality of patient care." Mars, 1997, at 249.

See also Dowell, 1994, at 369–70; Starr, 1982, at 305–308 ff; Parker, 1996, at 161; Hayward, 1996, at 406; Morreim, 1999.

14. Bing v. Thunig, 143 N.E. 2d 3 (N.Y. 1957).

15. Bing v. Thunig, 143 N.E. 2d 3, 8 (N.Y. 1957).

16. Darling v. Charleston Community Memorial Hospital, 211 N.E. 2d 253 (Ill. 1965).

17. Johnson v. Misericordia Community Hospital, 301 N.W. 2d 156 (Wisc. 1981).

18. The court continued: "Additionally, it should: (1) solicit information from the applicant's peers, including those not referenced in his application, who are knowledgeable about his education, training, experience, health, competence and ethical character; (2) determine if the applicant is currently licensed to practice in this state and if his licensure or registration has been or is currently being challenged; and (3) inquire whether the applicant has been involved in any adverse malpractice action and whether he has experienced a loss of medical organization membership or medical privileges or membership at any other hospital. . . . This is not to say that hospitals are *insurers* of the competence of their medical staff, for a hospital will not be negligent if it exercises the noted standard of care in selecting its staff." Johnson v. Misericordia Community Hospital, 301 N.W. 2d 156, 174–75 (Wisc. 1981).

19. For more detailed discussion, see Allred, Tottenham, 1996; Sage, 1997; Chittenden, 1991, at 468–73; Trueman, 2000.

20. Thompson v. Nason Hosp., 591 A.2d 703 (Pa. 1991).

21. Thompson v. Nason Hosp., 591 A.2d 703, 707 (Pa. 1991). See also Walls v. Hazelton State General Hosp., 629 A.2d 232 (Pa.Cmwlth 1993); Welsh v. Bulger, 698 A.2d 581 (Pa. 1997); Simmons v. Tuomey Regional Medical Center, 498 S.E.2d 408 (S.C.App. 1998), aff'd as modified, 533 S.E.2d 312 (S.C. 2000); Johnson v. Misericordia Community Hospital, 301 N.W. 2d 156 (Wisc. 1981).

22. Shannon v. McNulty, 718 A2d 828 (Pa Super 1998) (HMO held liable for corporate negligence after it allegedly provided inadequate telephone advice and inadequate physician care to a pregnant woman who believed she was in premature labor). Other cases similarly allege corporate negligence. See, e.g., Lupo v. Human Affairs Intern., Inc. 28 F.3d 269 (2nd Cir. 1994); Herrera v. Lovelace Health Systems, Inc., 35 F.Supp.2d 1327 (D.N.M . 1999); Fritts v. Khoury 933 F.Supp. 668 (E.D.Mich. 1996).

23. Wickline v. State of California, 192 Cal. App. 3d 1630 (1987) (dicta); Wilson v. Blue Cross of Southern Cal., 271 Cal. Rptr. 876, 833 (Cal. App. 2 Dist. 1990); Long v. Great West Life & Annuity Ins., 957 P.2d 823 (Wyo. 1998). See also Helvestine, 1989, at 174 ff; Allred, Tottenham, 1996, at 462.

In contrast, in Gafner v. Down East Community Hosp., 735 A.2d 969 (Me. 1999), the Supreme Court of Maine refused to accede to plaintiffs' request "to recognize a duty on the part of a hospital to adopt rules and policies controlling the actions of independent physicians practicing within its walls" (735 A.2d 976).

24. See Allred, Tottenham, 1996; Chittenden, 1991, at 468–73; Trueman, 2000; Havighurst, 1997, at 601–3; Hall, 1988, at 458 (discussing Darling v. Charleston Community Memorial Hospi-

tal, 211 N.E. 2d 253 (Ill. 1965), opening the door to direct negligence on the part of hospitals); Shannon v. McNulty, 718 A2d 828 (Pa Super 1998); Kampmeier v. Sacred Heart Hospital, 1966 WL 220979 (E.D. PA); Wickline v. State of California, 192 Cal. App. 3d 1630 (1987); Wilson v. Blue Cross of Southern Cal., 271 Cal. Rptr. 876 (Cal. App. 2 Dist. 1990); McClellan v. Health Maintenance, 604 A.2d 1053 (Pa. Super. 1992), appeal denied, 616 A.2d 985 (1992); Steineke v. Share Health Plan, 518 N.W. 2d 904 (Nev. 1994) (see dissent); Foster v. BCBS Mich, 969 F.Supp. 1020 (E.D.Mich 1997); Jones v. Chicago HMO, 730 NE2d 1119 (Ill. 2000). But see St. Luke's Episcopal Hosp. v. Agbor, 952 S.W.2d 503 (Tex. 1997) (hospital found not liable for negligent credentialing based on explicit state statute; because this case predated Texas' more recent statute holding health plans potentially liable for their medical decisions, it is unclear whether this decision still presents precedent).

   In some cases, a claim for direct negligence that might otherwise go forward is preempted by federal ERISA law. See Lancaster v. Kaiser Foundation Health Plan, 958 F.Supp. 1137 (E.D.Va. 1997); Andrews-Clarke v. Travelers Ins., Co., 984 F.Supp. 49 (D. Mass. 1997); Altieri v. Cigna Dental Health, Inc., 753 F.Supp. 61 (D.Conn. 1990); Elsesser v. Hospital of Philadelphia College, 802 F.Supp. 1286 (E.D.Pa. 1992) (preempting claims such as for misrepresentation, though not for ostensible agency); Kearney v. U.S. Healthcare, Inc., 859 F.Supp. 182 (E.D.Pa. 1994); Dearmass v. Av-Med, Inc., 865 F.Supp. 816 (S.D. Fla. 1994); Pacificare of Oklahoma, Inc. v. Burrage, 59 F.3d 151 (10th Cir. 1995). See also Sage, 1997, at 186.

   25. Wethly, 1996, at 821–24.

   26. Sage, 1997, at 173–74.

   27. Hospitals often employ physicians in specialties such as radiology, anesthesiology, and pathology. Some HMOs, in particular the "staff-model" HMOs, employ virtually all their physicians. See Sloan v. Metro Health Council, 516 N.E. 2d 1104 (Ind. App. 1 Dist. 1987); Schleier v. Kaiser Foundation Health Plan, 876 F.2d 174 (D.C. Cir. 1989); Haas v. Group Health Plan, Inc. 875 F.Supp. 544 (S.D.Ill. 1994); Allred, Tottenham, 1996.

   28. See, e.g., Chase v. Independent Practice Ass'n, 583 N.E. 2d 251, 255 (Mass. App. Ct. 1991); Raglin v. HMO Illinois, Inc., 595 N.E. 2d. 153 (Ill. App. 1. Dist. 1992); Overstreet v. Doctors Hospital, 237 S.E.2d 213 (Ga.App.1 Div., 1977); Hodges v. Doctors Hospital 234 SE2d 116 (Ga. App. 2 Div. 1977); Schleier v. Kaiser Foundation Health Plan, 876 F.2d 174, 177 (D.C. Cir. 1989); State. Emp. Sec. v. Reliable Health Care, 983 P.2d 414 (Nev. 1999); Mduba v. Benedictine Hospital, 384 N.Y.S. 2d 527, 529 (App. 3d Dept 1976). See also Trueman, 2000, at 235. Regarding the definition of employment more generally, see Nationwide Mut. Ins. Co. v. Darden, 503 U.S. 318 (1992); NLRB v. United Insurance Col, 390 U.S. 254 (1968).

   It is interesting to note that, in *AmeriHealth Inc./AmeriHealth HMO,* the National Labor Relations Board investigated whether independent-practice physicians affiliated with an MCO were actually employees eligible to unionize. Physicians claimed that they were "so integrated with and controlled by AmeriHealth that they meet the statutory definition of employees, which, in turn, is based on the common law definition of 'servants'" (Leibenluft, p. 8). En route to concluding that these physicians could not claim to be employees, the NLRB Regional Director found, among other things, that the HMO lacked substantial control over the physical conduct of the physicians, that it did not control their access to patients, that the physicians retained their economic separateness from the HMO, and that they retained wide entrepreneurial discretion regarding how to run their practices and make their profits. See *AmeriHealth Inc./AmeriHealth HMO,* Case-4–RC- 19260, 326 N.L.R.B. No 55 (Aug. 28, 1998) and *AmeriHealth Inc./AmeriHealth HMO,* Case-4-RC (Reg'l Dir. Decision (May 24, 1999)); discussed in: Leibenluft, 1999. See also *AmeriHealth Inc./AmeriHealth HMO and United Food and Commercial Workers Union, Local 56,* No. 4-RC-19260 (N.L.R.B. Oct. 18, 1999). See also Hirshfeld, 1999, at 58–59

   29. Petrovich v. Share Health Plan of Illinois, Inc., 719 NE 2d 756, 770 (Ill. 1999).

   30. See, e.g., Insinga v. LaBella, 543 So.2d 209 (Fla. 1989); Clark v. Southview Hosp. & Family Health Ctr., 628 N.E. 2d 46 (Ohio 1994); Sword v. NKC Hospitals, Inc., 714 NE2d 142 (Ind. 1999).

   31. Baptist Memorial Hosp. System v. Sampson, 969 S.W.2d 945, 949 (Tex. 1998). See also Insinga v. LaBella, 543 So.2d 209 (Fla. 1989); Clark v. Southview Hosp. & Family Health Ctr., 628 N.E. 2d 46 (Ohio 1994); James by James v. Ingalls Memorial Hosp., 701 N.E.2d 207 (Ill.App. 1 Dist. 1998); Sword v. NKC Hospitals, Inc., 714 NE2d 142 (Ind. 1999); Pamperin v. Trinity Memorial, 423 N.W.2d 848 (Wis. 1988); Kashishian v. Port, 481 N.W.2d 277 (Wis. 1992).

   However, a few courts have held that not even these are required. In a case involving allegedly incompetent care from emergency room physicians, one court held that a hospital has nondelegable duties toward patients in the sense that even if it can delegate its activities to another agent (in this case, the rendering of emergency care), it cannot delegate its own liability for faulty care. "'The real effect of finding a duty to be nondelegable is to render not the duty, but the liability, not delegable; the person subject to a nondelegable duty is certainly free to delegate the duty, but will be liable to third parties for any negligence of the delegatee, regardless of any fault on the part of the delegator.'" Simmons v. Tuomey Regional Medical Center, 498 S.E.2d 408, 412 (S.C.App. 1998), aff'd as modified, 533 S.E.2d 312 (S.C. 2000) (hospital owes nondelegable, but not absolute, duty to render competent service to emergency room patients).

A Texas appellate court similarly held that a hospital will automatically bear liability for the negligence of its emergency room physicians. See Sampson v. Baptist Memorial Hosp. System, 940 S.W. 2d 128 (Tex. App.-San Antonio, 1996). That ruling, however, was overturned by the state's supreme court, as noted above, in Baptist Memorial Hosp. System v. Sampson, 969 S.W.2d 945 (Tex. 1998)(rejecting the idea that a hospital has a nondelegable duty "solely because it opens its doors for business," at 949).

In contrast, in Butkiewicz v. Loyola Univ. Medical Center, 724 N.E.2d 1037 (Ill. App. 1 Dist. 2000), an Illinois appellate court found that although a patient might reasonably have believed an independent radiologist to be an employee of a hospital, ostensible agency did not apply because the patient used this hospital at his doctor's recommendation rather than having relied on any representations made by the hospital.

32. See, e.g., Boyd v. Albert Einstein Med. Center, 547 A.2d 1229 (Pa. Super. 1988); Independence HMO, Inc. v. Smith, 733 F.Supp. 983 (E.D.Pa. 1990), Albain v. Flower Hospital, 553 N.E.2d 1038 (Ohio 1990); Elsesser v. Hospital of Philadelphia College, 802 F.Supp. 1286 (E.D.Pa. 1992); DeGenova v. Ansel, 555 A.2d 147 (Pa. Super. 1988) (against an insurer); Paterno v. Albuerne, 855 F.Supp. 1263 (S.D.Fla. 1994); Kearney v. U.S. Healthcare, Inc., 859 F.Supp. 182 (E.D.Pa. 1994); Dearmass v. Av-Med, Inc., 865 F.Supp. 816 (S.D. Fla. 1994); Independence HMO, Inc. v. Smith, 733 F.Supp. 983 (E.D.Pa. 1990); Jackson v. Roseman, 878 F.Supp. 820 (D.Md. 1995); Prihoda v. Shpritz, 914 F.Supp. 113 (D.Md. 1966) . See also Dunn v. Praiss, 606 A.2d 862 (N.J. Super.A.D. 1992); Dunn v. Praiss, 656 A.2d 413 (N.J. 1995); McClellan v. Health Maintenance, 604 A.2d 1053 (Pa. Super. 1992), appeal denied, 616 A.2d 985 (1992); Petrovich v. Share Health Plan of Ill., Inc. 696 NE2d 356 (Ill. App. 1998); Jones v. Chicago HMO Ltd. of Illinois, 703 N.E.2d 502 (Ill. App. 1 Dist. 1998) aff'd in part, rev'd in part, 730 NE2d 1119 (Ill. 2000); Negron v. Patel, 6 F.Supp.2d 366 (E.D.Pa. 1998); Clark v. Southview Hosp. & Family Health Ctr., 628 N.E. 2d 46, 54 (Ohio 1994); Sloan v. Metropolitan Health Council, 516 N.E. 2D 1104, 1109, (Ind. Ct. App. 1987).

But see: Raglin v. HMO Illinois Inc., 595 N.E. 2d 153 (Ill. App. 1 Dist. 1992)(denying claim for vicarious liability on ground that HMO did not control physicians); Chase v. Independent Practice Ass'n, 583 N.E. 2d 251, 255 (Mass. App. Ct. 1991) (finding no vicarious liability in IPA-type HMO); Ricci v. Gooberman, 840 F.Supp. 316, 317 (D.N.J. 1993).

ERISA has sometimes preempted ostensible agency claims. See, e.g., Nealy v. U.S. Healthcare HMO., 844 F.Supp. 966 (S.D.N.Y. 1994); Pomeroy v. Johns Hopkins Medical Services, Inc., 868 F.Supp. 110 (D.Md. 1994); Hull v. Fallon, 188 F.3d 939 (8th Cir. 1999).

In other instances, courts held that ERISA does not preempt such a claim. See Dukes v. U.S. Healthcare, Inc., 57 F.3d 350 (3rd Cir. 1995); In Re U.S. Healthcare, Inc., 193 F.3d 151 (3rd Cir. 1999), cert. denied 120 SCt 2687 (2000); Lancaster v. Kaiser Foundation Health Plan, 958 F.Supp. 1137 (E.D. Va. 1997); Prihoda v. Shpritz, 914 F.Supp. 113 (D.Md. 1996); DeGenova v. Ansel, 555 A.2d 147 (Pa. Super. 1988); Independence HMO, Inc. v. Smith, 733 F.Supp. 983 (E.D.Pa. 1990); Elsesser v. Hospital of Philadelphia College, 802 F.Supp. 1286 (E.D.Pa. 1992); Boyd v. Albert Einstein Med. Center, 547 A.2d 1229 (Pa. Super. 1988); Schleier v. Kaiser Foundation Health Plan, 876 F.2d 174 (D.C. Cir. 1989); Stroker v. Rubin, 1994 WL 719694 (E.D.Pa. 1994).

33. Allred, Tottenham, 1996, at 483 ff.; Chittenden, 1991; Trueman, 2000. See also Petrovich v. Share Health Plan of Illinois, 696 N.E.2d 356, 360–61 (Ill. App. 1 Dist. 1998); Jones v. Chicago HMO Ltd. of Illinois, 703 N.E.2d 502, 504 (Ill. App. 1 Dist. 1998), aff'd in part, reversed in part, Jones v. Chicago HMO, 730 NE2d 1119 (Ill. 2000); McEvoy v. Group Health Co-Op., 570 N.W. 2d 397 (Wis. 1997).

34. There are exceptions. In Brandon v. Aetna Services, Inc., 46 F.Supp.2d 110 (D.Conn. 1999), the plaintiff alleged "that Defendants committed malpractice by engaging in the practice of medicine or psychiatry 'by undertaking to make decisions about what psychiatric and psychological treatment was and was not appropriate for Mr. Brandon,' and then failing to exercise the degree and skill ordinarily exercised by psychiatrists and psychologists in Connecticut or Vermont by failing or refusing to 'approve and pay for at least six months of treatment . . .'" (at 112). The district court held this claim to be preempted by ERISA. Other exceptions in which the plaintiff tried to claim that the plan literally practiced medicine include Corcoran v. United Healthcare, Inc., 965 F2d 1321 (5th Cir 1992), cert denied 113 SCt 812 (1992); Kuhl v. Lincoln Nat. Health Plan, 999 F.2d 298

(8th Cir. 1993) cert. denied 510 U.S. 1045, 114 S.Ct. 694 (1994); Williams v. Good Health Plus, Inc., 743 S.W.2d 373, 378 (Tex.App.–San Antonio 1988); Roessert v. Health Net, 929 F.Supp. 343 (N.D.Cal. 1996); Garrison v. Northeast Georgia Medical Center, Inc., 66 F.Supp2d 1336 (N.D.Ga. 1999); Williams v. California Physicians' Service, 85 Cal.Rptr.2d 497 (Cal.App. 3 Dist. 1999); Wilson V. Chestnut Hill Healthcare, 2000 WL 204368 (E.D.Pa., 2000).

35. The common law prohibition on corporate practice of medicine is largely a product of the 1930s. Concerns about corporate hucksterism, lay control over treatment decisions, division of professional loyalties, and the like prompted a line of court decisions prohibiting corporations from hiring physicians, attorneys, dentists, optometrists, and other professionals as employees. See Mars, 1997; Dowell, 1994; Starr, 1982, at 305–308 ff; Parker, 1996; Hayward, 1996; Morreim, 1999, at 944–950.

Leading cases include People v. United Medical Service, 200 N.E. 157 (Ill. 1936); People v. Pacific Health Corporation, 82 P.2d 429 (Cal. 1938) (citing "evils of divided loyalty and impaired confidence" at 430); Dr. Allison, Dentist, Inc. v. Allison, 196 N.E. 799 (Ill. 1935); Parker v. Board of Dental Examiners, 14 P.2d 67 (Cal. 1932); People v. Merchants' Protective Corporation, 209 P. 363 (Cal. 1922); Teseschi et al. v. Mathis, 183 A. 146 (N.J.1936); State v. Bailey Dental Co. 234 N.W. 260 (Iowa 1931); Bennett v. Indiana State Board of R. and E., 7 N.E.2d 977 (Ind. 1937); Bartron v. Codington County, 2 N.W.2d 337 (So.Dak. 1942); Semler v. Dental Examiners, 294 U.S. 608 (1935).

36. For further discussion, see Morreim, 1999. See also Starr, 1982; Chase-Lubitz, 1987; Rosoff, 1987; Mars, 1997; Dowell, 1994; Parker, 1996; Clousson, Butz, 1996, at 192; Hayward, 1996; Hall, 1988, at 511–18; Hirshfeld, Harris, 1996, at 11–12.

37. " 'The test of the relationship is the right to control. It is not the fact of actual interference with the control, but the right to interfere that makes the difference between an independent contractor and a servant or agent. . . . An independent contractor has been said to be 'one who, exercising an independent employment, contracts to do a piece of work according to his own methods and without being subject to the control of his employer, except as to the result of his work.' " Daw's Critical Care v. Dept. of Labor, 622 A.2d 622, 631 (Conn.Super. 1992) (citations omitted).

"Indicia that characterize control in an employment relationship for purposes of NRS 612.085(1) include, but are not limited to, whether the employer has the right to direct the daily manner and means of a person's work, whether the worker is required to follow the putative employer's instructions, and whether the worker can refuse work offered without ramification." State. Emp. Sec. v. Reliable Health Care, 983 P.2d 414, 417 (Nev. 1999); Mduba v. Benedictine Hospital, 384 N.Y.S. 2d 527 (App. 3d Dept 1976).

See also Charter Peachford Behavioral v. Kohout, 504 SE2d 514, 525 (Ga. App. 1998); Jacobson, Pomfret, 1998, at 1062.

38. In Conrad v. Medical Bd. of State of Cal., 55 Cal. Rptr 2d 901 (Cal.App. 4 Dist. 1996), the California Appellate Court struck down a hospital district's effort to hire physicians, citing the corporate practice ban. "The doctrine is intended to ameliorate 'the evils of divided loyalty and impaired confidence' which are thought to be created when a corporation solicits medical business from the general public and turns it over to a special group of doctors, who are thus under lay control" (at 903). In this case, employment agreements would have required the physician-employees "to meet targets of 4,600 patient encounters per year. If the physician does not meet the target, and if 45 percent of the fees generated by the physician are less than his or her base salary, then the employment contract will not be extended. The employment contract also provides for an incentive fund which represents additional compensation which the physician may receive from the surplus funds remaining after the employee-physicians' base salaries are deducted from a certain percentage of the collections made by the hospital's adult medicine division, the physicians' employer" (at 905).

In Washington state, a partnership featuring a physician, nurse, and business manager was found to have been an illegal, unenforceable arrangement (Morelli v. Ehsan, 756 P.2d 129 (Wash. En Banc 1988)), while a Texas appeals court invalidated a partnership between a physician and two nonphysicians for operating a hospital emergency department (Flynn Bros., Inc. v. First Medical Associates, 715 S.W.2d 782 (Tx. App. 1986)). See also Garcia v. Texas State Board of Medical Examiners, 384 F.Supp. 434 (W.D.Tex. 1974): "The relationship between the licensed optometrist and his unlicensed employer is that of master and servant. The master is in a position where he may dictate to his servant the manner of conducting his business, the kind and nature of the goods to be sold and furnished to the patient, in order to procure the most favorable financial gain to the employer. And this may be done without regard to the public health, since the employer is a non-resident and beyond the jurisdiction of the courts of this state, and not licensed." Chase-Lubitz at 470–474; Parker, 1996, at 166–67.

39. Rosoff, 1987, at 494–497; Mars, 1997, at 252; Parker, 1996, at 161; Hayward, 1996, at 410. See also Los Angeles County v. Ford, 263 P.2d 638 (Cal. App. 2 Dist. 1953); Cal. Med. Assn. V. Regents of University, 94 Cal. Rptr.2d 194 (Cal. App. 2 Dist. 2000).

40. "Any act or omission alleged to constitute negligence against HealthAmerica necessarily involves the practice of medicine, which HealthAmerica is barred from doing by statute." Williams v. Good Health Plus, Inc., 743 S.W.2d 373, 378 (Tex.App.–San Antonio 1988). See also Sage, 1997, at 177. See also Sword v. NKC Hospitals, Inc., 714 NE2d 142, 149 (Ind. 1999) (summarizing early doctrines holding that hospitals could not be liable for negligence of independent contractor physicians because the former had no right to control the conduct of the latter).

41. See, for instance, Kuhl v. Lincoln Nat. Health Plan, 999 F.2d 298 (8th Cir. 1993) cert. denied 510 U.S. 1045, 114 S.Ct. 694 (1994). The health plan for a patient needing complex surgery for heart problems initially denied precertification to do the surgery at an out-of-plan hospital that was better equipped to perform the procedure. Delays in eventual certification ultimately were followed by the patient's deterioration and death. The Eighth Circuit held that all state-based claims were preempted by ERISA but responded to plaintiff's argument that the health plan had exercised its own medical judgment. "The Kuhls attempt to avoid ERISA preemption by suggesting that Lincoln National's actions with respect to Buddy Kuhl went beyond the mere administration of benefits. They assert that Lincoln National not only refused to precertify payment for Buddy Kuhl's operation, but 'cancelled' the operation and undertook treatment of Buddy Kuhl according to its own medical opinions." Id., at 303. However, the court found that " '[a]rtful pleading by characterizing Lincoln National's actions in refusing to pay for the surgery as "cancellation" or by characterizing the same administrative decisions as "malpractice" does not change the fact that plaintiffs' claims are based on the contention that Lincoln National improperly processed Kuhl's claim for medical benefits.' . . . [W]e are compelled to agree with the district court. Lincoln National became involved in the cancellation . . . only after the Barnes Hospital staff requested a precertification review. Lincoln National's admission that it 'cancelled' the surgery cannot be stretched to imply that Lincoln National went beyond the administration of benefits and undertook to provide Buddy Kuhl with medical advice." Id., at 303.

See also Corcoran v. United Healthcare, Inc., 965 F2d 1321 (5th Cir 1992), cert denied 113 SCt 812 (1992); Garrison v. Northeast Georgia Medical Center, Inc., 66 F.Supp2d 1336 (N.D.Ga. 1999). But see Roessert v. Health Net, 929 F.Supp. 343 (N.D.Cal. 1996) (holding that ERISA did not preempt claims and remanding substantive issues regarding corporate medical practice to state courts).

42. See, e.g., Murphy v. Board of Medical Examiners, 949 P.2d 530 (Ariz.App.Dist.1 1997).

43. Ortolon, 1997, at 27.

44. As noted by some commentators, "[c]overage disputes are most appropriately viewed as an insurance-purchasing decision by a pool of subscribers, not a medical-treatment decision by an individual patient. The denial of coverage does not prevent the doctor from rendering care; it merely determines that, in the insurer's judgment, the subscriber pool has chosen not to pay for the particular treatment. Thus, where the parties leave the scope of coverage undefined, a particular case is rationally decided by asking only what range of treatment options the purchasers would have chosen to insure at the time they signed up, not what treatment they want to receive now that the insurance has been paid and their illness is manifest." Hall, Anderson, 1992, at 1676.

45. St. Francis Reg. Med. Ctr. v. Weiss, 869 P.2d 606, 616 (Kan. 1994).

46. Decisions that have favored plaintiffs include Nesseim v. Mail Handlers Ben. Plan, 792 F. Supp. 674, 675 (D.S.D. 1992) (later reversed, see Nesseim v. Mail Handlers Ben. Plan, 995 F.2d 804 (8th Cir. 1993)); Calhoun v. Complete Health Care, Inc., 860 F.Supp. 1494, 1499 (S.C.Ala. 1994); Pirozzi v. Blue Cross-Blue Shield of Virginia, 741 F.Supp. 586 (E.D. Va. 1990); Wilson v. Group Hospitalization, 791 F.Supp. 309 (D.D.C. 1992); Taylor v. BCBSM, 517 N.W.2d 864 (Mich.App. 1994); Bailey v. Blue Cross/Blue Shield of Va., 866 F.Supp. 277 (E.D.Va. 1994); Bailey v. Blue Cross/Blue Shield of Va., 67 F.3d 53 (4th Cir. 1995); Arkansas BCBS v. Long, 792 S.W.2d 602 (1990); Blue Cross and Blue Shield v. Brown, 800 S.W. 2d 724 (Ark. App. 1990); DiDomenico v. Employers Co-op. Industry Trust, 676 F.Supp. 903 (N.D. Ind. 1987); Leonhardt v. Holden Business Forms Co., 828 F. Supp. 657 (D. Minn. 1993).

Other decisions cite plain contractual language to uphold a denial of coverage. These include ERISA cases in which courts declined to hold that a denial was "arbitrary and capricious." See Johnson v. Dist. 2 Marine Eng. Beneficial Ass'n, 857 F.2d 514 (9th Cir. 1988); Spain v. Aetna Life Ins. Co., 11 F.3d 129 (9th Cir. 1993), cert. denied 511 U.S. 1052, 114 S.Ct. 1612 (1994); Sweeney

v. Gerber Products Co. Med. Benefits Plan, 728 F.Supp. 594, (D.Neb. 1989); Loyola University of Chicago v. Humana Ins. Co., 996 F.2d 895 (7th Cir. 1993); Fuja v. Benefit Trust Life Ins. Co., 18 F.3d 1405, 1412 (7th Cir. 1994); McGee v. Equicor-Equitable HCA Corp., 953 F.2d 1192 (10th Cir. 1992); Harris v. Mutual of Omaha Companies, 992 F.2d 706, 713 (7th Cir. 1993); Arrington v. Group Hospitalization & Med. Serv., 806 F.Supp. 287, 290 (D.D.C. 1992); Barnett v. Kaiser Foundation Health Plan, Inc., 32 F.3d 413 (9th Cir. 1994); Farley v. Benefit Trust Life Ins. Co., 979 F.2d 653 (8th Cir. 1992); Thomas v. Gulf Health Plan, Inc., 688 F. Supp. 590 (S.D. Ala. 1988); Doe v. Group Hospitalization & Medical Services, 3 F.3d 80 (4th Cir. 1993).

47. See above, Chapter 3, § B-2.

48. No. 219692 (Cal. Super. Ctl, 28 December 1993). See also Meyer, Murr, 1994, at 36. See above, Chapter 2, § C-1.

49. This particular case is complex, with serious questions about the fairness of the procedures by which the health plan made its decision. Meyer, Murr, 1994, at 36.

50. Studdert, Brennan, 2000. The jury award was later allegedly reduced in a settlement whose terms were not made public.

51. Associated Press. "Breast Cancer Procedure Bogus," *Memphis Commercial Appeal*, March 11, 2000, A-5. It might also be noted that during the heyday of using ABMT for breast cancer, many hospitals and physicians made enormous sums of money from the treatment. See Kolata, Eichenwald, 1999.

52. 452 S.E.2d 589 (N.C. Ct. App.), *aff'd*, 464 S.E.2d 44 (N.C. 1995). See above, Chapter 2.

53. It is worth noting that credible allegations of negligence also were lodged against the family that failed to bring the boy back in a timely fashion for scheduled follow-up care, that the treating physician was negligent in failing to monitor and prescribe appropriately for the patient's condition, and that the patient had the option to transfer to a state-run facility—an offer the family refused. See Muse v. Charter Hosp. Winston-Salem Inc., 452 S.E.2d 589, 595–97, 599–600 (Judge Orr's dissent) (N.C.App. 1995).

54. Leahy, 1989.

55. Leahy, 1989, at 1520.

56. A recent California case demonstrates a willingness, at least in the dicta of a concurring opinion, to acknowledge that an unfortunate result need not overturn an otherwise desirable policy. In Creason v. Department of Health Services, 957 P.2d 1323 (Cal. 1998), the state's screening program for newborns had failed to detect the plaintiff's congenital lack of a thyroid gland. The California Supreme Court denied the cause of action based on statutory interpretation, but Justice Kennard added an important piece of reasoning in his concurring opinion. "[T]o impose civil liability on the Department here and in any similar future case may well threaten the continuation of a generally beneficial statewide program that has screened millions of California babies for disabling congenital disorders. . . . 'Far more persons would suffer if government did not perform these functions at all than would be benetifed by permitting recovery in those cases where the government is shown to have performed inadequately.' . . . The facts of this case are heartrending, and the desire to afford the stricken child and her parents some measure of comfort and financial assistance is strong. But these considerations alone cannot dictate the outcome in this case." 957 P.2d 1333. Further discussion of courts' emerging willingness to accept the broader policy importance of enforcing health plans' contractual limits will be presented in Chapter 10.

57. Fault has been a cornerstone of American tort law ever since Massachusetts Chief Justice Lemuel Shaw asked in 1850 whether Mr. Kendall was at fault when he accidentally struck Mr. Brown while separating two fighting dogs. Brown v. Kendall, 60 Mass. (6 Cush.) 292 (1850). See also White, 1980, at 14–16; Williams, 1984, at 554–63. See also Coleman, 1982, at 373; Epstein, 1997, at 361; Harper, James, 1961; Keeton, O'Connell, 1975; Wasserstrom, 1961.

Because of the admitted difficulties in ascribing fault fairly, a number of commentators have recommended various no-fault approaches to medical malpractice. For further discussion see Horwitz, Brennan, 1995; Johnson, Brennan, Newhouse, et al., 1992; King, 1992; White, 1988; Epstein, 1988; Petersen, 1995; O'Connell, 1986: 49: 125–141; Tancredi, 1986; O'Connell, 1977; Johnson, Brennan, Newhouse, et al., 1992; Weiler, Newhouse, Hiatt, 1992.

A variation on this theme concerns enterprise liability, in which large enterprises such as hospitals or health plans bear all liability for error, regardless of fault. For further discussion, see Abraham, Weiler, 1994 ; Sage, Jorling, 1994; Sage, 1997; Furrow 1997, at 498–509. See also Chapter 5, § A-2.

58. Coleman, 1982, at 380.

59. For further discussion of cases in which reasonableness has perfused tort doctrine, see Morreim, 1987, at 1759–60.

60. United States v. Carroll Towing Co., 159 F.2d 169 (2d Cir. 1947). For further discussion see Morreim, 1985–86, at 1052; Morreim, 1987, at 1758–59. Note that this appeal to Hand's generally economic approach to tort law is not tantamount to embracing the more purely economic theories of tort offered by Posner and Danzon. That is, we need not resolve tort issues simply by asking who can best afford to pay for the damages. See Gafner v. Down East Community Hosp., 735 A.2d 969, 978 (Me. 1999) (rejecting the notion that liability should be placed "on the party most able to pay"). See also Morreim, 1985–86, at 1052, n. 39.

61. Klisch v. Meritcare Medical Group, Inc., 134 F.3d 1356, 1360 (8th Cir. 1998)(citing Ouelette v. Subak, 391 N.W.2d 810, 816 (Minn. 1986)). See also Morlino v. Medical Center, 706 A.2D 721, 731 (N.J. 1998); Brannen v. Prince, 421 S.E.2d 76, 80 (Ga. App. 1992); Deyo v. Kinley, 565 A.2d 1286 (Vt. 1989); Jones v. Chidester, 610 A.2d 964 (Pa. 1992); Parris v. Sands, 25 Cal. Rptr. 2d 800 (Cal. App. 2 Dist. 1993); Riggins v. Mauriello, 603 A.2d 827 (Del. 1992); Tefft v. Wilcox, 6 Kan. 46 (1870); Aiello v. Muhlenberg R. Med. Ctr., 733 A.2d 433, 438 (N.J. 1999).

62. This is health plans' duty of "contributive justice." See Morreim, 1995(a), at 250.

CHAPTER 4

1. Epstein, 1976, at 126; King, 1986, at 131, 146; Feldman, Ward, 1979, at 79; Holder, 1978, at 1ff.; Green, 1988, at 235. See also Chew v. Meyer, 527 A.2d 828, 832 (Md. App. 1987); Hammonds v. Aetna Casualty & Surety Company, 243 F. Supp. 793, 801 (Ohio 1965).

2. Gilmore, 1974; Feinman, Feldman, 1985, at 883 n.16; Huber, 1988, at 34; Feldman, Ward, 1979, at 79, 88; Epstein, 1976, at 119, 126; Green, 1988.

3. Insurance is best understood in terms of spreading risk in order to limit losses for those who incur what is usually a personally unexpected, even if statistically predictable, adverse event. Robert Jerry defines a contract of insurance as "an agreement in which one party (the insurer), in exchange for a consideration provided by the other party (the insured), assumes the other party's risk and distributes it across a group of similarly situated persons, each of whose risk has been assumed in a similar transaction." Jerry, 1996, at 17. The Supreme Court describes the "business of insurance" according to: (1) whether the practice regulated has "the effect of transferring or spreading a policyholder's risk"; (2) whether the practice serves as "an integral part of the policy relationship between the insurer and the insured"; and (3) whether "the practice [is] limited to entities within the [insurance] industry". Unum Life Ins. Co. of America v. Ward, 119 S.Ct. 1380, 1386, 1389–90 (1999) (citing Metropolitan Life Ins. Co. v. Massachusetts, 471 U.S. 724, 743 [1984]). For further discussion of how the McCarran-Ferguson Act defines the business of insurance, see Pilot Life Ins. Co. v. Dedeaux, 481 U.S. 41, 48–49 (1986); Hemphill v. Unisys Corp., 855 F.Supp. 1225 (D.Utah 1994); Baker, 1994.

4. Starr, 1982, at 295, 363–78; Butler, Haislmaier, 1989, at 6–17; Havighurst, 1995, at 111–115.

5. Light, 1983, at 1316; Thurow, 1984, at 1570; Thurow, 1985. For a more detailed discussion of this historical picture and relevant bibliographical citations, see Morreim, 1991(a).

6. Wing, 1986, at 618–622, 625–627; Enthoven, Kronick, 1989; Butler, Haislmaier, 1989; Roe, 1981; Delbanco, Meyers, Segal, 1979.

7. Hall, Anderson, 1992, at 1644–47; Anderson, Hall, Steinberg, 1993.

8. Some plans, for instance, began to list precisely which sorts of transplant they do and do not cover. See, e.g., Healthcare America Plans, Inc. v. Bossemeyer, 953 F.Supp. 1176 (D.Kan. 1996) affd w/o opin. 166 F.3d 347; Bailey v. Blue Cross/Blue Shield, 866 F. Supp. 277 (E.D. Va. 1994), aff'd, 67 F.3d 53 (4th Cir. 1995).

9. For a useful discussion of the "reasonable expectations" doctrine from which judge-made insurance emerged, see Swisher, 2000.

For further discussion of judge-made insurance in the health care context see, e.g., Abraham, 1981; Ferguson, Dubinsky, Kirsch, 1993. Indeed, courts need not become involved if insurers simply agree to provide benefits under only the threat of litigation. Peters, Rogers, 1994; Hall, Anderson, 1992; James, 1991; Havighurst, 1995, at 22; Kalb, 1990; Huber, 1988; Anders, 1994; Holoweiko, 1995, at 171–2.

In other cases, federal or state governments mandate the use of a new technology, obviating even the need to threaten litigation. For example, nearly half a dozen states plus the federal government have mandated HDC/ABMT for breast cancer. Holoweiko, 1995; ECRI, February 1995, at 10. The federal government did likewise. "On September 10, 1994, the United States Office of Personnel Management (OPM) 'mandat[ed] immediate coverage of HDC/ASCR for all diagnoses for which it is considered standard treatment and, in addition, specifically for breast cancer, multiple myeloma, and epithelial ovarian cancer' for the approximately 200 insurers participating in the Federal Health Benefits program, which covers nine million federal employees." ECRI, February 1995, at 10. See also Hoffman, 1999; Korobkin, 1999.

10. Hall, Smith, Naughton, et al., 1996, at 1063.

11. Morreim 1995(a).

12. For instance, numerous suits have been brought by plaintiffs seeking coverage for autologous bone marrow transplant (ABMT), particularly for advanced breast cancer. See, e.g., Goepel v. National Mail Handlers Union, 36 F.3d 306 (3d Cir. 1994); Fuja v. Benefit Trust Life Ins. Co., 18 F.3d 1405 (7th Cir. 1994); Harris v. Blue Cross Blue Shield, 995 F.2d 877 (8th Cir. 1993); Nesseim v. Mail Handlers Benefits Plan, 995 F.2d 804 (8th Cir. 1993); Harris v. Mutual of Omaha Cos., 992 F.2d 706 (7th Cir. 1993); Bailey v. Blue Cross/Blue Shield, 866 F. Supp. 277 (E.D. Va. 1994), aff'd, 67 F.3d 53 (4th Cir. 1995); Calhoun v. Complete Health Care, Inc., 860 F. Supp. 1494 (S.D. Ala. 1994), aff'd, 61 F.3d 31 (11th Cir. 1995); Arrington v. Group Hospitalization & Med. Serv., 806 F. Supp. 287 (D.D.C. 1992); Wilson v. Group Hospitalization & Med. Servs., Inc., 791 F. Supp. 309 (D.D.C. 1992), appeal dismissed, 995 F.2d 306 (D.C. Cir. 1993); Pirozzi v. Blue Cross-Blue Shield, 741 F. Supp. 586 (E.D. Va. 1990); Sweeney v. Gerber Products Co. Med. Benefits Plan, 728 F. Supp. 594 (D. Neb. 1989); Thomas v. Gulf Health Plan, Inc., 688 F. Supp. 590 (S.D. Ala. 1988).

13. Mimbs v. Commercial Life Ins. Co., 832 F. Supp. 354, 358 (S.D. Ga. 1993) (footnote omitted). See also Conrad, Seiter, 1995, at 191: "Because lack of coverage frequently translates, at least as a practical matter, to lack of access to care, prospective and concurrent utilization review can expose a health plan to liability claims of a kind from which indemnity plans are largely insulated." The major exception to this practice is the Emergency Medical Treatment and Active Labor Act (EMTALA), which forbids hospitals with emergency departments from requiring assurance of payment before screening and stabilizing patients in an emergency condition. See 42 U.S.C. § 1395dd (1994).

14. See Loyola Univ. of Chicago v. Humana Ins. Co., 996 F.2d 895 (7th Cir. 1993); Reilly v. Blue Cross and Blue Shield United, 846 F.2d 416 (7th Cir. 1988); Blue Cross and Blue Shield v. Brown, 800 S.W.2d 724 (Ark. Ct. App. 1990); Sarchett v. Blue Shield, 729 P.2d 267 (Cal. 1987).

15. For example, in Mimbs v. Commercial Life Insurance Co., 832 F. Supp. 354 (S.D. Ga. 1993), an insurer refused to verify for a hospital that the patient had insurance to cover expenses for heart surgery. The patient's surgery was delayed for more than a month, allegedly causing a permanent deterioration in his condition that, in turn, forced him to sell his business. In other examples, patients' estates have brought wrongful death suits on the grounds that the health plan's refusal to pay for or provide a certain treatment caused the patient's death. See Dukes v. U.S. Healthcare, Inc., 57 F.3d 350 (3d Cir. 1995); Kuhl v. Lincoln Nat'l Health Plan, 999 F.2d 298 (8th Cir. 1993); Spain v. Aetna Life Ins. Co., 11 F.3d 129 (9th Cir. 1993); Corcoran v. United Healthcare, Inc., 965 F.2d 1321 (5th Cir. 1992); Nealy v. U.S. Healthcare HMO, 844 F. Supp. 966 (S.D.N.Y. 1994); Dunn v. Praiss, 606 A.2d 862 (N.J. Super. Ct. App. Div. 1992).

16. As Havighurst notes, a classic problem in contract law is "to determine the proper approach for courts to adopt in interpreting incomplete or ambiguous contracts. Some rules of interpretation have evolved. One example . . . is the principle of *contra proferentem,* which requires the ambiguities . . . to be construed against the . . . drafter of the contract, in an effort to honor the 'reasonable expectations' of the insured." Havighurst, 1995, at 182.

17. "Ambiguities in the plan should be resolved against the insurer." Bucci v. Blue Cross-Blue Shield of Connecticut, 764 F. Supp. 728, 730 (D.Conn. 1991). "If a court finds that an insurance policy is ambiguous, . . . an ambiguous policy will be construed in favor of the insured." Katskee v. Blue Cross/Blue Shield, 515 NW2d 645, 647 (Neb. 1994). See also McLaughlin v. Connecticut General Life Ins. Co., 565 F. Supp. 434, 440 (N.D. Cal. 1983). For further discussion and case citations see Havighurst, Blumstein, Brennan, 1998, at 1223–30. See also I.V. Serv. v. Trustees of Am. Consulting Engineers, 136 F.3d 114 (2nd Cir. 1998) (finding ambiguity in contract terms as applied to AIDS patient receiving off-label drug treatment for neutropenia that occurred as a result of other drugs with which the patient was being treated). The court noted that it is important to look at "how the Plan language has been interpreted by the Plan administrators in the past; and (2) who drafted the contract terms" (at 120). For further discussion of ambiguities in the context of insurance law, see Swisher, 2000, at 735–42.

18. Commonly, "medically necessary means medically appropriate. It excludes experimental care, nonstandard treatments, treatment without any known benefit, and treatment such as cosmetic surgery not intended to relieve a medical condition." Hall, Smith, Naughton, et al., 1996, at 1055. "Under the test of 'medical necessity,' which serves almost universally as the contractual touch-

stone of plan coverage, the criteria used to check the spending discretion of providers are almost exclusively medical, not economic." Havighurst, 1995, at 15.

19. Coverage categories might include inpatient care and outpatient care (including hospital and health professional services for both emergency and nonemergency situations); care for mental illness and substance abuse; prescription drugs; laboratory, radiology, and diagnostic services; home health care and hospice services; durable medical equipment; rehabilitation; and the like. Not all plans cover all categories, and some place monetary caps on certain categories, such as mental health services. Also, for care within their covered categories, plans typically carve out exceptions, most commonly for services that are "experimental" or "innovative."

20. Havighurst, 1995

21. See Havighurst, 1995, at 14–16, 110–19.

22. Daniels, Sabin, 1998; Morreim 1997(b); Morreim, 2000(a); Hall, Anderson, 1992, at 1683–93; Bergthold, 1995, at 183; Mariner, 1994, at 1516.

23. See James, 1991, at 365 (discussing DiDomenico v. Employers Coop. Indus. Trust, 676 F. Supp. 903 [N.D. Ind. 1987], which involved a health care plan that refused to cover "experimental" transplants but failed to determine which transplants were experimental); Barber, 1996, at 399–406 (surveying cases involving disputes over health care plans' vague or nonexistent definitions of "experimental" treatments excluded from coverage); Bergthold, 1995; Havighurst, 1995, at 15, 110 ff.; Holder, 1994; Holoweiko, 1995, at 180; Steinberg, Tunis, Shapiro, 1995; Havighurst, Blumstein, Brennan, 1998, at 1223–30.

When employers directly contract for services with providers such as physicians and hospitals rather than going through established health plans, benefit specification may be even less explicit.

24. For further discussion see Chapter 8, § B-1.

25. See Morris v. Metriyakool, 344 N.W.2d 736, 756 (Mich. 1984) (Ryan, J., concurring). ("A contract of adhesion is a contract which has some or all of the following characteristics: the parties to the contract were of unequal bargaining strength; the contract is expressed in standardized language prepared by the stronger party to meet his needs; and the contract is offered by the stronger party to the weaker party on a 'take it or leave it' basis"; citation omitted). *Id.*

"[T]he stronger party drafts the contract, and the weaker has no opportunity, either personally or through an agent, to negotiate concerning its terms." Madden v. Kaiser Found. Hosps., 552 P.2d 1178, 1185 (Cal. 1976). See also Wheeler v. St. Joseph Hospital, 133 Cal. Rptr. 775 (Cal. App. 1977); McLaughlin v. Connecticut General Life Ins. Co., 565 F. Supp. 434, 447–48 (N.D. Cal. 1983).

For further discussion of contracts of adhesion, see Havighurst 1986(a), at 166–170; Morreim, 1997(b), at 45–46; Anderson, Hall, Steinberg, 1993, at 1636 (defining contracts of adhesion as "contracts . . . in which the subscriber cannot effectively bargain with the insurer to change specific terms"); Ferguson, Dubinsky, Kirsch, 1993, at 2120 ("[C]ourts generally hold that printed insurance contracts, in contrast to other types of business contracts, are to be interpreted most strongly against the party preparing the form on the grounds that an insured must sign such a contract or otherwise forego the service."); Gottsegen, 1981, at 140–41 (describing court's tendency to "recognize that insurance policies are not genuinely negotiated agreements, but contracts of adhesion written by the insurer and available only on a take-it-or-leave-it basis"); Kalb, 1990, at 1125–26 (recognizing and counseling against courts' tendency to classify insurance contracts as contracts of adhesion); Havighurst, Blumstein, Brennan, 1998, at 1223–30; Swisher, 2000, at 758–762.

26. Tunkl v. Regents of University of California, 383 P.2d 411 (Cal. 1963); Olson v. Molzen, 558 S.W. 2d 429 (Tn. 1977); Emory University v. Porubiansky, 282 S.E. 2d 903 (Ga. 1981); Ash v. New York University Dental Center, 564 N.Y.S.2d 308, 311 (A.D. 1 Dist. 1990); Meiman v. Rehabilitation Center, Inc., Ky. 444 S.W. 2d 78 (Ky. 1969); Cudnick v. William Beaumont Hospital, 525 N.W.2d 891 (Mich. App. 1994); Wheeler v. St. Joseph Hospital, 133 Cal. Rptr. 775 (Cal. App. 1977).

In contrast, courts will sometimes let exculpatory contracts stand. In Massengill v. S.M.A.R.T., 996 P.2d 1132 (Wyo. 2000), for instance, a member of a sports and fitness club was held to the terms of an exculpatory contract he signed upon enrolling in the club. In evaluating a negligence exculpatory clause, courts should consider four factors: " '(1) whether a duty to the public exists; (2) the nature of the service performed; (3) whether the contract was fairly entered into; and (4) whether the intention of the parties is expressed in clear and unambiguous language' " (996 P.2d 1136). In this case, the arrangement was entirely voluntary and did not concern any public duty.

27. In Wheeler v. St. Joseph Hospital, 133 Cal. Rptr. 775 (Cal. App. 1977), a California appellate court found that although arbitration agreements were not in principle against public policy, a

hospital's requirement that patients agree to arbitration as a condition of admission constituted an unenforceable adhesion contract.

Note that in some other cases courts upheld arbitration clauses—but only when the court felt the clause was not adhesory. See, e.g., Madden v. Kaiser Found. Hosps., 552 P.2d 1178, 1185 (Cal. 1976); Erickson v. Aetna Health Plans of Cal., 84 Cal.Rptr.2d 76 (Cal.App. 4 Dist. 1999); Morris v. Metriyakool, 344 N.W.2d 736, 756 (Mich. 1984). In these cases courts have been careful to note that the definition of adhesion was not met: the health plan's enrollees did have bargaining power, and they did have alternative choices. See also Daly, 1995; Havighurst, 1995, at 124, 272 ff.; Mehlman, 1993, at 356.

28. One study pegs the figure at 84%. Blendon, Brodie, Benson, 1995, at 243; American College of Physicians, 1996, at 845.

Another study concluded that 78% of firms offer just one plan, although often with multiple products, such as a POS version of an HMO (point-of-service, permitting expanded choices for added fees). Berenson, 1997, at 173.

Yet another study found that "[surveys have estimated that 44–58 percent of workers who have insurance are given no choice of plans. However, even persons who have options may be denied effective choice. For example, an employer may drop an employee's plan from the available list, forcing him or her to change." In this study, 42% of respondents said they had no choice of health plan when they enrolled in their current health plan. Of those with choices, 20% said they had too little choice; 31% said employer forced them to change health plans in the past 5 years. Overall, 63% had no choice, inadequate variety, or a forced change of health plans. Gawande, Blendon, Brodie, 1998, at 186–88.

From a somewhat different vantage point, a study looking at workers rather than employers found that 48% of employees have only one health plan available, while 23% have only two plans to choose from, and 12% have three plans to choose from. Etheredge, Jones, Lewin, 1996 at 94.

29. Interesting arguments lie on both sides of this issue. If one views health care as essentially a gift, an "extra" that the employer voluntarily adds on to the employee's wages, then it is not so odd to suppose that the health plan's duties are to the employer more than to the patient—and that it is the employer, not the patient, who is shortchanged by a plan's failure to deliver adequate resources.

On the other hand, one might suppose that the employee pays for and owns the health care package, even though the employer does the actual contracting work in order to secure the tax advantages of employment-based health care and to gain the price advantage of the employer's bargaining power. In this scenario the health plan owes its duties to the employee (subscriber), more than to the employer. Even if the employee had little or no choice among plans, it is still likely that because of the two economic advantages of work-based health benefits, the plan is better and/or cheaper than anything the employee could have afforded on her own. Hence, there may still be good reason to enforce an employment-based contract even if the employee had little choice among plans.

30. See Gleason, 1995, at 1483; Mariner, 1995.

31. Holder, 1994, at 19; Holoweiko, 1995.

32. Employee Retirement Income Security Act, 29 U.S.C. §§ 1001–1461 (1994). ERISA will be discussed extensively in Chapter 11.

33. See, e.g., Firestone Tire & Rubber Co. v. Bruch, 489 U.S. 101, 115 (1989); Barnett v. Kaiser Found. Health Plan Inc., 32 F.3d 413, 415–16 (9th Cir. 1994).

34. See Salley v. E.I. DuPont de Nemours & Co., 966 F.2d 1011, 1014 (5th Cir. 1992); Reilly v. Blue Cross & Blue Shield United, 846 F.2d 416, 419 (7th Cir. 1988); Leonhardt v. Holden Bus. Forms Co., 828 F. Supp. 657, 665 (D. Minn. 1993).

35. See, e.g., Bucci v. Blue Cross-Blue Shield of Connecticut, 764 F. Supp. 728 (D.Conn. 1991); Doe v. Travelers Ins. Co., 971 F.Supp. 623 (D.Mass. 1997) (upheld, 167 F.3d 53 (1st Cir. 1999)); Leonhardt v. Holden Business Forms Co., 828 F. Supp. 657 (D. Minn. 1993); Calhoun v. Complete Health Care, Inc., 860 F.Supp. 1494 (S.C.Ala. 1994); Wilson v. CHAMPUS, 65 F.3d 361 (4th Cir. 1995). For further discussion, see Morreim, 1997(b); Morreim 1998(b).

36. Reciprocally, when contracts are clearly written and fairly enforced, courts are much more likely to enforce them. See Chapter 11; see also Morreim, 1995(a).

37. Furthermore, in cases in which a health plan denies a resource that by contract the patient should have received, such cheering is entirely appropriate.

38. Contracts with such widespread, important, concealed provisions are generally not enforceable as the "meeting of the minds" required for bona fide contracts. See, eg, DeMott, 1988, at 903 (noting some protections built into contract law: "the classical rules of offer and acceptance, by requiring that an acceptance precisely mirror the terms of the offer to which it responds, delay

contract formation and thereby create opportunities for reflection and exit from improvident commitments") (footnotes omitted).

39. For further discussion, see Morreim, 1991(a), Chapter 7; Morreim 1995(b); Morreim, 1994(a).

40. For further discussion, see Morreim 1995(c).

41. Retchin, Brown, Yeh, 1997; Webster, Feinglass, 1997; Retchin, Penberthy, Desch, et al., 1997; Goldzweig, Mittman, Carter, et al., 1997; Obstbaum, 1997; Batavia, 1999. See also Adelson v. GTE Corp., 790 F. Supp. 1265 (D.Md. 1992); Bedrick v. Travelers Insur. Co., 93 F.3d 149 (4th Cir, 1996).

For further discussion and additional citations documenting the ways in which managed care finances may be eroding the coverage available for quality of life–oriented care, see Morreim, 2000(b).

42. Morreim, 1995(a).

43. Pitsenberger, 1999, at 323.

A third scenario raises an interesting public policy challenge—one that will be identified but not explored in depth here. In some instances a contract will clearly state that a particular intervention is not covered, but a court may conclude that no acceptable health plan should deny this or that particular kind of coverage. That is, the courts overrule the health plan by reason of public policy rather than on grounds of contract. In Blue Cross and Blue Shield v. Brown, 800 S.W. 2d 724 (Ark. App. 1990), for instance, an Arkansas appellate court overturned an insurer's provision that denied coverage for inpatient services when a patient terminates his or her own admission against medical advice. The court invalidated the exclusion on the ground that it was contrary to public policy. "'This policy exclusion would divest the insured of benefits already accrued, for which no reasonable basis exists. We conclude that the exclusion of benefits prior to an AMA [against medical advice] discharge is against public policy.'" 800 S.W. 2d at 725–26, citing Arkansas Supreme Court in Arkansas BCBS v. Long, 792 S.W.2d 602 (1990).

44. Grumet, 1989. See also Ogrod, 1997; Light, 1992, at 2505–06; Kenagy, Berwick, Shore, 1999; Mayer, Cates, 1999; Kassirer, 1995.

45. Wynia, Cummins, VanGeest, et al., 2000; Novack, Detering, Arnold, et al., 1989.

46. Morreim, 1991(b); Freeman, Rathore, Weinfurt, et al., 1999.

CHAPTER 5

1. See, e.g., BMW v. Gore, 116 S.Ct. 1589, 1598 (1996): "Elementary notions of fairness enshrined in our constitutional jurisprudence dictate that a person receive fair notice not only of the conduct that will subject him to punishment, but also of the severity of the penalty that a State may impose."

2. For further discussion of that reorganization see Morreim, 1999, at 944–950; Landon, Wilson, Cleary, 1998; Morreim, 1997(b), at 8–16; Iglehart, 1992; Iglehart, 1995; Kletke, Emmons, Gillis, 1996.

3. American Medical Association v. United States, 317 U.S. 519 (1943).

4. Chase-Lubitz, 1987, at 475. The FTC found several anticompetitive effects of the corporate ban: "First, the provisions sought to limit price competition among doctors by fixing the adequacy of compensation and by prohibiting competitive bidding. Second, the provisions inhibited competition by limiting hospitals, prepaid health plans, and lay entities to the traditional fee-for-service method of compensation and by proscribing their use of salaries and other more cost-efficient payment methods. Last, the provisions restricted arrangements between physicians and nonphysicians and, therefore, prevented the creation of more economical business structures" (at 476–77). See American Medical Association v. F.T.C. 638 F. 2d 443 (2nd. Cir. 1980), aff'd per curiam 455 U.S. 676 (1982); United States v. Oregon Medical Society, 343 U.S. 326 (1952); American Medical Association v. United States, 317 U.S. 519 (1943).

See also Rosoff, 1987, at 493; Mars, 1997, at 268; Dowell, 1994, at 370; Parker, 1996, at 167.

5. Mars, 1997, at 251–52.

6. Mars, 1997, at 265–66. See also Dowell, 1994, at 372: In the corporate employment context, the "management agreement should clearly acknowledge the physician will have complete control over matters of diagnosis, treatment, and medical judgment." See also Hayward, 1996, at 428.

7. Tenn. Code Ann. §§ 63–6–204, 63–6–225 & 63–11–205. See also Mars, 1997, at 276–77.

8. Hayward, 1996, citing So. Dak. statute at 428: S.D. Codified Laws Ann. § 36–4–8.1 (Supp. 1995).

In like manner, the Texas HMO Act stipulates that the act does not "authorize any person to regulate, interfere, or intervene in any manner in the practice of medicine or any healing art." Williams v. Good Health Plus, Inc., 743 S.W.2d 373, 375 (Tex.App.–San Antonio 1988).

The Louisiana State Board of Medical Examiners has officially opined that "a corporation may not necessarily be said, by the mere fact of employing a physician to practice medicine, and by that fact alone, to be itself practicing medicine. As contemplated by the Medical Practice Act, the essence of the practice of medicine is the exercise of independent medical judgment in the diagnosing, treating, curing or relieving of any bodily or mental disease, condition, infirmity, deformity, defect, ailment, or injury in any human being . . .' If a corporate employer seeks to impose or substitute its judgment for that of the physician in any of these functions, or the employment is otherwise structured so as to undermine the essential incidents of the physician patient relationship, the Medical Practice Act will have been violated. But if a physician employment relationship is so established and maintained as to avoid such intrusions, it will not run afoul of the Medical Practice Act." Board of Medical Examiners. Statement of Position: Corporate Practice of Medicine; Applicability of Louisiana Medical Practice Act to Employment of Physician by Corporation Other than a Professional Medical Corporation. September 24, 1992, p. 2 (re. La.Rev. Stat. §§ 37:1261–1292). See also Mt. Sinai Hospital v. Zorek, 271 NYS2d 1012, 1016 (NY Civ Ct 1966).

9. In a bit of irony it may be noted that this proposal, in essence, says that health plans and hospitals should be able to employ physicians as long as they do not truly satisfy the legal definition of an "employer," i.e., one who controls and directs the actions of the employee. As noted in Daw's Critical Care v. Dept. of Labor, 622 A.2d 622, 631 (Conn.Super. 1992), " '[t]he test of the relationship is the right to control. . . .' "

Some courts might find such a move odd. "The very nature of a radiologist's function requires the exercise of independent professional judgment. Accordingly, a hospital is not in a position to, and generally does not, exercise control over a radiologist's performance of his or her professional activities." Pamperin v. Trinity Memorial, 423 N.W.2d 848, 848 (Wis. 1988). Similarly, as noted by the Wisconsin Supreme Court, "Mount Sinai may have required that physicians supplied by MPP be members of Mount Sinai's staff, and required the physicians to comply with the policies, by-laws, rules, and regulations of Mount Sinai. That does not indicate that a master–servant relationship existed any more than it did in Pamperin. . . . Mount Sinai did not reserve control and there are no facts alleged to indicate that they had the right of control over the discretion and specific professional techniques in performing medical procedures employed by Dr. Port." Kashishian v. Port, 481 N.W.2d 277, 280 (Wis. 1992).

10. Muse v. Charter Hosp. Winston-Salem Inc., 452 S.E.2d 589 (N.C.App. 1995), aff'd 464 SE2d 44. See Chapter 2, and Chapter 3 § C.

11. Muse v. Charter Hosp. Winston-Salem Inc., 452 S.E.2d 589, 594 (N.C.App. 1995), aff'd 464 S.E.2d 44. Interestingly, other potentially relevant causal factors were dismissed by the court. The patient could have been transferred to a state facility but was not. Instead, he was doing reasonably well at discharge and went on a week-long vacation with family, after which he began outpatient treatment. Questions were raised about the quality of physicians' care, both in the inpatient and subsequent outpatient settings. Nevertheless, the court still held that the hospital was the cause of the boy's subsequent suicide because it had interfered with medical judgment.

12. A strikingly similar view is expressed in dicta by the Seventh Circuit. "We must remember that doctors, not insurance executives, are qualified experts in determining what is the best course of treatment and therapy for their patients. Trained physicians, and them [sic] alone, should be allowed to make care-related decisions (with, of course, input from the patient). Medical care should not be subject to the whim of the new layer of insurance bureaucracy now dictating the most basic, as well as the important, medical policies and procedures from the boardroom." Herdrich v. Pegram, 154 F.3d 362, 377 (7th Cir. 1998), reversed, Pegram v. Herdrich, 120 U.S. 2143 (2000).

See also Wickline v. State of California, 192 Cal. App. 3d 1630, 1645 (1987): Although "[t]hird party payors of health care services can be held legally accountable when medically inappropriate decisions result from defects in the design or implementation of cost containment mechanisms . . . the physician who complies without protest with the limitations imposed by a third party payor, when his medical judgment dictates otherwise, cannot avoid his ultimate responsibility for his patient's care. He cannot point to the health care payor as the liability scapegoat when the consequences of his own determinative medical decisions go sour" (dicta, emphasis added).

See also Pappas v. Asbel, 675 A.2d 711, 716 (Pa.Super. 1996): "Considerations of cost containment of the type which drive the decision making process in HMO's did not exist for employee welfare plans when ERISA was enacted." Aff'd, 724 A.2d 889 (Pa. 1998), vacated, 120 S.Ct. 2686.

See also Mt. Sinai Hospital v. Zorek, 271 NYS2d 1012, 1016 (NY Civ Ct 1966): "Once the treating doctor has decided on a course of treatment for which hospitalization is necessary, his judgment cannot be retrospectively challenged."

13. For a more detailed discussion of capitation and other risk-sharing arrangements, see Chapter 6 § B-2.

14. In Pegram v. Herdrich, 120 U.S. 2143, 2150 (2000), the plaintiff argued that physician-owned HMOs posed conflicts of interest incompatible with the loyalty duties of ERISA fiduciaries. The Supreme Court held that such risk-bearing arrangements are not inherently unacceptable but left the door open to legislative constraints on such arrangements. See Chapter 10 § B-1 and Chapter 11 § C-2–a.

15. See Morreim, 2000(c), at 705–706.

16. A number of courts have found that it is legitimate for health plans, at least under some conditions, to deny coverage for resources that a physician might otherwise like to use. See, e.g., Sarchett v. Blue Shield of California, 729 P. 2d 267, 272–73 (Cal. 1987); Lockshin v. Blue Cross of Northeast Ohio, 434 N.E. 2d 754, 756 (Ohio App. 1980); Free v. Travelers Ins. Co., 551 F. Supp. 554, 560 (D. Md.1982); Blue Cross & Blue Shield of Ky. v. Smither, 573 S.W.2d 363, 365 (Ky. App. 1978). But see Van Vactor v. Blue Cross Ass'n, 365 N.E. 2d 638 (Ill. 1977).

17. Abraham, Weiler, 1994; Sage, Hastings, Berenson, 1994; Abraham, Weiler,1994(b). For an excellent discussion of historical and current concepts of enterprise liability, see Sage, 1997.

18. Sage, 1997, at 159–64, 169–70, 191; Havighurst, 1997, at 603–6, 622.

19. Havighurst, 1997, at 587. They should thus bear all liability "for personal injuries and other losses arising from care rendered by health care providers to enrollees under the contract between the health plan and the purchaser of coverage." Havighurst, 1997, at 626. Enterprise liability, in other words, would be a form of automatic vicarious liability. *Id.*, at 617. Enterprise liability might also be described in terms of "nondelegable" duties (at 614). For further discussion of the notion of nondelegable duties, see also Walls v. Hazelton State General Hosp., 629 A.2d 232 (Pa.Cmwlth 1993); Sampson v. Baptist Memorial Hosp. System, 940 S.W.2d 128 (Tex.App.–San Antonio 1996); Thompson v. Nason Hosp., 591 A.2d 703 (Pa. 1991); Simmons v. Tuomey Regional Medical Center, 498 S.E.2d 408 (S.C.App. 1998), aff'd as modified, 533 S.E.2d 312 (S.C. 2000); Chittenden, 1991, at 464–65.

Sage discusses the merits of the idea, though he does not so heartily endorse it. Sage, 1997. Brewbaker discusses a related notion, suggesting that health plans should be held to an implied warranty on the quality of their care. Brewbaker distinguishes implied warranties from enterprise liability mainly insofar as the latter, but not the former, restricts liability exclusively to the health plan or some other single entity. Under this approach, physicians could still be liable alongside the health plan. See Brewbaker, 1997, at 147–48.

20. Havighurst, 2000, at 8.

21. Havighurst, 2000, at 9.

22. Havighurst, 2000, at 8.

23. Sage, 1997, at 164, 166; Havighurst, 1997, at 589, 599; Havighurst, 2000, at 10–20.

24. Sage, 1997, at 167, 196; Havighurst, 1997, at 599–600; Havighurst, 2000, at 14–17.

25. Sage, 1997, at 166.

26. Havighurst, 1997, at 590–91. As troubling questions about MCOs' quality of care are pressed, "a strong backlash against HMOs and other managed care plans is threatening to move many decisions out of the hands of competing health plans and into the hands of Congress or state legislatures" (at 591).

27. Havighurst, 1997, at 588.

28. Havighurst, 1997, at 594–95.

29. McDonald, 1996.

30. See Gold, Hurley, Lake, 1995; McDonald, 1996; Trauner, Chesnutt, 1996; Felsenthal, 1996.

31. Horn, Sharkey, Tracy, et al., 1996; Streja, Hui, Streja, et al., 1999; Soumerai, McLaughlin, Ross-Degnan, et al., 1994; Soumerai, Ross-Degnan, Avorn, et al., 1991; Soumerai, Ross-Degnan, Fortess, et al., 1993; Schroeder, Cantor, 1991; Horn, Sharkey, Phillips-Harris, 1998.

32. Goldfarb, 1995, at 546; Shapiro, Wenger, 1995; Bree, Kazerooni, Katz, 1996; Feldstein, Wickizer, Wheeler, 1988; Field, Gray, 1989; Rosenberg, Allen, Handte, et al., 1995; Kleinman, Boyd, Heritage, 1997; Zalta, 1991; Kapur, Joyce, van Vorst, et al., 2000.

33. Gerber, Bijlefeld, 1996; Kirsner, Federman, 1996; Gerbert, Maurer, Berger, et al., 1996.

34. Havighurst proposes that health plans need not inevitably bear all liability. They can negotiate to share risk with providers if this seems prudent. See Havighurst, 2000. Although in principle such an option is available, in practice it can be very difficult for physicians, particularly those in small group practices, to negotiate the terms of their contracts with large health plans. The more

dominant a particular plan is in a given market, the less leverage physicians have. Indeed, this discrepancy of bargaining power, whether real or perceived, has driven increasing numbers of physicians to inquire into the possibility of unions and collective bargaining. Yacht, 2000; Cohen, 2000; Quinn, 2000; Azevedo, 1997; Lowes, 1998; Roemer, 1998; Marcus, 1984; Mangan, 1995.

35. Havighurst himself has noted the connection between risk and control in an earlier work, suggesting that hospitals might willingly accept increased liability in order to gain the power of increased control. He notes hospitals' response to the case of Darling v. Charleston Community Memorial Hospital, 211 N.E. 2d 253 (Ill. 1965), in which a liability was imposed on a hospital for its physician staff's failures: "More surprising than the legal result in that case was the widespread reaction to it, which suggested that hospital managers had been waiting for some excuse to demand more cooperation and quality assurance from their medical staffs." Havighurst, 1984, at 1079. In this way, hospitals' governing boards and staff committees gained legitimacy. The upshot, however, is that risk is closely connected with the need to exert control.

36. See Chapter 1, n. 2; Chapter 2, n. 59.

37. For further discussion of defensive medicine, see Chapter 2, n. 83.

38. As noted in Chapter 2, the strongest predictor of whether a physician will be sued is often the extent to which patients feel that they are being treated with honesty, respect, and personal interest. See Beckman, Markakis, Suchmen, et al., 1994, at 1368–69; Hickson, Clayton, Githens, et al., 1992, at 1362; Hickson, Clayton, Entman, et al., 1994, at 186; Huycke, Huycke, 1994, at 797; Levinson, 1994, at 1620; Anderson, 1995, at 39, 42; Kam, 1995, at 42, 44.

39. Physician groups have already raised a number of these concerns. Havighurst, 1997, at 628; Sage, 1997, at 170 (n. 46); Kassirer, 1995.

40. The case of Helling v. Carey, 519 P.2d 981 (Wash. 1974), was discussed briefly in Chapter 2 § B-3-a. In that case the Washington Supreme Court rewrote the standard of care to supplant a physician-based standard it considered to be inadequate. A young woman visited her ophthalmologist repeatedly for eye problems, but her underlying glaucoma was discovered too late to save her sight. Because glaucoma is almost completely confined to older patients, physicians did not routinely test patients under age forty. The court saw fit to change the standard of care, contradicting prevailing practice.

> The precaution of giving this test to detect the incidence of glaucoma to patients under 40 years of age is so imperative that irrespective of its disregard by the standards of the opthalmology [sic] profession, it is the duty of the courts to say what is required to protect patients under 40 from the damaging results of glaucoma. We therefore hold, as a matter of law, that the reasonable standard that should have been followed under the undisputed facts of this case was the timely giving of this simple, harmless pressure test and that, in failing to do so, the defendants were negligent, which proximately resulted in the blindness sustained by the plaintiff for which the defendants are liable.

519 P.2d 983.

Interestingly, the court's judgment was not as wise as it presumed. Once one recognizes that the tonometry test used to detect glaucoma has very poor sensitivity and specificity (that is, it has high numbers of both false-positives and false-negatives), and once these are brought to the under-40 population that has a very low incidence of glaucoma, the actual value of the test is astonishingly low, and cumulative costs are stunningly high. On one analysis, if the test were routinely used for patients under age 40, for every one patient whose glaucoma was correctly diagnosed by the test, some 17,500 other young people would have test results that falsely indicated the presence of glaucoma. If the test were repeated on this group, the number of false-positives would be reduced to 12,250. In all, "twenty-eight rounds of tonometry tests, 83,348 separate tests, would be required to reduce the number of false positives to fewer than two. At a mean charge of $25 per test, this series of tests would cost $2,083,700." Fortess, Kapp, 1985, at 217.

41. Havighurst, 1997, at 616.

42. Morreim, 2000(a).

43. Brennan, Leape, Laird, et al., 1991.

44. Anderson, 1995; Kam, 1995; Levinson, 1994; Levinson, Roter, Mullooly, et al., 1997; Lawthers, Localio, Lair, et al., 1992; Shapiro, Simpson, Lawrence, et al., 1989; Sommers, 1985; Rice, 1995; Menken, 1992, at 58.

45. Bennett v. Indiana State Board of R. and E., 7 N.E.2d 977, 981 (Ind. 1937). Similarly, the South Dakota Supreme Court feared an "undue emphasis on mere money making, and commercial exploitation of professional services. . . . Such an ethical, trustworthy and unselfish professionalism as the community needs and wants cannot survive in a purely commercial atmosphere." Bartron v. Codington County, 2 N.W.2d 337, 346 (So.Dak. 1942).

46. In re. Co-operative Law Co., 92 N.E. 15, 16 (N.Y. 1910).

47. Physicians and plans, of course, are hardly the only players in the delivery of health care. Employers, other kinds of providers and, above all, patients have a key role to play. However, physicians have the legally crucial power of prescription and with it a virtual monopoly over access to many diagnostic and therapeutic interventions. Health plans, including employers when plans are self-funded, have a rather similar near monopoly over access to the funding that is prerequisite to most health care. Because these two entities play such a crucial role, attention here will focus on them.

48. See, generally, Morreim, 2000(a); Morreim, 1998.

49. For a useful introduction, with references, concerning the defining characteristics of professions, see Ozar, 1995.

50. Morreim, 1998, at 331.

51. According to one estimate, some seventy-five national organizations have developed about 1800 sets of guidelines. Gabel, 1997, at 142.

52. As noted by Feinstein, clinical research, as opposed to basic science and laboratory research, has long been looked down upon as being somehow inferior "applied" work. As a result, until recently funding has focused mainly on the latter and not on the former. Feinstein, 1994. And as noted by other commentators, those who use guidelines "cannot help but notice that guideline developers must often reckon with research that is modest in rigor, discordant, or nonexistent. Although most guidelines are an amalgam of evidence and expert opinion, methods of integrating knowledge and experience into guidelines, particularly when data are sparse, are neither as mature nor as transparent as methods of incorporating research results." Cook, Giacomini, 1999, at 1950.

53. A number of factors make such research difficult. Unlike a drug, the effectiveness of an invasive procedure is heavily dependent on providers' varying skills, including improvements in skill with repetition of the procedure. As it is difficult to measure or control for such variation, the research is less reliable. Further, in surgery it is impossible to do fully blinded studies, as required in the classic randomized, double-blind, controlled trial, since of course the surgeon will know which procedure he is performing. Placebo controls, another common feature of "gold-standard" science, are usually not accepted in this realm given the high risks of "sham" surgery. Moreover, patients are not as willing to be randomized in the case of surgical or invasive procedures as they are for drug trials. See Frader, Caniano, 1998; Freeman, Vawter, Leaverton, et al., 1999; Macklin, 1999.

54. Dalen, 1998, at 2180.

55. Dalen, 1998, at 2179.

56. Hall, 2000; Rapoport, Teres, Steingrub, et al., 2000; Bernard, Sopko, Cerra, et al. , 2000.

57. Bennett, 1993; Merkatz, Temple, Sobel, et al., 1993.

58. Soumerai, Ross-Degnan, Fortess, et al., 1993; Balas, Kretschmer, Gnann, et al., 1998; Kassirer, Angell, 1994, at 669; Evans, 1995, at 59; Epstein, 1995, at 58, 59; Feinstein, 1994, at 800; Krimsky, 1999, at 1475; Perry, Thamer, 1999, at 1870.

"These guidelines activities are uncoordinated, however, and different agencies sometimes issue different guidelines on the same topic. Occasionally, their recommendations conflict. At least some of these differences are probably attributable to the vastly different methods used to create the guidelines. Methodological differences include the types of people selected to be in the expert group, methods used to collect and synthesize evidence, methods used to structure the group discussion and arrive at consensus, and degree to which recommendations are linked directly with the evidence behind them." Power, 1995. See also Holoweiko, 1995, at 181.

Economic analysis in particular may require "unique methodologic choices, such as which types of costs to include (direct, indirect, intangible, induced), which perspective to apply (that of society, payer, provider, patient), which design to adopt (cost-identification, cost-benefit, cost-effectiveness, cost-utility), from where to obtain costs (indemnity database, managed care or capitated database, hospital cost systems, Medicare, Medicaid), and whether to collect resource consumption data prospectively or retrospectively through various modeling techniques." Task Force on Principles for Economic Analysis of Health Care Technology, 1995, at 61–62.

In designating endpoints of study, one study might take survival alone as the mark of success, while another might focus on survival without major neurological deficits. Whyte, Fitzhardinge, Shennen, et al., 1993; Allen, Donohue, Dusman, 1993.

59. Hornberger, Wrone, 1997; Ray, 1997; Iezzoni, 1997.

60. "Even when measures are aggregated, statistical power may be insufficient to detect a significant improvement in outcomes. For example, in a modestly sized health plan with 25,000 members, one might estimate that 150 persons will have diabetes and use insulin. Even if all 150 participated in a program that reduced the number of diabetes-related complications by 50% through improved

diet, exercise, and appropriate use of insulin, the statistical power would be too low to document the program value compared with complication rates with a previous program." Epstein, Sherwood, 1996, at 833. See also Durham, 1998, at 114.

For further discussion of the scientific problems behind health plans' practice guidelines, see Eddy, 1993(b); Woolf, Lawrence, 1997; American College of Physicians, 1994; Hillman, Eisenberg, Pauly, et al., 1991; Kessler, Rose, Temple, et al., 1994; Brody, 1995; Stelfox, Chua, O'Rourke, et al., 1998; Rennie, 1997; Anders, 12/15/94, B-6; Task Force on Principles for Economic Analysis of Health Care Technology, 1995; Kassirer, Angell, 1994, at 669; Evans, 1995, at 59; Garber, 1994, at 124; King, 1/10/95, at A-1; Pearson, Goulart-Fisher, Lee, 1995, at 943–44; Epstein, Sherwood, 1996.

61. Stelfox, Chua, O'Rourke, et al., 1998; Gosfield, 1994, at 79; Brody, 1995.

62. King, 1995, at A-1. As another example, a study of clot lysis in patients who have suffered heart attack might, if funded by the manufacturer of one particularly expensive drug, incorporate methodological or analytic techniques that might tend to favor that drug. Brody, 1995.

As another example, many of the early studies of high-dose chemotherapy with autologous bone marrow transplant (HDC/ABMT) for breast cancer also showed sobering scientific deficits. For instance, treatment-related deaths (death within one month after transplant) were

> frequently disregarded; these patients were reported as 'unevaluable' because they 'did not survive long enough to exhibit a clinical response.' In many cases, omitting these patients led to higher response rates. Eliminating early deaths is inappropriate (particularly when they may have been caused by the treatment) and not standard for trial design or analysis.

ECRI, February 1995, at 7.

Other methodologic problems were rampant. Some studies lacked controls entirely, others included only those patients who had already shown they were responsive to chemotherapy, and still other studies neglected to keep track of key patient characteristics, such as the number of metastatic sites or estrogen receptor status. *Id.*

Interestingly, one more recent study of the same treatment also had serious problems, as its principal investigator admitted to having falsified data in order to please the cancer community. See Weiss, Rifkin, Stewart, et al., 2000.

63. Kessler, Rose, Temple, et al., 1994, at 1351.

64. "The HTA [health technology assessment] activities of many for-profit and not-for-profit research organizations are based almost exclusively on funding from the private sector (e.g., pharmaceutical, biotechnology, and medical device manufacturers). These assessments are commissioned generally to fulfill the needs of the funding organizations. . . . In a recent report, Rettig concludes that managed care organizations have strong incentives to support and conduct HTA in the current health care environment. The major downside to these independent and often proprietary assessments is that they often fail to lead to consistency in coverage and, therefore, technologies are available to patients based on the vicissitudes of their particular insurer. . . . The most likely causes of wide variance in results are the use of evidence of inferior quality or incomplete scope, applying inadequate resources, or allowing self-interest to affect the outcome in favor of the health plan." Perry, Thamer, 1999, at 1870–71.

Another type of industry-driven outcomes research is post-marketing studies of FDA-approved products. Typically, this research is undertaken to demonstrate which pharmaceuticals or other products are most cost-effective. Yet such research has no official requirements for scientific rigor, and studies sometimes are more of a marketing device than a bona fide research effort. The only requirement is that the results of such studies not be used in official marketing. Hillman, Eisenberg, Pauly, et al., 1991. See also Nelson, Quiter, Solberg, 1998; Friedberg, Saffran, Stinson, et al., 1999; Krimsky, 1999.

65. One study found that the majority of guidelines in peer-reviewed medical literature in fact do not mention costs at all, and only 14% provided any estimates about costs of various options for care. Shaneyfelt, Mayo-Smith, Rothwangl, 1999, at 1904. See also Culpepper, Sisk, 1998, at 80.

66. Holder, 1994, at 19; see also Rosenbaum, Frankford, Moore, et al., 1999, at 231.

"Most health insurers and managed care plans rely on ad hoc opinion by experts; only in a few instances are there HTA [health technology assessment] programs or structured processes for coverage decision making." Perry, Thamer, 1999, at 1870.

67. Rosenbaum, Frankford, Moore, et al., 1999, at 231 (citing: M&R: Healthcare management guidelines. New York: Milliman and Robertson, 1996–1998). In 1999 a suit was filed against M&R. Two pediatricians, whom M&R cited as the authors of its pediatric hospitalization guidelines, alleged not only that they did not write the guides, but that the guides are dangerous and

inappropriate for pediatric care. Cleary v. Yetman, No. 99-56719 (Tex. Dist. Ct. Harris Cty., 333d Dist. Filed Nov. 1999). See Martinez, 2000; Page, 2000.

68. Ross, 1998.

69. For a useful overview of the major methodological problems of 279 guidelines published in peer-reviewed medical literature, see Shaneyfelt, Mayo-Smith, Rothwangl, 1999. As noted by Shaneyfelt et al.: "Guidelines published in the peer-reviewed medical literature during the past decade do not adhere well to established methodological standards" (at 1900).

70. Shaneyfelt, Mayo-Smith, Rothwangl, 1999, at 1904.

71. In scientific research, evaluation of diseases and treatments "generally requires a priori hypotheses, randomization (to eliminate selection bias and confounding), homogeneous patients at high risk for the outcome, experienced investigators who follow a protocol, a comparative measure such as a placebo (if ethical), and intensive follow-up to ensure compliance. Under these circumstances, if a treatment proves to be better than a placebo (or a comparative measure), one can be reassured that the treatment can work. However, questions may remain about the ability of the treatment to work adequately in a broader range of patients and in usual practice settings in which both patients and providers face natural barriers to care." Epstein, Sherwood, 1996, at 833. See also Feinstein, Horwitz, 1997; Wells, Sturm, 1995, at 80.

"Clinical trials are not real life. To assess efficacy in as unconfounded a manner as possible, trials sometimes exclude certain patients (e.g., the elderly, the very young, those too sick, or those taking certain other medications). Any special vulnerability to adverse events in those groups will be missed." Friedman, Woodcock, Lumpkin, et al., 1999, at 1733.

72. Epstein, Sherwood, 1996.

"The failure to account for the effects of comorbid and associated conditions on the clinical outcome of chronic diseases is reflected in the common disjunction that occurs between the efficacy of an intervention, such as a drug used in a clinical trial, and the lack of effectiveness of the same drug used in clinical practice. For example, as many as 60% to 80% of patients with heart failure have been excluded from clinical trials of angiotensin-converting enzyme inhibitor therapy owing to comorbid and associated conditions that tend to oabscure the efficacy of the drug in improving functional capacity or prognosis. This standard practice in research has a rational basis. However, the clinician must treat 100% of the patients with heart failure, not just the 20% to 40% who are free of comorbidities and associated conditions. Moreover, the clinical effectiveness of drug therapy is often limited by the very comorbid and associated conditions for which patients were excluded from drug trials." DeBusk, West, Miller, et al., 1999, at 2740.

One result of this misfit between the original study's narrowly identified participants and the ordinary folk who later use the drug is that sometimes even well-researched new drugs and procedures must be quickly withdrawn from the market, as they suddenly produce undesirable results and side-effects that were not seen during the research period. Between September 1997 and September 1998, five FDA-approved drugs were removed from the market because of unexpected side-effects or interactions with other drugs. In the case of one, mibefradil (Posicor), by the time the drug was removed, it "was known to interact with 26 different drugs, a number and diversity that could not, in practical terms, be addressed by standard labeling instructions or additional public warnings." Friedman, Woodcock, Lumpkin, et al., 1999, at 1729.

73. Gellins, Rosenberg, Moskowitz, 1998, at 694. See also Feinstein, 1994.

74. Leape, 1995; Woolf, 1993(a), at 2646; Power, 1995; Feinstein, 1994.

75. Tannock, 1987; Gifford, 1996, at 42.

76. Sometimes patients' preferences are not included even when they clearly should be, for example, in the management of angina or benign prostatic hypertrophy. See Hlatky, 1995; Nease, Kneeland, O'Connor, et al., 1995, at 1185; Rodwin, 1994, at 156; Stevens, 1993, at 88–89.

See also Hayward, Wilson, Tunis, et al., 1995; King, Lembo, Weintraub, et al, 1994; Feinstein, Horwitz, 1997, at 532–33; Ross, 1998; Shaneyfelt, Mayo-Smith, Rothwangl, 1999, at 1904.

77. See Chapter 2, § B-3, at n. 88.

78. Shekelle, Kahan, Bernstein, et al., 1998, at 1888.

79. "'Medicine abounds with situations in which alternative clinical strategies are available with no scientific evidence indicating which is preferable'" Hall, 1988, at 480. See also Katz, 1984, at 165–206; Fox, 1957; Gorovitz, Macintyre, 1975; Eddy, 1984, at 74–75.

80. Morreim, 1990; Katz, 1984; Eddy, 1984.

Mark Hall views the situation in strong terms. "To a large extent, this preservation of professional autonomy is unjustified. Unquestionably, sound medical practice requires a degree of restriction on interference with the details of medical treatment, whether from a lay or professional source. The scientific foundations of medicine justify some group autonomy and its judgmental nature justifies some individual autonomy. It is wrong, however, to insist on absolute freedom from control. When the unknown value of medical procedures leaves a broad range of acceptable methods of patient management and medical practice—the current situation with the great bulk of medicine—it is difficult to maintain that influencing physicians to exercise their judgment conservatively is inappropriate. To the extent that restrictions on institutional influence lack a strong quality-of-care justification, they serve primarily to protect the vested interests of physicians." Hall, 1988, at 535.

81. "Underuse is the failure to provide a health care service when it would have produced a favorable outcome for a patient. . . . Overuse occurs when a health care service is provided under circumstances in which its potential for harm exceeds the possible benefit. . . . Misuse occurs when an appropriate service has been selected but a preventable complication occurs and the patient does not receive the full potential benefit of the service." Chassin, Galvin, National Roundtable on Health Care Quality, 1998, at 1002.

See also Bodenheimer, 1999(b); Schuster, McGlynn, Brook, 1998; Chassin, 1998.

82. Schuster, McGlynn, Brook, 1998, at 520–21. The analysis reviews a large number of studies that report on quality of health care in the United States.

83. Avorn, Solomon, 2000; Gold, Moellering, 1996, at 1445–46; Gonzales, Steiner, Lum, et al., 1999; Joshi, Milfred, 1995; McKay, 1996; Hueston, 1997; Fraser, Stogsdill, Dickens, et al., 1997; Nyquist, Gonzales, Steiner, et al., 1998; Schwartz, Mainous, Marcy, 1998; Chassin, Galvin, National Roundtable on Health Care Quality, 1998; Gonzoles, Steiner, Sande, 1997; Culpepper, Sisk, 1998; Dowell, Marcy, Phillips, et al., 1998; Dowell, Marcy, Phillips, et al., 1998(b); Fix, Strickland, Grant, 1998.

84. Lange, Hillis, 1998. "Although the patients enrolled in the United States were more likely than their Canadian counterparts to undergo coronary angiography (68 percent vs. 35 percent, respectively) and subsequent revascularization (31 percent vs. 12 percent), the incidence of reinfarction and death during more than three years of follow-up was similar. The chief predictors of the decision by U.S. physicians to use coronary angiography were a relatively young age of the patient and the availability of a catheterization facility. Furthermore, there was marked regional variation within the United States in the rates of use of angiography and revascularization, which was not explained by differences in the characteristics of the patients or the incidence of complications of myocardial infarction" (at 1838). Rather, excessive use is probably related to the more widespread availability of facilities and trained personnel in the United States (at 1839). See also Fisher, Welch, 1999.

There is a counterargument, however. At least one study has shown that although the U.S. level of coronary bypass surgery may not always lead to improved survival, it has been associated with improved quality of life and reduction of symptoms of angina. See Hamm, Reimers, Ischinger, et al., 1994. In comparisons between the U.S. and Canada, higher rates of the surgery in the US were associated with improved quality of life. See Mark, Naylor, Phil, et al., 1994; Tu, Naylor, Kumar, et al., 1997. By the same token, Canadians also had to wait a significantly longer period of time to receive surgery, thus by implication living with angina symptoms for a longer period. See McGlynn, Naylor, Anderson, et al., 1994.

85. Over the past two decades, a number of studies have shown that aggressive therapy featuring angiography and revascularization does "not reduce the incidence of nonfatal reinfarction or death as compared with the more conservative, ischemia-guided approach" and that the incidence of adverse events is similar, if not greater, in the aggressively managed patients. Lange, Hillis, 1998, at 1839.

86. When a certain class of drugs has been "used to suppress largely asymptomatic arrhythmias, the result was a 2.5-fold increase in mortality;" and a two-year followup of some patients who had undergone angioplasty for coronary artery disease (including many with only mild disease) showed that the angioplasty "had reduced symptoms only in the group with severe angina, yet doubled the risk of nonfatal myocardial infarction (MI) or death overall." Fisher, Welch, 1999, at 447.

87. Fisher, Welch, 1999, at 447.

88. The study focused on the appropriateness of decisions made by utilization reviewers. Another panel of experts disagreed, deeming only about 30% of the tubes to be unwarranted. See Kleinman LC et al., 1997. See also Kleinman, Kosecoff, Dubois, et al., 1994 (finding in another study of the same issue that at least 23% of proposed tube placements were inappropriate and 35% were equivocal).

89. The drugs included stimulants, antidepressants, clonidine, and neuroleptics. Zito, Safer, dosReis, et al., 2000; Coyle, 2000.

90. Oberfield, 1999; Rose, 1995; Finkelstein, Silvers, Marrero, et al., 1998; Cuttler, Silvers, Singh, et al., 1996; Bercu, 1996.

91. Krumholz, Murillo, Chen, et al., 1997; Pashos, Normand, Garfinkle, et al., 1994; Frances, Go, Dauterman, et al., 1999.

92. Wang, Stafford, 1998, at 1901–1906. See also Newcomer, 1998; Burton, 1998; Winslow, 1998; Frances, Go, Dauterman, et al., 1999; Califf, O'Connor, 2000, at 1336.

93. Ironically, of those for whom the drugs were prescribed, a third actually had contraindications for β-blocker use. Donohoe, 1998, at 1598. See also Burton, 1998; Deedwania, 1997.

94. Donohoe, 1998, at 1597.

Another study investigated whether physicians prescribe treatments appropriately for patients with acute MI. This includes giving aspirin; appropriately withholding calcium channel blockers for those with impaired left ventricular function; prescribing ACE inhibitors at discharge; using thrombolytics or angioplasty for reperfusion; prescribing beta-blockers at discharge; and advising patients to quit smoking. The study found that aspirin was used 86% during hospitalization and 78% after; calcium channel blockers were appropriately withheld 82% of the time; use of ACE inhibitors at discharge was only 60%; reperfusion was 67%; beta-blocker prescription at discharge was 50%; and smoking cessation advice was 42%. Researchers concluded: "Substantial geographic variation exists in the treatment of patients with AMI [acute MI], and these gaps between knowledge and practice have important consequences. Therapies with proven benefit for AMI are underused despite strong evidence that their use will result in better patient outcomes." O'Connor, Quinto, Traven, et al., 1999, at 627.

95. Bratzler, Raskob, Murray, et al., 1998, at 1909.

Another example: Although it has been known for many years that prenatal administration of corticosteroids for fetuses at risk of premature delivery can greatly reduce mortality and morbidity, physicians' actual adherence to this recommendation was low until highly focused educational efforts were undertaken. "Antenatal corticosteroid therapy reduces the risk of infant mortality by approximately 30%, of neonatal respiratory distress syndrome by approximately 50%, and of both intracranial hemorrhage and periventricular leukomalacia by approximately 70%. . . . Despite evidence of its effectiveness, use of corticosteroid therapy in eligible infants remained relatively low through the 1990s. Of particular importance, the therapy was used less often when GA [gestational age] was less than 28 weeks, compared with GA between 28 and 34 weeks. Yet these very low-GA infants were precisely the group that would most likely benefit from antenatal corticosteroids." Leviton, Goldenberg, Baker, et al., 1999, at 46.

96. Legorreta, Christian-Herman, O'Connor, et al., 1998; Hartert, Windom, Peebles, et al., 1996; Havranek, Graham, Pan, et al., 1996, at S-10; see also Donohoe, 1998, at 1599.

97. Weiner, Parente, Garnick, et al., 1995; Leape, 1995; Harris, 1996; Newcomer, 1998; Epstein, Sherwood, 1996; Donohoe, 1998, at 1600; Burton, 7/8/98.

98. Moser, 1998. As Furberg notes regarding the question whether drugs called calcium agonists (CAs) should be used for hypertension:

> The documentation on efficacy and safety is limited to small, short-term clinical trials, typically a few hundred patients treated for 2 to 3 months. Pharmaceutical companies have used skillful marketing based on concepts and mechanisms of action to promote these agents and have avoided for more than a decade calls for large-scale, randomized clinical trials to determine the effect of these drugs on major cardiovascular disease end points. Clinicians have chosen to prescribe CAs without proper evidence of health efficacy and long-term safety."

Furberg, 1995, at 2157. See also Lederle, Applegate, Grimm, 1993; Goodwin, Goodwin, 1984.

99. Avorn, Chen, Hartley, 1982; Orlowski, Wateska, 1992; Schwartz, Soumerai, Avorn, 1989.

100. Donohoe, 1998, at 1600. See also Broadhead, 1994; Rost, Smith, Matthews, et al., 1994; Bungard, Ghali, Teo, et al., 2000 (noting that, in cases in which patients should receive warfarin therapy for atrial fibrillation, only 15%-44% are prescribed the drug; at 42); Samsa, Matchar, Goldstein, et al., 2000 (finding that only a third of patients with this condition received the anticoagulent drug warfarin).

Of note, the use of breast-conserving surgery is rising in some areas, though not always with the use of adjunctive radiation therapy. See Riley, Potosky, Klabunde et al., 1999; Du, 1999.

101. At the beginning of the study, "handwashing compliance before and after defined events was 9% and 22% for health care workers in the medical ICU and 3% and 13% for health care workers in the cardiac surgery ICU, respectively. After the education/feedback intervention program, handwashing compliance changed little. . . ." Of note, after an alcohol-based waterless handwashing antiseptic was made easily available by each bed, handwashing compliance improved to 48%. Still, that is less than half the desirable level. Bischoff, Reynolds, Sessler, et al., 2000, at 1017.

102. Havranek, Graham, Pan, et al., 1996, at S-10; Burton, 1998; Asch, Sloss, Hogan, Et al., 2000.

One study focused on physicians in United HealthCare plans at three sites, looking for whether: [1] physicians measured potassium levels in patients on diuretics; [2] more than one H2 agonist was (inappropriately) prescribed for patients with peptic ulcer disease; [3] insulin-dependent diabetics had their A1C levels measured; and [4] insulin-dependent diabetics received an annual eye exam. Across the three plans, the figures were: [1]: 41%, 50%, 47%; [2]: 21%, 18%, 20% [i.e., instances in which patients received the wrong thing]; [3]: 26%, 26%, 23%; and [4]: 46%, 43%, 62%. The chief medical officer of the plan concluded: "'Mediocre' is the best word to describe the clinical performance revealed in these measures.'" Newcomer, 1998, at 35.

103. Newcomer, 2000, at 60 (citations omitted).

104. Newcomer, 2000, at 60 (citations omitted).

105. Prescriptions for Cox-2 inhibitors "account[ed] for 40 percent of all prescriptions in this class, but only 14 percent of patients receiving the drugs have arthritis. More than 75 percent of UnitedHealth Group's patients take the medicines for less than two months. The risk of ulcers for short-term pain therapy is minimal, and pain relief is no better than it was with older alternatives. Rather than customizing treatment options for this short-term therapy group, physicians have simply used the new drug for all indications." Newcomer, 2000, at 60.

106. Evans, Pestotnik, Classen, et al., 1998.

107. Burton, Troxclair, Newman, 1998; see also Lundberg, 1998.

Another study comparing autopsy findings to premortem diagnoses found that in a third of the cases, autopsy detected an unexpected pathological diagnosis directly contributing to the patient's death. Additional unexpected diagnoses were found in nearly 80% of the cases. Durning, Cation, 2000. See also Mort, Yeston, 1999 (finding a 41% rate of discrepancies between pre- and postmortem diagnoses in a surgical intensive care unit; of these errors, 85% were undiagnosed infectious processes).

108. Hadorn, 1992.

109. Mangione, Nieman, 1997, at 721.

110. "Most guidelines . . . have not been successful in changing physician behavior." Landon, Wilson, Cleary, 1998, at 1379. As evidence, Landon cites: Weingarten, Riedinger, Hobson, et al., 1996.

Physicians do not always stay up to date via the commonly presumed means of browsing medical journals, attending professional meetings, and conferring regularly with colleagues. Naylor, 1998, at 1392. See also Lewis, Lasater, Ruoff, 1995; Grimshaw, Russell, 1993; Cabana, Rand, Powe, et al., 1999; Furrow, 1994, at 403 ff.; Poses, Cebul, Witgon, et al., 1992; Gifford, Holloway, Frankel, et al., 1999; Stross, 1999.

In one of the more sobering studies of physicians' failure to adhere to guidelines of good care, the SUPPORT "study attempted to influence decisions for seriously ill patients by providing physicians with more accurate prognostic estimates and information about their patients' views about cardiopulmonary resuscitation, content of advance directives, and endeavored to enhance communication about these topics by using trained nurse facilitators to engage the physicians about these matters. These interventions, conducted in actual clinical settings in several major teaching hospitals, had no effect on the decision-making process in these units." Elstein, Christensen, Cottrerll, et al., 1999, at 63. See also Schroeder 1999; The SUPPORT Principal Investigators, 1995 (finding that many patients die in pain, not consulted about their wishes).

111. For example, organized medicine's support for the early corporate bans allegedly was at least partly based on fears about lost revenues and increased competition. Starr, 1982, at 15–27.

A number of antitrust suits chastising organized medicine for its resistance to HMOs and to contract medicine point out that, at least sometimes, when certain business practices have been condemned as unethical or as bad medicine, underlying concerns have reflected economic interests. In American Medical Association v. United States, 317 U.S. 519 (1943), the Supreme Court held that the American Medical Association (AMA) was guilty of antitrust violations as it opposed prepaid group practice and forbade its members to interact with physicians in such arrangements. The AMA "conspired to boycott Group Health in order to prevent it from marketing medical services in competition with petitioners' doctor members" (at 523).

In another antitrust case against the AMA, the Court held that the organization's long-term opposition to chiropractic was not just rooted in concerns for public health; it was also rooted in the desire to eliminate competition. Wilk v. American Medical Ass'n, 895 F.2d 352 (7th Cir. 1990) (cert. denied 111 S.Ct. 513 (1990)). Citing the district court's ruling with approval, the Court noted that "the AMA was not motivated solely by such altruistic concerns. Indeed, the court found that the AMA intended to 'destroy a competitor,' namely chiropractors. It is not enough to carry the day to argue that competition should be eliminated in the name of public safety" (at 361).

In Virginia Pharmacy Bd. v. Va. Consumer Council, 425 U.S. 748 (1976), the Supreme Court struck down a rule of the state pharmacy board, declaring it to be unethical to advertise drug prices. The Court noted wide variations in prices and suggested that secrecy about prices served more to keep prices high than to protect consumers. See also Goldfarb v. Virginia State Bar, 421 U.S. 773 (1975).

The Court acknowledges, at certain points, that the professions may have certain ethical tenets that differ from business. But in none of these cases does the Court deem such a possibility to be a justification of anticompetitive activity. See Goldfarb v. Virginia State Bar, 421 U.S. 773, 786 (1975); National Society of Professional Engineers v. United States, 435 U.S. 679, 696 (1978).

112. Leape, Brennan, Laird, et al., 1991; Brennan, Leape, Laird, et al., 1991.

Leape notes that a 1% rate of negligent errors may seem acceptable, but "a 1% failure rate is substantially higher than is tolerated in industry, particularly in hazardous fields such as aviation and nuclear power. As W.E. Deming points out . . ., even 99.9% may not be good enough: 'If we had to live with 99.9%, we would have: 2 unsafe plane landings per day at O'Hare, 16 000 pieces of lost mail every hour, 32 000 bank checks deducted from the wrong bank account every hour.'" Leape, 1994. See also Feinstein, 1997.

113. The study looked at all medication-prescribing errors in a teaching hospital from January 1, 1987, through December 31, 1995. During that period the rate of errors per written order, per admission, and per patient-day all increased significantly. Lesar, Lomaestro, Pohl, 1997. Another study found that fatal adverse drug reactions (whether or not the product of either error or negligent error) rank between the fourth and sixth leading cause of death in the United States. Lazarou, Pomeranz, Corey, 1998.

See also Bootman, Harrison, Cox, 1997; Lesar, Briceland, Stein, 1997; Avorn, 1997; Bates, Spell, Cullen, 1997; Classen, Pestotnik, Evans, et al., 1997; Lesar, Briceland, Stein, 1997; Bates, Cullen, Laird, et al., 1995; Leape, Bates, Cullen, et al., 1995; Bates, 1998.

114. Institute of Medicine, 1999; Nuland, 1999, A-22.

115. Feinstein, 1997, at 1286. Feinstein goes on to note: "The combination of shortened durations of time for both the patient in hospital and the house officer on a service has reduced the house officer's sense of continuity of care within the hospital . . . and has increased the difficulties of maintaining rigorous patterns of supervision and discussion" (at 1287).

116. For some of these functions, other kinds of practitioners can serve equally well, including advanced practice nurses and physicians' assistants.

117. *Differential diagnosis* is a term commonly used in clinical medicine to indicate the various diagnoses that might be possible given the patient's initial signs, symptoms, history, and the like. Further diagnostic evaluation then helps the physician to whittle down this list to one or a small number of working diagnoses, on the basis of which treatment options can be considered.

118. "The very nature of a radiologist's function requires the exercise of independent professional judgment. Accordingly, a hospital is not in a position to, and generally does not, exercise control over a radiologist's performance of his or her professional activities." Pamperin v. Trinity Memorial, 423 N.W.2d 848, 848 (Wis. 1988).

119. Several courts have distinguished between purely business functions and more clinically oriented activities. See, e.g., Women's Medical Center v. Finley, 469 A.2d 65, 73 (N.J. Super.A.D. 1983). Other courts have rejected the distinction, including Parker v. Board of Dental Examiners, 14 P.2d 67 (Cal. 1932)

120. This does not entail, of course, that health plans will use only one single set of guidelines. Different large purchasers such as employers may want different levels of coverage, and these, in turn, may require variations in the guidelines that the health plan applies to beneficiaries' care.

121. Luft observes that 1% of the population consumes 30% of all medical care costs, while the bottom 50% accounts for only 3% of expenditures. Luft, 1995, at 26. Also of note, "85% of Americans spend less than $3000 a year on medical care, and 73% have less than $500 a year in claims." Editorial, 1994.

122. Morreim, 2000(a). See also Marrie, Lau, Wheeler, et al., 2000.

123. Daniels, Sabin, 1998; Sabin, Daniels, 1994; Holoweiko, 1995; Reiser, 1994; Grimes, 1993; Steinberg, Tunis, Shapiro, 1995; Bergthold, 1995. See also Bucci v. Blue Cross-Blue Shield of Connecticut, 764 F. Supp. 728 (D.Conn. 1991). The insurer used five-factor "Technical Evaluation

Criteria" used by a Blue Cross Blue Shield plan for evaluating new technologies. "Summarized, the criteria are (1) government regulatory approval; (2) evidence which permits conclusions as to the effect on patient health; (3) demonstrated improvement of the patient's health; (4) demonstration of medical benefit at least equal to that offered by established alternative treatment; and (5) improvement other than in investigational settings" (at 731). However, the court rejected the criteria as invalid on the ground that they were subjective in nature and imprecise.

124. If one person in Plan X receives bone marrow transplant that is then denied to another person with the same disease in the same plan, the latter patient can easily complain of unjust treatment, perhaps even at the cost of his life. Meyer, Murr, 1994; Sage, 1996; Morreim, 2000(a).

125. See Chapter 5, § B-2.

126. Daniels, Sabin, 1998.

127. "The *Clinical Practice Guidelines Directory* (http://www.ama-assn.org) serves as a repository of guidelines on more than 2000 topics from more than 90 organizations. It is easy to use and can quickly point a reader toward the sources of guidelines on relevant topics. The U.S. Preventive Services Task Force Guide to Clinical Preventive Services (http://lww.com) is an evidence-based source of preventive care recommendations. . . . Another resource available on the Internet is the National Guideline Clearinghouse, which includes guidelines that meet specific criteria for being evidence-based. The Agency for Health Care Policy and Research, in partnership with the American Association of Health Plans and the American Medical Association, has invited developers of practice guidelines, including professional societies, to submit guidelines for possible inclusion in the National Guideline Clearinghouse. Guidelines must contain systematically developed statements that satisfy the Institute of Medicine's definition of a guideline; be developed under the auspices of a medical organization; be derived from a systematic review of the relevant literature and science; have been developed, reviewed, or revised in the past 5 years; and be available in English." Weingarten, 1999, at 455. The Web site for the National Guideline Clearinghouse is http://www.guideline.gov. See also the "Clinical Evidence" guidelines, published by British Medical Journal, available at www.clinicalevidence.org.

128. Combining efforts and resources will probably produce better results than the less well-funded, potentially biased investigations of any one health plan. Fortunately, some collaborative research and guidelines construction is already underway. A large number of major corporations have pooled funds to create the Foundation for Accountability (FAcct), an organization that is conducting outcomes studies on a variety of conditions. The research looks not only at standard morbidity and mortality, as many such studies do, but also investigates quality of life, return to normal functions of living, and other matters important to a broader view of medical outcomes. Terry, 1996.

In an analogous effort, the Managed Care Outcomes Study, funded by six MCOs and the National Pharmaceutical Council, recently published a study indicating that excessively stringent formulary limits tend perversely to increase patient visits to outpatient offices, emergency rooms, and hospitals and to raise overall costs of care. Horn, Sharkey, Tracy, et al., 1996. In the same vein, the HMO Research Network coordinates twelve research organizations located within integrated health care organizations. Durham, 1998.

The Ambulatory Sentinel Practice Network (ASPN) looks at common clinical dilemmas of everyday practice and has created guidelines, e.g., for CT scanning in new-onset headache, whether and when to do dilation and curettage after uncomplicated miscarriage, whether there should be hospitalization of every woman with pelvic inflammatory disease, and whether to prescribe a 10-day antibiotic course for every child with otitis media. See Nutting, Beasley, Werner, 1999. For further discussion see Morreim, 1997(b), at 49–52; Morreim, 2000(a).

129. A physician in the office may only have 10–15 minutes with a patient. "Yet, in that time, the physician may also need to call the MCO to authorize a specialty referral, consult a directory to determine which specialist is on the MCO panel, refer to a managed care formulary to choose a drug, and even take a call from a hospital nurse urging the physician to discharge another patient before the end of the day. Under these circumstances, it is difficult to keep the physician focused on the many initiatives each MCO employs to achieve . . . improved quality and reduced costs." Leider, 1998, at 583.

130. "[T]he most common cause of serious medication errors with respect to antibiotics is a failure to note a patient's known allergy, a mistake that can be addressed at the institutional level by devoting greater resources to eliciting information, developing more effective charting and communication among providers, and maintaining a work environment that promotes attentiveness." Sage, Jorling, 1994, at 1021. See also Leape, Cullen, Clapp, et al., 1999; Bates, Gawande, 2000.

131. Balas, Weingarten, Garb et al., 2000; Morris, 2000; Marrie, Lau, Wheeler, 2000; Durieux, Nizard, Ravau, et al., 2000; Evans, Pestotnik, Classen, et al., 1998; Natsch, Kullberg, Meis, et al., 2000; Avorn, Solomon, 2000; Classen, 1998; Hunt, Haynes, Hanna, et al., 1998; Wells, Sherbourne, Schoenbaum, et al., 2000; Garibaldi, 1998; Fraser, Stogsdill, Dickens, et al., 1997; Overhage, Tierney, McDonald, 1996; Elson, Connelly, 1995; Avorn, Soumerai, Taylor, et al., 1988; Bates, Leape, Cullen, et al., 1998 ; Raschke, Gollihare, Wunderlich, et al., 1998; Soumerai, Avorn, 1990; Hunt, Haynes, Hanna, et al., 1998; Morhane, Matthias, Nagle, et al., 1998; Gawande, 1998; Furrow, 1994.

132. Soumerai, McLaughlin, Gurwitz, et al., 1998; Leider, 1998.

133. Grandinetti, 1997; Suchman, Eiser, Goold, et al., 1999; Enthoven, Singer, 1995.

134. In this one might disagree, at least somewhat, with the Pennsylvania Supreme Court in Thompson v. Nason Hosp., 591 A.2d 703 (Pa. 1991). A hospital was sued for its physicians' failure to recognize the dangers posed by some medications a patient had taken prior to being injured in a motor vehicle accident. In an amicus brief the state's hospital association argued "that it is neither realistic nor appropriate to expect the hospital to conduct daily review and supervision of the independent medical judgment of each member of the medical staff of which it may have actual or constructive knowledge" (at 708). The court disagreed, however, holding that "It is well established that a hospital staff member or employee has a duty to recognize and report abnormalities in the treatment and condition of its patients. . . . If the attending physician fails to act after being informed of such abnormalities, it is then incumbent upon the hospital staff member or employee to so advise hospital authorities so that appropriate action might be taken. [citing *Darling*] . . . When there is a failure to report changes in a patient's condition and/or to question a physician's order which is not in accord with standard medical practice and the patient is injured as a result, the hospital will be liable for such negligence" (at 709).

Up to a point, a hospital (or health plan) surely may be expected to "control" its employees by establishing policies, by periodically checking on compliance with those policies, and by having procedures in place to address failures to adhere to those policies. However, it is neither feasible nor reasonable to expect an institution to be aware of, anticipate, or avert each and every instance of inadequate conduct on the part of its employees and staff members. Such levels of scrutiny would require constant one-on-one supervision of every physician at every moment. If courts want nevertheless to impose liability, even when the institution had and implemented proper policies and could not have avoided the adverse outcome, then it might be plausible to suppose that such a court is more interested in finding a party affluent enough to pay for injuries than in apportioning damages according to fault.

135. In Gafner v. Down East Community Hosp., 735 A.2d 969 (Me. 1999), the Supreme Court of Maine explicitly refused to extend hospitals' corporate liability beyond credentialing to include dictating the clinical details of care. Critical of the Pennsylvania Supreme Court's approach in Thompson v. Nason, the Maine court quoted Justice Flaherty's dissent in that case, which established broad duties for hospitals to supervise medical staff. Calling the decision a " 'monumental and ill-advised change,' " Flaherty noted that it places " 'financial burdens upon hospitals for the actions of persons who are not even their own employees. At a time when hospital costs are spiraling upwards to a staggering degree, this will serve only to boost the health care costs that already too heavily burden the public' " (cited in *Gafner*, 735 A.2d 978). Flaherty noted that the *Thompson* decision provides no guidance regarding " 'the extent to which hospitals must now monitor staff physicians, nor did it articulate the standard of care to which hospitals must adhere' " (cited in *Gafner*, 735 A.2d 978).

136. It is important that such assessments be properly risk rated so that they do not unfairly penalize physicians whose only "fault" is that they care for the sickest patients. For further discussion of the hazards and cautions related to physician profiling, see Hofer, Hayward, Greenfield, et al., 1999; Bindman, 1999; Kassirer, 1994; Salem-Schatz, Moore, Rucker, et al., 1994.

137. American College of Physicians, 1994, at 423.

138. American College of Physicians, 1994, at 426.

139. Laffel, Berwick, 1992; Blumenthal, 1996; Leape, Woods, Hatlie, et al., 1998; Kahn, 1995; Berwick 1996(b); Berwick 1996(c).

140. In some cases health plans' medical judgments may improve upon attending physicians' judgments. This is rooted partly in the fact that so many ordinary physicians' actual practices are not well founded on scientific research and can very widely, without any particular relation to patients' underlying illnesses.

An example comes from a recent Sacramento case. The attending physician for a woman with an ostensibly localized cancer of the cervix (squamous cell cancer in situ) wanted to treat her with hysterectomy, i.e., removal of the entire uterus as well as the cervix, even though her cancer appeared to be completely confined to the original site. Humana, the patient's HMO, recommended an alternative. Removing just the affected cone of the cervix would be not only less expensive, but equally effective in terms of removing the cancer and distinctly safer, with decreased risks of bleeding, adverse anesthesia reactions, abdominal pains, and infections. If a pathologist's review of the removed tissue showed that the cancer was confined to the excised cone, nothing further would need to be done; if the review showed the cancer was not confined, hysterectomy could then be undertaken. Philp, 1998.

"When it comes to hysterectomies, hundreds of thousands of women have been saved from needless surgeries by health insurers and medical researchers who had the courage to challenge [their peers'] practice patterns. Back in 1975, when insurers rarely scrutinized surgery proposals, American doctors performed 725,000 hysterectomies. Experts throughout the 1980s suggested that many hysterectomies every year [were unnecessary]. What's more, studies out of Dartmouth University have proven that doctors in certain sections of the country are far more likely to recommend surgery than doctors elsewhere. One's zip code rather than one's medical condition can be a better predictor of whether a doctor will recommend surgery." Philp, 1998. Relying on its own physicians and on an independent panel, the MCO thus offered a medical judgment that it deemed not just to be more consistent with the patient's contract, but medically superior to the attending physician's opinion. As the case turned out, however, the patient elected to follow her physician's more aggressive approach and paid $14,000 out of pocket for the hysterectomy. Pathological review showed that her cancer was confined to the cone of the cervix. Nevertheless, the patient sued the MCO and won a jury verdict of $13.1 million. Philp, 1998. For further discussion, see Lowes, 2000.

141. For instance, if asthmatic patients do not fare as well as they should, the MCO might need to reexamine its own disease management guidelines, or it might need to monitor its physicians' performance more closely. In either case, the decisions it makes at that point will be based at least partly on medical judgments and could have a significant impact on patients' care and outcomes. Hence, the plan may be practicing medicine.

142. Garibaldi, 1998.

CHAPTER 6

1. In an earlier work on this subject, I proposed a Standard of Medical Expertise (SME) that applied to physicians and a Standard of Resource Use (SRU) that generally applied to health plans. See Morreim, 1985–86. The distinction was further explicated in Morreim, 1991(a).

More recent work builds on but modifies that distinction, broadening expertise concerns to encompass health plans, while reciprocally applying resource issues to providers such as physicians. See Morreim, 1997(b).

2. Crane, 1997.

3. Ricci v. Gooberman, 840 F. Supp. 316, 316 (D.N.J. 1993).

4. Kohn, Corrigan, Donaldson, eds., 1999, at 51.

5. See, e.g., Haas v. Group Health Plan, Inc., 875 F. Supp. 544, 546 (S.D. Ill. 1994).

6. Pellegrino, Thomasma, 1981.

7. Pacificare of Oklahoma, Inc. v. Burrage, 59 F.3d 151, 154 (10th Cir. 1995).

8. Institutions such as hospitals, as another form of provider, also can be assessed for expertise. Corporate negligence, for instance, can occur when a hospital fails to exercise due care in credentialing and supervising its physician staff. Corporate negligence doctrine initially arose regarding hospitals' duties to grant or extend privileges only to physicians who could provide adequate quality of care. See Insinga v. LaBella, 543 So. 2d 209, 214 (Fla. 1989).

9. Henderson, Siliciano, 1994, at 1398.

10. Nealy v. U.S. Healthcare HMO, 844 F. Supp. 966 (S.D.N.Y. 1994); 711 N.E.2d 621 (N.Y. 1999).

11. Nealy v. U.S. Healthcare HMO, 844 F. Supp. 966, 969 (S.D.N.Y. 1994). Similarly in another case, delays and denials of treatment arose due to the fact that the patient received a new identification number. See American Health Care Providers, Inc. v. O'Brien, 886 S.W.2d 588, 589 (Ark. 1994).

12. Jones v. Chicago HMO, 730 N.E.2d 1119 (Ill. 2000).

13. Jones v. Chicago HMO, 730 N.E.2d 1119, 1132 (Ill. 2000).

14. Jones v. Chicago HMO, 730 N.E.2d 1119, 1129, 1134 (Ill. 2000).

15. Payton v. Aetna/US Healthcare, Sup Ct New York, Index No. 100440/99, March 22, 2000 (Judge Herman Cahn); discussed in Trueman, 2000, at 221–22.

16. Initially the HMO did not respond. Later it concluded that Mr. Payton was covered but did not actually authorize inpatient treatment as requested. Subsequently the plan decided that Payton had not purchased the necessary rider to his insurance contract for this treatment to be covered. Thereafter the plan gave conflicting instructions about how to file a grievance. After Mr. Payton filed a grievance with the Consumer Services Bureau of the State Insurance Department, the Health Care Bureau of the State Attorney General's Office advised the HMO that his contract "plainly" covered inpatient substance abuse treatment. Payton v. Aetna/US Healthcare, Sup Ct New York, Index No. 100440/99, March 22, 2000 (Judge Herman Cahn); discussed in Trueman, 2000, at 221–22.

17. Payton v. Aetna/US Healthcare, Sup Ct New York, Index No. 100440/99, March 22, 2000, at p. 6.

18. Crum v. Health Alliance Midwest, Inc., 47 F.Supp.2d 1013 (C.D.Ill. 1999).

19. For further discussion of ERISA, see Chapter 11.

20. See also McDaniel v. Blue Cross & Blue Shield of Alabama, 780 F.Supp. 1360 (S.D.Ala. 1991); see related decision at 780 F.Supp. 1363 (S.D. Ala. 1992). The plaintiff was advised by her physician to undergo a complete hysterectomy, for which she then requested preauthorization in compliance with her insurer's requirements. She received a letter of approval, underwent the surgery, and then requested reimbursement. Only then did UM nurses actually look at the patient's records, whereupon they discovered that Mrs. McDaniel's medical problem pre-existed the effective date of her insurance coverage. Despite earlier authorizations, coverage was then denied on the ground that the policy did not cover preexisting conditions. As the district court concluded, this health plan committed a breach of its expertise duties by failing to exert the effort necessary to give the enrollee an accurate answer to her question. The plan was required to pay for the hysterectomy even though, under contract, it would not otherwise have been obligated to cover it. McDaniel v. Blue Cross & Blue Shield of Alabama, 780 F.Supp. 1360 (S.D.Ala. 1991) (finding that failure to fully review medical records before issuing preauthorization constituted breach of duty of care); related decision at 780 F.Supp. 1363 (S.D. Ala. 1992) (holding that denial of coverage was arbitrary and capricious, and that letter authorizing treatment could mislead enrollee to believe that eligibility for benefit depended only on employer's timely payment of premiums).

21. Sanus/New York v. Dube-Seybold-Sutherland, 837 S.W.2d 191 (Tex.App.—Houston [1st Dist.] 1992).

22. See Wickline v. California, 239 Cal. Rptr. 810, 819 (Cal. Ct. App. 1986); Wilson v. Blue Cross, 271 Cal. Rptr. 876, 884 (Cal. Ct. App. 1990).

23. See Schleier v. Kaiser Found. Health Plan, 876 F.2d 174, 176 (D.C. Cir. 1989); Dearmas v. Av-Med, Inc., 865 F. Supp. 816, 818 (S.D. Fla. 1994); Kearney v. U.S. Healthcare, Inc., 859 F. Supp. 182, 184 (E.D. Pa. 1994); Ricci v. Gooberman, 840 F. Supp. 316, 316 (D.N.J. 1993); Elsesser v. Hospital of the Phila. College of Osteopathic Med., 802 F. Supp. 1286, 1289–1290 (E.D. Pa. 1992); Independence HMO, Inc. v. Smith, 733 F. Supp. 983, 986 (E.D. Pa. 1990); Raglin v. HMO Ill., Inc., 595 N.E.2d 153, 154–55 (Ill. App. Ct. 1992); Harrell v. Total Health Care, Inc., 781 S.W.2d 58, 59–60 (Mo. 1989); Dunn v. Praiss, 656 A.2d 413, 417 (N.J. 1995); Albain v. Flower Hosp., 553 N.E.2d 1038, 1041–42 (Ohio 1990); McClellan v. Health Maintenance Org., 604 A.2d 1053, 1057–59 (Pa. Super. Ct. 1992); Boyd v. Albert Einstein Med. Ctr., 547 A.2d 1229, 1231 (Pa. Super. Ct. 1988).

24. See Chittenden, 1991, at 453–85; Conrad, Seiter, 1995, at 194; Tiano, 1990, at 91–98; Wiehl, et al., 1993, at 12–15; Rice, 1996, at 193–94.

25. Grumet, 1989; Ogrod, 1997; Light, 1992, at 2505–06; Kenagy, Berwick, Shore, 1999; Mayer, Cates, 1999; Kassirer, 1995.

26. As noted in Chapter 4, such categories might include (or not) inpatient care, outpatient care, mental illness and substance abuse, prescription drugs, home health care, durable medical equipment, rehabilitation, and the like.

27. For instance, most commercial plans refuse to pay for research or experimental services, cosmetic procedures, long-term custodial care, and the like.

28. See McGann v. H&H Music Co., 946 F.2d 401, 406–07 (5th Cir. 1991); cf. Pisciotta v. Teledyne Indus., Inc., 91 F.3d 1326, 1330 (9th Cir. 1996) ("In general, welfare benefits are not subject to vesting requirements under ERISA. Employers may adopt, modify or terminate welfare benefit plans.") (citing Curtiss-Wright Corp v. Schoonejongen, 514 U.S. 73, 78 (1995)).

29. See, e.g., American College of Physicians, 1996, at 845–47 (1996); Goldsmith, 1994, at 26; Pincus, 1995, at 33; Slomski, 1995, at 194; Terry, 1995, at 54.

30. See Alexander v. Choate, 469 U.S. 287, 303 (1985).

31. Note that this approach does not grant physicians license to waste resources or to pursue "infinitesimal" benefits regardless of cost. It means only that if the expected benefit is of significant value to the patient and there is no obstacle to undertaking the intervention, then the physician ordinarily should not act unilaterally to deny patients resources.

32. See Trauner, Chesnutt, 1996, at 159.

In some cases a physician may have to phone for approval for every intervention costing more than $200 and, perhaps, wait long periods only to speak with a utilization clerk lacking the education or medical sophistication to understand the question. Or an HMO may drop a physician for ordering an ambulance to transport an unconscious patient. See McDonald, 1996, at 181, 184. In other cases, tight pharmaceutical formularies may greatly restrict the drugs physicians can prescribe.

In the same vein, an MCO may contract with hospitals and other facilities far from members' homes, potentially exacerbating an illness or injury while a patient is en route to the distant site. See Felsenthal, 1996.

33. See, e.g., Chew v. Meyer, 527 A.2d 828 (Md. Ct. Spec. App. 1987). See additional discussion in Chapter 7.

34. See Wickline v. State, 192 Cal. App. 3d 1630, 1645 (1987). A California court of appeal found that although third party payors can be held liable when their cost containment systems result in medically inappropriate care, physicians nevertheless remain responsible for the care they give their patients and have an obligation to contest economically inappropriate decisions by third-party payors.

35. See Azevedo 1996(b), at 43, 47; Larson, 1996, at 44.

36. See Morreim, 1997(c), at 333.

37. For further discussion, see Morreim, 2000(c), at 705–706; Berwick, 1996; Frank, McGuire, Newhouse, 1995; Robinson, Casalino, 1995; Friedman, 1996; Kerr, Mittman, Hays, et al., 1995; Gold, Hurley, Lake, et al., 1995.

38. See Woolhandler, Himmelstein, 1995, at 1706. See also Ogrod, 1997; Azevedo, 1996.

39. Pegram v. Herdrich, 120 U.S. 2143 (2000).

40. See Balanced Budget Act of 1997, Pub. L. No. 105-33, §4041, 111 Stat. 251, 276 (amending Social Security Act §1855, 42 U.S.C. §1395w-21); Overbay, Hall, 1996. See also Morreim 1998(b).

41. Robinson, 1999, at 1259.

42. Robinson, 1999, at 1259.

43. See Morreim. 1991(b), at 444; Novack, Detering, Arnold, et al., 1989, at 2983–85; Freeman, Rathore, Weinfurt, et al., 1999; Wynia, Cummins, VanGeest, et al., 2000.

44. For further discussion of the difference between conflicts of obligation and conflicts of interest, see Morreim 1998(b).

45. These arrangements particularly raise issues of contributive justice. See Morreim 1995(a), at 248.

46. Tefft v. Wilcox, 6 Kan. 46, 61–62 (Kan. 1870).

47. The physician must "have and use the knowledge, skill and care ordinarily possessed and employed by members of the profession in good standing." Keeton, Dobbs, Keeton, et al., 1984, at 187. "'Wisconsin law holds that a physician (general practitioner or specialist) is liable in an action for medical negligence if he or she fails to exercise that degree of care and skill which is exercised by the average practitioner in the class to which he or she belongs, acting in the same or similar circumstances.'" Johnson v. Agoncillo, 515 NW2d 508, 510 (Wis.App. 1994). "A physician must act with that degree of care, knowledge and skill ordinarily possessed and exercised in similar situations by the average member of the profession practicing in the field." Aiello v. Muhlenberg R. Med. Ctr., 733 A.2d 433, 437 (N.J. 1999). See also Morlino v. Medical Center, 706 A.2D 721, 734 (N.J. 1998) (describing the standard of care as "the degree of care, skill, and diligence . . ." required of a physician) (citing Rogers v. Meridian Park Hosp., 772 P.2d 929, 933 (1989).

48. Havighurst 1986(a), at 149.

49. Havighurst 1986(a), at 161. See also Havighurst 1986(b); Epstein, 1997, at 359–80, 413–16; Epstein, 1986; Epstein, 1976.

50. Epstein, 1976, at 94–95; Epstein, 1997, at 360.

51. The case of Muse v. Charter Hospital, Inc., 452 S.E.2d 589 (N.C.App. 1995), previously discussed in Chapter 2, illustrates the point. The provider—in this case a hospital—was required to provide resources (hospital care) despite the fact that the insurer had no obligation to pay for them. See id. at 594–95.

52. Similarly, even if health plans can rightly be expected to provide reasonably efficient administration and overall surveillance for quality of care, they should not face tort liability for individual physician errors that they could not have spotted—and should not have spotted if keeping an appropriate distance from day-to-day clinical decisions.

53. To propose that expertise should be addressed under tort, while resource disputes should be managed within contract, does not mean that each case must be litigated entirely in one or the other. Many of health care's complex battles will have elements of each, but this is no different from the many other lawsuits in which plaintiffs allege contract-based claims alongside tort claims.

CHAPTER 7

1. These latter duties can also concern resources and will be discussed further below.

2. See, e.g., Taylor v. Hill, 464 A.2d 938, 942 (Me. 1983); Shilkret v. Annapolis Emergency Hosp. Ass'n, 349 A.2d 245, 248–54 (Md. 1975); McCormack v. Lindberg, 352 N.W.2d 30, 36 (Minn. Ct. App. 1984).

3. Note, however, that when expertise is the sole focus, there is likely to be less variation in beliefs about what is good practice than under the currently broader realm of malpractice litigation in which resources also figure into the equation.

For optimal evolution of medical knowledge and skills, perhaps courts should grant greater deference to medical literature and explicit professional consensus than heretofore. For example, some of the many guidelines now flourishing throughout health care focus on medical expertise and could be incorporated into litigation by judicial notice or by being introduced into evidence by a party. Anesthesia guidelines, for instance, emphasize the importance of regularly monitoring vital signs—efforts that require conscientiousness more than elaborate technologies. Evidence indicates that these guides have significantly reduced the incidence of intraoperative hypoxic injuries. Such professional guidelines arguably have a legitimate place in litigation. See, e.g., Eichorn, 1989; Goldsmith, 1992; Woolf 1993(a), at 2649. See also Allred, Tottenham, 1996, at 537. See also Leahy, 1989, at 1506 (suggesting that professional guidelines be incorporated into the [expertise] standard of care via judicial notice).

4. Chew v. Meyer, 527 A.2d 828 (Md. Ct. Spec. App. 1987).

5. Chew v. Meyer, 527 A.2d 828, 832 (Md. Ct. Spec. App. 1987).

6. Murphy v. Godwin, 303 A.2d 668, 673 (Del. Super., 1973). The court went on to explain that this duty is fiduciary in character, a duty of care "'that includes and comprehends a duty to aid the patient in litigation, to render reports when necessary and to attend court when needed.'" 303 A.2d 674, citing Alexander v. Knight, 197 A.2d 142, 146 (1962)(dictum). Accordingly, plaintiffs' claim for negligent nonfeasance could go forward.

In Wickline v. State of California, 192 Cal. App. 3d 1630 (1987), a California appellate court noted that "the physician who *complies without protest* with the limitations imposed by a third party payor, when his medical judgment dictates otherwise, cannot avoid his ultimate responsibility for his patient's care" (at 1635, dicta, emphasis added). A physician may be intimidated by a health plan's denial of coverage, but he is "not paralyzed . . . nor rendered powerless to act appropriately if other action was required under the circumstances" (at 1635). The court was not quite clear about what a physician should do but indicated that protesting an inappropriate utilization review denial was at least one action the court expected.

7. As one contract said, "'Physician shall agree not to take any action or make any communication which undermines or could undermine the confidence of enrollees, potential enrollees, their employers, their unions, or the public' . . . 'Physician shall keep the Proprietary information [payment rates, utilization review procedures, etc.] and this Agreement strictly confidential.'" Woolhandler, Himmelstein, 1995, at 1706.

Such nondisparagement clauses, however, are either gone or rapidly disappearing as the federal government restricts their use and as health plans themselves disavow them. See Miller, 1997, at 1104–05; Orient, 1994, at 159; Wooley, 1993, at 394; Morreim, 1991(c); Morain, 1995, at 39. See also Kassirer, 1995, at 50 (discussing the tension between a physician's obligation to provide appropriate care and his desire to maintain status as an authorized provider for HMOs).

8. Neade v. Portes, 710 N.E.2d 418 (Ill.App. 1999); rev'd, 739 N.E.2d 496 (Ill. 2000).

9. Shea v. Esensten, 208 F3d 712, (8th Cir. 2000) ("Shea II"). See also Moore v. Regents of the University of California, 793 P.2d 479 (Cal. 1990) (cert. denied 112 S. Ct. 2967 (1992)).

But see Pryzbowski v. U.S. Healthcare, Inc., 64 F.Supp.2d 361 (D.N.J. 1999). In this case a patient requesting additional surgery for her back pain alleged that her physician committed malpractice by failing to advocate on her behalf for more prompt resolution of her request. The federal district court held: "Plaintiff has failed to show that the defendants owed plaintiff a 'duty to advocate' so as to expedite the approval of her surgery. All she has offered in support of the alleged duty are the Hippocratic Oath and the Code of Medical Ethics." The court went on to note that even if there was a duty to advocate, the plaintiff had produced no evidence that the physicians failed to fulfill such a duty (64 F.Supp.2d 370). This case does not necessarily defeat the notion that physicians have reasonable duties of advocacy in certain settings, however. The court points to the meagre argumentation provided by the plaintiff to support either the existence or the breach of such a duty in the context of prodding a health plan to move faster.

10. The measure of due diligence should come from several sources. Partly it will be based on ordinary persons' expectations that physicians will be patients' advocates. As in most other tort litigation, those reasonable expectations will be supplied typically by a jury. Yet these judgments must also be informed by the realities of the health care marketplace. Hence, this litigation should also include testimony from those who experience the details of health plans' bureaucracies, routine requirements, and "hassle-factors." Other market realities can be supplied by health plans as administrators document what they expect of physicians and how other physicians in their plan fare under the same rules. For further discussion, see Morreim, 1991(a), Chapter 5.

11. Tabor v. Doctors Memorial Hospital, 563 So. 2d 233 (La. 1990).

12. See Grumet, 1989, at 607; Light, 1994, at 498–99; Light, 1992, at 2505–06.

13. See generally Rosenberg, Allen, Handte, et al., 1995, at 1328–29; Shapiro, Wenger, 1995, at 1353.

14. Such cases of a physician's failure to request resources must, of course, be distinguished from failures of expertise in which the physician simply did not know that the test or treatment would be useful or needed for the patient.

The scenario becomes more complicated when the physician makes only a token effort on behalf of a patient's resource request. In some health plans, for instance, a physician who does not believe that a particular test or treatment is needed or who believes that the plan will reject such a request can appear to meet the patient's demand for the resource by writing "the patient requests that. . . ." This wording acts as a signal telling the health plan that the request is not entirely serious, even while ostensibly complying with the patient's desire to request the treatment.

15. See Chapter 6 § B-2. Before focusing on physicians who directly hold substantial control over health plan resources, it should be noted in passing that some physicians hold a different sort of control. When a physician serves as a member of a health plan's management, e.g., by reviewing utilization appeals, he acts as an employee representing the health plan. Here, allegations about improper denials of resources should be lodged against the health plan that employs that physician and should ordinarily be managed as contract cases.

Hand v. Tavera, 864 S.W.2d 678 (Tex. Ct. App. 1993), raises interesting questions. The plaintiff arrived at an emergency room with a significant headache of several days' duration, and the emergency room physician believed that the problem was severe hypertension that could quickly lead to a stroke. Although the emergency room physician recommended hospitalization, the health plan's physician who was empowered to authorize such an admission denied the request in favor of symptomatic relief and outpatient management. Shortly after leaving the hospital, the patient suffered a stroke that had long-term adverse consequences. The Texas appellate court held that "when the health-care plan's insured shows up at a participating hospital emergency room, and the plan's doctor on call is consulted about treatment or admission, there is a physician–patient relationship between the doctor and the insured . . . and the doctor owes the patient a duty of care." *Id.,* at 679–80. The health plan's contract with the physician brings the patient and the review physician together "just as surely as though they had met directly and entered the physician–patient relationship." *Id.,* at 679.

The decision is interesting but appears to conflate several different issues. On the one hand, there may be reason to suppose that a physician who serves as the plan's primary care utilization manager does indeed have a relationship with those patients for whose care he stands as a personal gatekeeper. In that event, any deficiencies in expertise or effort could indeed be accountable in a tort suit. On the other hand, to the extent that the physician was acting as the plan's resource administrator, the patient's complaint should be regarded as a contractual question.

16. "[T]he precise nature of the fiduciary relationship remains a source of confusion and dispute. Legal theorists and practitioners have failed to define precisely when such a relationship exists, exactly what constitutes a violation of this relationship, and the legal consequences generated by such a violation." Cooter, Freedman, 1991, at 1045–46 (footnotes omitted). As DeMott observes:

Fiduciary obligation is one of the most elusive concepts in Anglo-American law. Applicable in a variety of contexts, and apparently developed through a jurisprudence of analogy rather than principle, the fiduciary constraint on a party's discretion to pursue self-interest resists tidy categorization. Although one can identify common core principles of fiduciary obligation, these principles apply with greater or lesser force in different contexts involving different types of parties and relationships. Recognition that the law of fiduciary obligation is situation-specific should be the starting point for any further analysis.

DeMott, 1988, at 879.

17. See Morreim, 1991(c), at 296.
18. See Cooter, Freedman, 1991, at 1046.
19. See Morreim, 1991(c), at 296.
20. For further discussion of physicians' fiduciary duties to patients, see Cooter, Freedman, 1991, at 1045–47, 1054–55; DeMott, 1988, at 882, 906; Mehlman, 1990, at 365–414; Mehlman, 1993, at 390; Morreim, 1991(c), at 296–301.
21. Rodwin, 1995, at 242–46.
22. See, e.g., Hammonds v. Aetna Cas. & Sur. Co., 243 F.Supp. 793, 801–01 (N.D. Ohio 1965); Moore v. Regents of the Univ. of Cal., 793 P.2d 479, 483 (Cal. 1990); Lockett v. Goodill 430 P.2d 589, 591 (Wash. 1967); Miller v. Kennedy, 522 P.2d 852, 860–61 (Wash. Ct. App. 1974), aff'd, 530 P.2d 334 (Wash. 1975). See generally Morreim, 1991(c), at 289–301; Liner, 1997, at 527.
23. See Azevedo, 1996(b), at 47. Admittedly, the conflict is not absolute. Poor-quality care can actually be against physicians' long-range interests in that it may cause illnesses to become more serious and therefore more costly. Nevertheless, the conflict of interest is clearly present and powerful.
24. Engalla v. Permanente Medical Group, 43 Cal Rptr 2d 621, 638 (Cal. App. 1 Dist. 1995) (citing: Foley v. Interactive Data Corp, 765 P.2d 373 (1988). See also Davis v. Blue Cross of Northern California, 600 P.2d 1060 (Cal. 1979) (discussing the "special nature of the insurer–insured relationship and the resultant duties which an insurer owes to its insureds", at 1065); Egan v. Mutual of Omaha Ins. Co., 598 P. 2d 452, 456 (Cal. 1979) ("'[the insurer] must give at least as much consideration to the latter's interest as it does to its own'"); Hartford Acc. & Indem. v. Mich. Mut. Ins., 462 N.Y.S.2d 175, 178 (A.D.1 Dept. 1983); Scott v. Dime Sav. Bank of New York, FSB, 886 F.Supp. 1073, 1078 (S.D.N.Y 1995), affd w/o opin. 101 F.3d 107 (2d Cir. 1996), cert. denied 520 U.S. 1122 (1997); McLaughlin v. Connecticut General Life Ins. Co., 565 F. Supp. 434, 451 (N.D. Cal. 1983)(citing Egan v. Mutual of Omaha approvingly as it said "'The obligations of good faith and fair dealing encompass qualities of decency and humanity inherent in the responsibilities of a fiduciary'" (Egan, 620 P.2d 141, 141 (Cal. 1979)); Potvin v. Metropolitan Life Ins. Co., 997 P.2d 1153, 1159 (Cal. 2000) (referring to "an insurance company with fiduciary obligations to its insureds"). See also Jerry, 1996, at 151–61, 903.
25. See DeMott, 1988, at 900:

[T]he presence of a fiduciary obligation significantly affects the conduct of litigation by affecting the allocation of burdens of proof. If a suit challenges a transaction between fiduciary and a beneficiary, the fiduciary has the burden of proving that it dealt candidly and fairly with the beneficiary. If the issue is, in contrast, merely whether a party has breached a contractual obligation, the party alleging the breach has the burdens of proof. *Id.* (footnote omitted).

See also Mehlman, 1993, at 368.
26. See Cooter, Freedman, 1991, at 1055–56:

The special obligations imposed on fiduciaries by the duty of loyalty help raise the enforcement probability. To overcome difficulties in proof, the law infers disloyalty from its appearance, presuming that a fiduciary will appropriate the principal's asset when it is in her self-interest to do so. This inference alters the usual rules of tort liability by shifting the burden of proof from a plaintiff to a defendant or by prohibiting completely the act in question.

Id. (footnotes omitted). See also Doe v. Roe, 681 NE2d 640, 645–46 (Ill.App.1 Dist. 1997).
27. A somewhat analogous phenomenon arises in the special setting of ERISA health plans. Ordinarily, when the benefits administrator in an ERISA plan is a fiduciary with obligations to administer the plan in the best interests of the beneficiaries, courts will grant considerable deference to the decisions of such administrators. However, considerably less deference is accorded when the health plan is in a conflict of interest, as in this case when the plan makes money by denying

services to beneficiaries. See Firestone Tire & Rubber Co. v. Brush, 489 U.S. 101, 115 (1989); Pitman v. Blue Cross & Blue Shield, 24 F.3d 118, 123 (10th Cir. 1994); Doe v. Group Hospitalization & Med. Servs., 3 F.3d 80, 85 (4th Cir. 1993); Brown v. Blue Cross & Blue Shield, 898 F.2d 1556, 1562–67 (11th Cir. 1990); Bucci v. Blue Cross-Blue Shield, 764 F.Supp. 728, 730 (D. Conn. 1991). Clearly, such a conflict applies to physicians who govern health care resources under personal financial risk. Accordingly, it is reasonable to expect that courts will not treat lightly the benefit denials of gatekeeper physicians. For further discussion see Chapter 11.

28. Weatherly v. Blue Cross Blue Shield Ins. Co., 513 N.W.2d 347, 353 (Neb. Ct. App. 1994) (quoting Braesch v. Union Ins. Co., 464 N.W.2d 769, 774–75 (Neb. 1991)).

29. Weatherly v. Blue Cross Blue Shield Ins. Co., 513 N.W.2d 353.

30. Weatherly v. Blue Cross Blue Shield Ins. Co., 513 N.W.2d 354.

31. See Pellegrino, Thomasma, 1981 at 24, 250; Pellegrino, 1987, at 1939 (1987).

32. Some authors propose an alternative to current bad faith case law that might be worth considering. Since bad faith cases have sometimes resulted in awards that many observers regard as excessive and thereby foster an unpredictability that can make it difficult for health plans to predict and price their risk level accurately, these commentators propose limited statutory remedies instead. See Baker, 1994, at 1424–25; Gergen, 1994, at 1255–57; Jerry, 1986, at 272, 319–20; Jerry, 1994, at 1342. One state permits winners to collect attorneys' fees, for instance, and an even stronger remedy imposes an 18 percent per annum penalty for delay in payment of insurance claims. See Tex. Rev. Civ. Stat. Ann. art. 21–21 § 16(b)(1) (West 1991); Tex. Rev. Civ. Stat. Ann. art. 21–55 § 6 (West Supp. 1997).

A still stronger remedy would be to permit treble damages for bad faith in processing insurance claims. See Gergen, 1994, at 1256. In these commentators' view, damages such as these can afford injured plaintiffs substantial extra compensation when their injuries are the product of major procedural failures. At the same time, they do not inject the kind of actuarial instability that can make it difficult for health plans to offer packages to consumers that have reasonable premium prices for their defined benefits. In essence, the proposal is analogous to the malpractice tort reforms that limit physicians' liability in states where legislators believe that excessive damage awards have introduced too much cost and unpredictability into the business of medicine and malpractice insurance. The idea is worth considering, though no stand will be taken here.

For further discussion of bad faith doctrine, see Fletcher v. Western Nat'l Life Ins.Co., 89 Cal. Rptr. 78, 92–94 (Cal. Ct. App. 1970); McEvoy v. Group Health Co-Op., 570 N.W. 2d 397 (Wis. 1997); Diamond, 1981, at 443–47; Louderback, 1982, at 192–96; Stern, 1983.

33. "Moreover, the remedies available to a beneficiary in litigation against a fiduciary differ from standard contract remedies. The beneficiary is entitled to restitution of any benefit realized by the fiduciary through the breach, or alternatively may recover any loss suffered as a result of the breach. In order to fully capture these benefits, expansive remedies, such as the imposition of a constructive trust, may be necessary." DeMott, 1988, at 900.

34. Cooter, Freedman, 1991, at 1069; see also Schoenholtz v. Doniger, 657 F.Supp. 899, 914 (S.D.N.Y. 1987) (citing state court decisions holding that beneficiaries may recover punitive damages against the trustees for breach of trust in cases of extreme disloyalty by fiduciary); George T. Bogert, Trusts § 157 (6th ed. 1987).

A somewhat related potential problem has recently been put to rest but could resurface in other forms in the future. It concerns a different sort of fiduciary, namely the ERISA administrator who exercises discretionary authority over the assets of an employee benefit plan. In Pegram v. Herdrich, 120 U.S. 2143 (2000), a woman whose treatment for appendicitis was delayed claimed that the physicians of Carle Clinic, who were in a full-risk arrangement, had breached their fiduciary duties as administrators of an ERISA health plan. When physicians also own the plan, plaintiff argued, they are mired in inescapable conflicts of interest that systematically threaten to deprive enrollees of benefits. Such arrangements should therefore be prohibited. The Supreme Court refused to invalidate such risk-bearing arrangements or even to agree that risk-bearing physicians were actually ERISA fiduciaries when they made treatment decisions. Such decisions that "mixed" treatment and eligibility determinations did not qualify as administrative fiduciary decisions. However, while the Court did not invalidate financial incentive arrangements, it did leave the door open to the possibility that Congress might want to do so.

A further, very distinctive risk could also arise when physicians' full-risk health plan is chosen by employers to serve as an employment benefit. As noted above, ERISA defines its fiduciaries in terms of the authority to make discretionary benefits decisions, eligibility determinations, and the like for the benefit of the plan's enrollees. Ordinarily, courts are very deferential to these fiduciaries' decisions because ERISA can force a fiduciary to bear personal responsibility for decisions of the wrong sort. However, such deference is distinctly reduced in those cases in which the ERISA fiduciary is in a conflict of interest. At this point, physicians who have formed their own PSO face a very distinctive problem. On the one hand, a major reason physicians may want to form such a PSO is to regain the clinical control they feel is imperative if they are to care for patients well without the annoying outside interference of utilization managers and the like. This decision-making control renders the physicians "fiduciaries" under ERISA's distinctive definition. On the other hand, these PSO physicians are clearly in conflicts of interest because they stand personally to lose or gain depending on how successfully they use resources for their PSO's enrollees. And, as noted, when fiduciaries are in conflicts of interest, courts are reluctant to defer very readily to decisions that deny a patient a resource to which he might plausibly be entitled. The net result is that because these physician–fiduciaries are in such systematic conflicts, the very resource control they seek is one thing of which they will have rather little. For futher discussion and a proposed resolution to this interesting dilemma, see Morreim 1998(b).

35. Orentlicher, 1996; Pearson, Sabin, Emanuel, 1998; Sugarman, Yarasbus, 1999; Anderson, Weller, 1999; Miller, Sage, 1999; Enthoven, Vorhaus, 1997; Morreim, 2000(c), at 723–24.

36. Bringing patients into the incentive structures may be one of the most powerful, least pernicious ways of containing costs while ensuring quality of care, so long as patients' incentives do not pose significant barriers to needed care. Morreim 1995(b).

37. If patients are fully apprised of the resource rules and incentive systems governing their health plans, then physicians' conflicts of interest would no longer be undisclosed, and they would no longer labor under the special legal hazards of fiduciaries in undisclosed conflicts. This approach would require considerably better information than patients typically receive. At present, subscribers are not ordinarily permitted access to their plans' guidelines (even physicians are often denied access), and many plans do not disclose information about physician incentives. See Woolhandler, Himmelstein, 1995; Orient, 1994, at 159; Kassirer, 1995, at 50; Morreim 1997(d); Wooley, 1993, at 394; Morain, 1995, at 39.

CHAPTER 8

1. See Chittenden, 1991, at 453–64; Conrad, Seiter, 1995, at 194; Tiano, 1990, at 80–98.

2. One of the MCOs, for instance, increased its enrollment from 30,000 to 300,000 virtually overnight. Its prior lack of a computerized billing system caused major delays and confusions in payments to physicians and hospitals. See Mirvis, Chang, Hall, et al., 1995, at 1236. Gottlieb, 1995.

3. See Mirvis, Chang, Hall, et al., 1995, at 1236. Gottlieb, 1995.

4. For further discussion of bad faith doctrine, see Chapter 7, § B-2.

5. Nutting, Beasley, Werner, 1999.

6. Wickline v. State of California, 192 Cal. App. 3d 1630 (1987).

7. Wickline v. State of California, 192 Cal. App. 3d 1630, 1645 (1987).

8. Wilson v. Blue Cross of Southern Cal., 271 Cal. Rptr. 876, 883 (Cal. App. 2 Dist. 1990).

9. Thompson v. Nason Hosp., 591 A.2d 703 (Pa. 1991).

10. Thompson v. Nason Hosp., 591 A.2d 703, 707 (Pa. 1991) (emphasis added); see also Welsh v. Bulger, 698 A.2d 581 (Pa. 1997).

11. Shannon v. McNulty, 718 A2d 828 (Pa Super 1998).

Various suits have assailed health plans for adopting guidelines that allegedly were medically faulty. In In re U.S. Healthcare, 193 F.3d 151, 162–63 (3d Cir. 1999), cert. denied 120 S.Ct. 2687 (2000), for instance, the Third Circuit permitted litigation to go forward in state courts, alleging that an ERISA health plan had acted with reckless indifference in adopting a guideline that discharged newborn infants within 24 hours.

12. Rosenbaum, Frankford, Moore, et al., 1999.

13. Berwick 1996(b); Berwick 1996(c); Laffel, Berwick, 1992; Blumenthal, 1996; Leape, Woods, Hatlie, et al., 1998; Kahn, 1995; Leape, 1995.

14. As noted by the Wisconsin Supreme Court:

> Through contractual arrangements with physicians and patients, HMOs are able to exert significant influence on, if not outright control over, the costs of treatment regimens administered to patients, thereby limiting waste. The fears attendant with such arrangements, however, revolve around the economic model of health care financiers focusing on reducing aggregate costs while failing to recognize and to protect adequately the medical needs of individual subscribers. This fear is particularly acute in the present high-cost medical econ-

omy where an adverse benefits ruling means not just that the financier will not provide payment, but also that the medical care itself is effectively denied.

McEvoy v. *Group Health Co-Op.*, 570 N.W. 2d 397, 403 (Wis. 1997).

15. Murphy v. Board of Medical Examiners, 949 P.2d 530 (Ariz.App.Dist.1 1997).

16. Murphy noted the patient's prior history of irritable bowel syndrome, her normal laboratory blood values, and the absence of evidence for stones on ultrasound examination (at 949 P.2d 530, 533 (Ariz.App.Dist.1 1997)). In this case the patient did not actually suffer an injury because she received the surgery and eventually also the reimbursement after the surgery revealed she did have gallstones.

17. Murphy v. Board of Medical Examiners, 949 P.2d 530, 535 (Ariz.App.Dist.1 1997).

18. Murphy v. Board of Medical Examiners, 949 P.2d 530, 536 (Ariz.App.Dist.1 1997). The court went on: "Dr. Murphy is not a provider of insurance. Instead, Dr. Murphy is an employee who makes medical decisions for his employer on whether surgeries or other non-experimental procedures are medically necessary. Such decisions are not insurance decisions but rather medical decisions because they require Dr. Murphy to determine whether the procedure is 'appropriate for the symptoms and diagnosis of the [c]ondition,' whether it is to be 'provided for the diagnosis,' care or treatment, and whether it is 'in accordance with standards of good medical practice in Arizona" (at 536).

Similarly, the Wyoming Supreme Court noted that, "[a]s described above, other courts have recognized that utilization review is medical decision-making, and a plan administrator that involves itself in a medical decision that amounts to a denial of treatment is making a medical decision." Long v. Great West Life & Annuity Ins., 957 P.2d 823, 828 (Wyo. 1998).

19. Morris v. Dist. of Col. Bd. of Medicine, 701 A.2d 364 (D.C.App. 1997).

20. Morris v. Dist. of Col. Bd. of Medicine, 701 A.2d 364, 367 (D.C.App. 1997) (court citing the words of the Board of Medicine).

In this case, however, the appellate court disagreed with the board on the ground that the defendant merely organized the physicians who actually performed the UR, did not have a vote, and did not on any occasion ask the committee to reconsider a decision. Morris v. Dist. of Col. Bd. of Medicine, 701 A.2d 364, 367 (D.C.App. 1997).

In Hand v. Tavera, 864 S.W.2d 678 (Tex.App.–San Antonio 1993), the plaintiff had gone to the emergency room (ER) with a three-day headache and a history of significant hypertension. The ER physician observed him for three hours and, noting that Hand's symptoms rose and fell with his blood pressure, concluded he needed to be admitted to the hospital. However, Dr. Tavera, the physician responsible to authorize admissions for Hand's HMO, determined that the patient could be treated on an outpatient basis. Hand went home and suffered a fatal stroke several hours later. Initially the defendant prevailed on the ground that no physician–patient relationship existed, hence no duty of care. But the decision was reversed on appeal. "[T]he contracts . . . show that the Humana plan brought Hand and Tavera together just as surely as though they had met directly and entered the physician–patient relationship. . . . In effect, Hand had paid in advance for the services of the Humana plan doctor on duty that night, who happened to be Tavera, and the physician–patient relationship existed. We hold that when the health-care plan's insured shows up at a participating hospital emergency room, and the plan's doctor on call is consulted about treatment or admission, there is a physician–patient relationship between the doctor and the insured." Hand v. Tavera, 864 S.W.2d 678, 679 (Tex.App.–San Antonio 1993). Without saying it in so many words, the court clearly felt that Dr. Tavera was practicing medicine, not merely making contractual coverage decisions.

21. Brandon v. Aetna Services, Inc., 46 F.Supp.2d 110 (D.Conn. 1999).

22. Brandon v. Aetna Services, Inc., 46 F.Supp.2d 110, 112 (D.Conn. 1999). In this case the substantive question was not resolved because the plaintiff's claims were preempted by ERISA.

23. Ortolon, 1997, at 27.

24. Adnan Varol, M.D. v. Blue Cross & Blue Shield, 708 F. Supp. 826 (E.D. Mich. 1989).

25. Assn. of Am. Physicians and Surgeons v. Weinberger, 395 F.Supp. 125 (N.D.Ill. 1975).

26. 395 F.Supp. 135.

27. 395 F.Supp. 134.

See also Szekely v. Florida Medical Association, 517 F.2d 345, 350 (5th Cir 1975): "Permitting HEW [Health, Education and Welfare Dept] to recoup funds paid out for medically unnecessary services does not constitute impermissible supervision of the practice of medicine, prohibited by § 1395" of the Medicare Act. See also Wickline v. State of California, 192 Cal. App. 3d 1630, 1645 (1987).

As noted by other commentators, "[c]overage disputes are most appropriately viewed as an insurance-purchasing decision by a pool of subscribers, not a medical-treatment decision by an individual patient. The denial of coverage does not prevent the doctor from rendering care; it merely determines that, in the insurer's judgment, the subscriber pool has chosen not to pay for the particular treatment. Thus, where the parties leave the scope of coverage undefined, a particular case is rationally decided by asking only what range of treatment options the purchasers would have chosen to insure at the time they signed up, not what treatment they want to receive now that the insurance has been paid and their illness is manifest." Hall, Anderson, 1992, at 1676.

28. See Williams v. Good Health Plus, Inc., 743 S.W.2d 373, 378 (Tex.App.–San Antonio 1988). In Pickett v. CIGNA Healthplan of Texas, Inc., 1993 WL 209858 (Tex.App.-Hous. 1st Dist., June 17, 1993), the plaintiff sued her physicians and her HMO for medical malpractice. The trial court granted summary judgment for the HMO and the appellate court affirmed because CIGNA did not actually provide care or employ the patient's physicians. Rather, it contracted with an independent practice association whose physicians provided the care. "The court looked to the Texas Medical Liability and Insurance Act, which defined a health care liability claim as 'a cause of action against a health care provider or physician for treatment, lack of treatment, or other claimed departure from accepted standards of medical care.' The court then looked at the definition of 'health care provider,' and found that CIGNA did not fall within it, noting further that HMOs in Texas do not comply with professional licensing requirements and thus, may not engage in the practice of medicine. The court concluded that CIGNA could not as a matter of law be liable for medical malpractice. Other courts have similarly held that an entity not licensed under the jurisdiction of the agency responsible for health care professionals is not a health care provider for purposes of medical malpractice claims." Garrison, 1998, at 804 (citations omitted).

See also Freedman v. Kaiser Found. Health Plan, 849 P.2d 811 (Colo. App. 1992). "The concept of respondeat superior cannot be invoked to make an HMO responsible for the medical malpractice of those independent contractor physicians that it is statutorily precluded from directing or controlling."

Propst v. Health Maintenance Plan, Inc., 582 N.E.D. 1142, 1143 (Ohio Ct.App. 1990) (appellate court agreeing with trial court that "health maintenance organizations . . . could not be considered to be practicing medicine (R.C. 1742.30). . . . Since the corporate defendants do not practice medicine, they may not be held liable under a complaint which sounds in medical malpractice").

Sova Drugs, Inc., v. Baines, 661 So.2d 393 (Fla.Dist.Ct.App. 1995) (pharmacy was not health care provider, hence not required to comply with Medical Malpractice Reform Act requirements of investigation and notice).

Schwartz v. Brownlee, 482 S.E.2d 827 (Va. 1997) (corporation, of which physician was president and sole shareholder, was not licensed as health care provider and thereby not entitled to statutory protection of $1 million malpractice cap).

See also Chittenden, 1991, at 454, 467–68.

This view, however, has been criticised. "One of the arguments HMOs most frequently raised was they simply were not making treatment decisions because that constitutes the practice of medicine. Managed care entities cannot practice medicine because the state bans the corporate practice of medicine, they argued. 'That is analogous to a speeder telling a cop he couldn't have been going 90 miles an hour because the speed limit is only 70,' Ms. Barron [lobbyist for Texas Medical Assn] said." Ortolon, 1997, at 27. See also Sloan v. Metro Health Council, 516 N.E. 2d 1104, 1106 (Ind. App. 1 Dist. 1987)(disagreeing with Iterman v. Baker, 15 N.E.2d 365 (Ind. 1938)).

29. St. Francis Reg. Med. Ctr. v. Weiss, 869 P.2d 606, 616 (Kan. 1994). Similarly, one of the early corporate practice cases notes that practice is "the diagnosis and treatment of ailments of human beings; the prescription of a form of treatment for the palliation of physical ailments of persons with the intention of receiving compensation therefor; and the maintenance of an office for the examination and treatment of persons afflicted or supposed to be afflicted by any ailment." People v. United Medical Service 200 N.E. 157, 163 (Ill. 1936).

See also Bartron v. Codington County, 2 N.W.2d 337, 341 (So.Dak. 1942), noting that to practice medicine is to "'recommend, prescribe or direct for the use of any person any drug, medicine, apparatus or other agency for the cure, relief or palliation of any ailment or disease of the mind or body, or for the cure or relief of any wound, fracture or bodily injury or deformity, after having received or with the intent of receiving therefor, either directly or indirectly, any . . . compensation, shall be regarded as practicing within the meaning of this article.'"

In the state of Washington, "practicing medicine includes activities such as diagnosing, advising, prescribing, curing, or administering drugs." [Wash. Rev. Code § 18.71.011 (1994)]. In Morris v. Dist. of Col. Bd. of Medicine, 701 A.2d 364, 367 (D.C.App. 1997), the District of Columbia Health

Occupations Revision Act of 1986 defines the practice of medicine as "'the application of scientific principles to prevent, diagnose, and treat physical and mental diseases, disorders, and conditions and to safeguard the life and health of any woman and infant through pregnancy and parturition.'" Hayward, 1996, at 424.

The Texas Medical Practice Act defines practicing medicine, in part, as publicly professing to be a physician or surgeon and professing to "diagnose, treat, or offer to treat any disease or disorder, mental or physical, or any physical deformity or injury by any system or method or to effect cures thereof," or actually engaging in these activities. Williams v. Good Health Plus, Inc., 743 S.W.2d 373, 375 (Tex.App.–San Antonio 1988).

See also Hall, 1988, at 453, as he refers to "physician licensing laws' all-encompassing definition of medical practice as diagnosing, treating, or prescribing for any physical or mental condition."

It may be noted that two of these definitions partly define medical practice in terms of an "intention of receiving compensation therefor" (St. Francis Reg. Med. Ctr. v. Weiss, 869 P.2d 606, 616, citing People v. United Medical Service 200 N.E. 157, 163) See also Bartron v. Codington County, 2 N.W.2d 337, 341 (So.Dak. 1942): "after having received or with the intent of receiving therefor, either directly or indirectly, any . . . compensation." This feature, present in earlier definitions, has largely been dropped from current statutes. Indeed, had it been retained, it would imply that physicians rendering charity care are not practicing medicine at all. Admittedly, many states have had good samaritan statutes to protect physicians who render care at the scene of an accident and charitable immunity statutes protecting hospitals that provide care for the poor. However, these statutes accomplish their public policy aims of encouraging care for the poor and desperate, not by denying that it is medical care in the first place, but by explicitly stating that those who render care in these circumstances will be immune from liability.

30. To be precise, states' licensing statutes can be seriously unclear. Most states define practice of medicine in terms of diagnosis, treatment, prescription, or prevention of human disease, ailment, injury, or other condition. Given such vagueness, it is not surprising to find states' interpretations can vary widely. In New Jersey, a "store owner was convicted of practicing medicine without a license when he advised customers on what foods they should eat after they had described their ailments." Andreson, 1998, at 439 (citing Pinkus v. MacMahon, 29 A.2d 885 (NJ 1943). Indiana deems tatooing to constitute the practice of medicine, while Texas is willing to consider publishing a book to be medical practice, and Ohio requires a medical license to perform acupuncture. Andreson, 1998, at 439–41.

31. See Chapter 3 § B-3.

32. In Ohio, for instance, "R.C. 1751.08(D) states plainly that a health insuring corporation holding a certificate of authority under R.C. Chapter 1751 'shall not be considered to be practicing medicine.' . . . Pursuant to this provision, . . . the health insuring corporation is not considered to be practicing medicine in the conduct of its utilization review program under R.C. 1751.77–86." Ohio Attorney General, Opinion 99–044; August 31, 1999, p. 4 of 15 (also citing Propst v. Health Maintenance Plan, 582 NE2d 1142 (Ohio Ct. App. 1990)).

The Ohio attorney general continued:

> It is sometimes stated that, if a health insuring corporation refuses to certify a health care service, the patient will be unable to obtain the service in question, even though her personal physician recommends it. It should be noted, however, that an adverse determination by a health insuring corporation means that the health insuring corporation will not pay for, reimburse, provide, deliver, arrange for, or otherwise make available the service in question. . . . It does not mean that the physician is precluded from providing the service or that the patient is precluded from obtaining the service from another source or through other means . . . A physician or other provider retains authority to provide whatever services are deemed appropriate for the patient, even if the services are not included under the plan of the health insuring corporation.

Ohio Attorney General, Opinion 99–044; August 31, 1999, pp. 3–4 of 15. Other attorneys general have opined similarly. See 60 N.C. Op. Att'y Gen 100, 1992 WL 525113 (N.C.A.G.)(Apr. 6, 1992); XXIV Kan. Op.Att'y Gen 49, Op. No. 90–130, 1990 WL 547153 (Kan.A.G. Nov. 28, 1990); Ark Op. Att'y Gen. No. 90–104, 1990 WL 358803 (Ark.A.G.(May 10, 1990); Miss. Op.Att'y Gen. No. 93–0088, 1993 WL 207349 (Miss.A.G.(May 18, 1993). For further discussion, see Andresen, 1998, at 444–446.

But see Murphy v. Board of Medical Examiners, 949 P.2d 530 (Ariz. App. 1997); La.Op.Att'y Gen. No. 98–491, 1999 WL 288869 (La.A.G.)(Apr. 27, 1999).

33. This was the defendant's argument in Murphy v. Board of Medical Examiners, 949 P.2d 530, 535 (Ariz.App.Dist.1 1997). Because the physician who performs utilization review for a third-party payor does not practice medicine, the argument concluded, he should not be subject to review by the Board of Medical Examiners. The Arizona appellate court disagreed.

As noted by the North Carolina Attorney General in 1992, a denial of coverage "does not prohibit the patient from seeking other funding sources or from seeking treatment without third-party benefits, and it does not prohibit the attending physician from providing the treatment. . . . Thus, the person performing the utilization review is not diagnosing, operating on, prescribing for, administering to or treating any ailment, injury or deformity, but is merely deciding whether or not third-party payment is available." 60 Op. N.C. Att'y Gen. 100 (1992), quoted in Andresen, 1998, at 444.

Partly in response to widespread opposition to intensive UR, many MCOs now use other forms of cost containment. Health plans have two basic ways to control costs: *rules* (by which the MCO applies UR criteria, sometimes in advance of treatment, to determine precisely what it will and will not cover) and *incentives* (through which financial risk is shifted back to physicians and other providers). For detailed descriptions, see Chapter 6 § B-2; Morreim, 1998; Hillman, 1991; Morreim, 1991(a). For MCOs a significant advantage of the latter approach is that as they transfer financial risk back to providers, they also transfer substantial clinical authority and with it the responsibility for the decisions that are then made. Note, however, that financial risk-shifting only partly permits health plans to bypass the micromanagement and UR that precipitate these questions about practicing medicine. Capitation arrangements frequently cover only a limited range of services, such as outpatient physician care and associated laboratory and radiologic studies. Most incentive arrangements reward physicians for being cost-conscious but still leave a significant level of financial risk with the health plan.

34. Corcoran v. United Healthcare, Inc., 965 F.2d 1321 (5th Cir. 1992), cert denied 113 S.Ct. 812 (1992).

35. Corcoran v. United Healthcare, Inc., 965 F.2d 1321, 1329 (5th Cir. 1992).

36. Corcoran v. United Healthcare, Inc., 965 F.2d 1321, 1330–31 (5th Cir. 1992).

37. Corcoran v. United Healthcare, Inc., 965 F.2d 1321, 1331 (5th Cir. 1992).

38. "[I]n a prospective system a beneficiary may be squarely presented in advance of treatment with a statement that the insurer will not pay. . . . A beneficiary in the latter system would be far less inclined to undertake the course of treatment that the insurer has at least preliminarily rejected. By its very nature, a system of prospective decisionmaking influences the beneficiary's choice among treatment options to a far greater degree than does the theoretical risk of disallowance of claim facing a beneficiary in a retrospective system. Indeed, the perception among insurers that prospective determinations result in lower health care costs is premised on the likelihood that a beneficiary, faced with the knowledge of specifically what the plan will and will not pay for, will choose the treatment option recommended by the plan in order to avoid risking total or partial disallowance of benefits." Corcoran v. United Healthcare, Inc., 965 F.2d 1321, 1332 (5th Cir. 1992).

39. Corcoran v. United Healthcare, Inc., 965 F.2d 1321, 1331 (5th Cir. 1992).

Another case capturing some of this debate is Petrovich v. Share Health Plan of Illinois, Inc., 193 F.3d 151 (3rd Cir. 1999). Although the plan was not literally accused of practicing medicine, plaintiffs claimed the plan was vicariously liable under the doctrine of "implied authority," in which a defendant exerts so much control over the otherwise independent contractor as to negate that independence. Share HMO argued "that the act of providing medical care is peculiarly within a physician's domain because it requires the exercise of independent medical judgment. Share thus maintains that, because it cannot control a physician's exercise of medical judgment, it cannot be subject to vicarious liability under the doctrine of implied authority" (at 770). In this case, as the Illinois Supreme Court held that the plan may well have exercised such close control over its physicians' decisions and conduct, it implied that the plan was practicing medicine. For further discussion see Trueman, 2000, at 215–226.

40. See, e.g., Wilson v. Blue Cross of Southern Cal., 271 Cal. Rptr. 876 (Cal. App. 2 Dist. 1990) (beneficiary's policy covered up to 30 days of inpatient psychiatric care per twelve-month period).

41. In *Wilson*, the patient had not exhausted all 30 days of his inpatient coverage; an outside utilization review entity suspended coverage on the gound that further inpatient care was not medically necessary. Wilson v. Blue Cross of Southern Cal., 271 Cal. Rptr. 876, 882–83 (Cal. App. 2 Dist. 1990).

42. As another example, an employee who has been discharged from his job may also lose health insurance. Such a loss will probably affect that person's health care and thereby his health, but one cannot thereby conclude that the employer had been practicing medicine. (This example from David Hyman, JD.)

43. Morris v. Dist. of Col. Bd. of Medicine, 701 A.2d 364 (D.C.App. 1997).

44. Morris v. Dist. of Col. Bd. of Medicine, 701 A.2d 364, 367 (D.C.App. 1997).

45. Morris v. Dist. of Col. Bd. of Medicine, 701 A.2d 364, 367 (D.C.App. 1997) (citations omitted).

Likewise, in his dissent in Long v. Great West Life & Annuity Ins., 957 P.2d 823 (Wyo. 1998), Justice Thomas argued: "It is clear . . . from the philosophical discussion that the premise for the assumed harm is that the insured will forego appropriate care because of the advanced advice that the carrier will not pay in full. The logical fallacy presented is that the carrier could be guilty of malpractice in a situation in which a physician could not. It would be fruitless to search for authority that a medical practitioner is guilty of malpractice because his patient decided not to pursue treatment because of the potential expense" (at 833).

In a similar vein, the California Supreme Court has held that insurers must have the power to determine which services they cover under the language of their contract, even if on occasion the insurer disagrees with the patient's own physician. Sarchett v. Blue Shield of California, 729 P. 2d 267 (Cal. 1987). See also Blue Cross & Blue Shield of Ky. v. Smither, 573 S.W.2d 363, 365 (Ky. App. 1978): "Since a large part of today's rising medical costs are borne by organizations which offer medical benefits plans, such as Blue Cross and Blue Shield, we believe these organizations should be entitled to some measure of protection and should be allowed to challenge decisions made by doctors."

46. Other examples of clearly nonmedical contract limits include explicit exclusions for preexisting conditions (see, e.g., England v. John Alden Life Ins. Col, 846 F.Supp. 798 (W.D.Mo. 1994)) or exclusions for specified services such as podiatry (see, e.g., Axelroth v. Health Partners of Alabama, 720 So.2d 880 (Ala. 1998)).

47. "Under the test of 'medical necessity,' which serves almost universally as the contractual touchstone of plan coverage, the criteria used to check the spending discretion of providers are almost exclusively medical, not economic." Havighurst, 1995, at 15. See also Hall, Smith, Naughton, et al., 1996, at 1055.

48. In the type of telemedicine most relevant to this discussion, a consulting physician at a geographic distance electronically gathers information about a patient, and then offers opinions and recommendations. Such electronic consultation can be particularly valuable for bringing sophisticated expertise to patients in isolated areas and for bringing specialized expertise to patients with unusual conditions. Clearly, in this setting the physician does no "hands-on" work whatever—until, perhaps, refined technologies become available for such interventions as remote robotic surgery. In the meantime, telemedicine represents a situation in which the physician's sole contribution is to provide his medical judgment.

Courts have been quite willing to find that a physician–patient relationship exists when the physician, located at a different geographic site, inserted medical judgments that changed the management of the case. In Hand v. Tavera, 864 S.W.2d 678, 679 (Tex.App.–San Antonio 1993), a Texas appellate court found that a health plan's UR physician did practice medicine when he advised that a patient visiting an emergency room could safely be managed with outpatient care rather than hospital admission. In other cases courts have found that a telephone conversation, such as one to make an appointment, is sufficient to create a physician–patient relationship. For a very useful discussion of potential liabilities surrounding telemedicine, see Kuszler, 1999. See also Terry, 1999.

In its recent opinion on corporate practice of medicine, the Louisiana Board of Medical Examiners offered a definition of medical practice that places a primacy on judgment. "As contemplated by the Medical Practice Act, the essence of the practice of medicine is the *exercise of independent medical judgment* in the diagnosing, treating, curing or relieving of any bodily or mental disease, condition, infirmity, deformity, defect, ailment, or injury in any human being. . . ." Board of Medical Examiners. Statement of Position: Corporate Practice of Medicine; Applicatility of Louisiana Medical Practice Act to Employment of Physician by Corporation Other than a Professional Medical Corporation. September 24, 1992, p. 2 (re. La.Rev. Stat. §§ 37:1261–1292) (emphasis added).

Note also that a comparable concept of medical practice appeared as early as the turn of the century. The Nebraska Supreme Court defined the medical practitioner as one "who undertakes to judge the nature of disease or to determine the proper remedy therefor, or to apply the remedy." Unfortunately, this view did not prevail, as a wide range of subsequent courts opined that the mere hiring of a physician constituted the practice of medicine. State Electro-Medical Institute v. Platner, 103 N.W. 1079, 1081 (Neb. 1905). See also the Kansas Supreme Court in 1890: "The practice of medicine may be said to consist in three things: *First,* in judging the nature, character, and symptoms of the disease; *second,* in determining the proper remedy for the disease; *third,* in giving or prescribing the application of the remedy to the disease. If the person who makes a diagnosis of a case also gives the medicine to the patient, he is, in our judgment, practicing medicine." Underwood v. Scott, 23 P. 942, 943 (Kan. 1890).

49. Murphy v. Board of Medical Examiners, 949 P.2d 530 (Ariz.App.Dist.1 1997).

50. Corcoran v. United Healthcare, Inc., 965 F.2d 1321 (5th Cir. 1992), cert denied 113 S.Ct. 812 (1992).

51. This example comes from Mount Sinai Hospital v. Zorek, 271 N.Y.S.2d 1012, 1016 (Civ. Ct. N.Y. 1966).

52. For example, some judgments about plastic surgery can lie on the border between medical judgments and difficult conceptual interpretations of contractual terms. Jeffrey, 1998.

53. A California Appellate court cites the Restatement 2d of Torts § 431: "'The actors' negligent conduct is a legal cause of harm to another if (a) his conduct is a substantial factor in bringing about the harm, and (b) there is no rule of law relieving the actor from liability. . . .'" Wilson v. Blue Cross of Southern Cal., 271 Cal. Rptr. 876, 883 (Cal. App. 2 Dist. 1990).

54. In other words, in certain situations an agent bears causal responsibility, or not, because she antecedently bore a duty of care. For example, the parent is the cause of a child's starvation not because the parent was the only one who failed to feed the child—when a child has starved, many people have failed to feed it—but because the parent is the one who antecedently had a duty to see to it that the child was fed. Thus, the parent and not some stranger down the street is the cause because of a prior duty. For further exploration of the relationship between causality and the duty of care, see Morreim, 1992(b).

55. Several states have recently enacted statutes stating or implying that health plans sometimes do practice medicine and creating a cause of action for medical malpractice when plans fail to exercise ordinary care when making medical decisions. These include Texas (TEXAS Civ. Prac & Rem. Code §§88.001–003); Georgia (Ga. H.B. 732, 145th Gen. Assembly, Reg. Sess. (Ga. 1999); Ga. S. Res. 210, 145th Gen. Assembly, Reg. Sess. (Ga. 1999)); Missouri (Mo. H.B. 335, § A, 89th Gen. Assembly, 1st Reg. Sess. (Mo. 1997) (codified as amended at Mo. Ann. Stat. § 354.505); California (Cal. Civ. Code § 3428 (West 1999)); Washington (2000 Wash. Legis. Serv. 6199 (West) (Second Substitute Senate Bill 6199, as amended by the House; passed by Senate 3/6/2000; passed by House of Representatives 3/3/2000)). Note that some of these statutes explicitly state that a health plan can defend a charge of malpractice by showing that it was not contractually obligated to provide the care in question. The Texas statute, for instance, provides that there is "no obligation on the part of the health insurance carrier, health maintenance organization, or other managed care entity to provide to an insured or enrollee treatment which is not covered by the health care plan of the entity." See TEXAS Civ. Prac & Rem. Code §§88.001–003, §88.002(d). Washington's statute, similarly, states that a defense to liability exists if the "health care service in question is not a benefit provided under the plan or the service is subject to limitations under the plan that have been exhausted." See new section 17, "Carrier Liability" (amending chapter 41.05 RCW).

56. Canterbury v. Spence, 464 F.2d 772 (D.C. 1972).

57. In addition to the Wisconsin Supreme Court and the *Corcoran* court, quoted above, several other courts have acknowledged the close connection between funding and the availability of care. One court took "judicial notice that, due to the high cost of major medical treatment, individuals who obtain such treatment typically depend upon insurance of some kind to cover much if not most of the bill. In the current health-care market, absent pre-claim verification of insurance coverage, patients may be forced to leave a hospital without receiving medical treatment—even though they are insured for the medical services they seek to obtain—because they lack other sufficient financial resources to pay the costs of treatment." Mimbs v. Commercial Life Ins. Co., 832 F.Supp. 354, 358 (S.D.Ga 1993) (health plan had incorrectly stated, in prospective UR, that the proposed care would not be covered).

In Long v. Great West Life & Annuity Ins., 957 P.2d 823, 827 (Wyo. 1998), the Wyoming Supreme Court noted that, "[a]lthough the attending physician is the ultimate decisionmaker regarding a patient's treatment, it is, as commentators note, naive to assume that a utilization reviewer's determination that recommended care is not medically necessary, and therefore not covered by insurance or the health plan, will not affect the treatment ultimately received by the patient."

Other courts have likewise "recognized the 'commercial realities' facing third-party payors of health care services, noting that in situations in which it is not clear whether a patient is covered by a health insurance plan, 'the provider wants to know if payment reasonably can be expected. Thus, one of the first steps in accepting a patient for treatment is to determine a financial source for the cost of care to be provided.'" Cypress Fairbanks Med. Ctr. v. Pan-American Life Ins., 110 F.3d

280, 282 (5th Cir. 1997) (citing Memorial Hosp v. Northbrook Life Ins., 904 F.2d at 246 (5th Cir '90)).

In Adnan Varol, M.D. v. Blue Cross & Blue Shield, 708 F. Supp. 826, 831 (E.D. Mich. 1989), the court noted that psychiatrists agreed to a utilization review program that gave an insurer "'the right to have significant and, perhaps, dominant influence in deciding what shall be accepted as the correct diagnosis and the proper treatment.'" The court disagreed with the psychiatrists, however, that this constituted unlicensed practice of medicine.

"Because lack of coverage frequently translates, at least as a practical matter, to lack of access to care, prospective and concurrent utilization review can expose a health plan to liability claims of a kind from which indemnity plans are largely insulated." Conrad, Seiter, 1995, at 191.

See also Morris v. Dist. of Col. Bd. of Medicine, 701 A.2d 364 (D.C.App. 1997): "'if health insurance is not available, a procedure very well might not be performed'" (at 367, citing the words of the Board of Medicine).

58. As proposed later in this chapter, contemporary tort law has a way to address cases when the health plan's causal role is small but real. Many states have now adopted concepts of proportionate fault in which each defendant's liability for the injury in question will be gauged according to the degree of its fault.

59. Menzel, 1990, at 145. For a case illustration regarding potentially material information about financial (non)coverage for care, see Kuczewski, DeVita, 1998. It might be worth noting in passing that the health plan need not make an error or a denial in order to be practicing medicine. On the definition presented here, an MCO can also be practicing medicine when, for instance, it correctly deems a test or treatment to be medically indicated and agrees to pay for it, thereby making that care possible for someone who would not otherwise receive it. Such cases are not particularly interesting to the legal system, but they are nonetheless examples of health plans practicing medicine.

60. For a prior exposition of these arguments, see Morreim, 2000(b).

61. "When a health plan agrees to cover health care services, the contract with the beneficiary generally specifies that the services must be paid for when they are reasonable and necessary for the diagnosis or treatment of an illness or injury suffered by the beneficiary." Hirshfeld, Harris, 1996, at 4. See also Bergthold, 1995, at 182; Mariner, 1994; Eddy, 1996, at 652; Anderson, Hall, Steinberg, 1993, at 1636–37; Hall, Anderson, 1992, at 1644–57.

62. "Usually, coverage hinges on the answers to two questions. First, is the proposed service a type that is covered? For example, radiography is covered as a type of diagnostic service. Second, even if the contemplated care is a type generally covered, is its use medically reasonable and necessary in this particular case and thus warranted? To answer the second question, the decision-making process should be individualized and factual." Rosenbaum, Frankford, Moore, et al., 1999, at 230.

63. As noted by Hirshfeld: "When a health plan agrees to cover health care services, the contract with the beneficiary generally specifies that the services must be paid for when they are reasonable and necessary for the diagnosis or treatment of an illness or injury suffered by the beneficiary." Hirshfeld, Harris, 1996, at 4.

64. Rosenbaum, Frankford, Moore, et al., 1999, at 230.

65. In some cases such listed services include procedures traditionally done by specialists, including dermatologic procedures such as skin biopsies, casting of undisplaced fractures, colposcopy, sigmoidoscopy, joint aspiration and injections, stress tests, and the like. Terry 1996(b); Cheney, 1995; Novak, 1998.

66. Glazer, 1992, at 362.

67. Steinberg, Tunis, Shapiro, 1995, at 144–45.

68. One of the most specific definitions comes from Florida's workmen's compensation law: "'Medically necessary' means any service or supply used to identify or treat an illness or injury which is appropriate to the patient's diagnosis, consistent with the location of service and with the level of care provided. The service should be widely accepted by the practicing peer group, should be based on scientific criteria, and should be determined to be reasonably safe. The service may not be of an experimental, investigative, or research nature, except in those instances in which prior approval . . . has been obtained.'" Mariner, 1994, at 1516–17. This more precise-looking definition is still almost hopelessly vague when one tries to define "appropriate," "widely accepted," "reasonably safe," "experimental," and the like.

See also Eddy, 1996, at 651–52; Helvestine, 1989, at 173.

69. Mariner, 1994, at 1516.

"[M]edically necessary means medically appropriate. It excludes experimental care, nonstandard treatments, treatment without any known benefit, and treatment such as cosmetic surgery not intended to relieve a medical condition." Hall, Smith, Naughton, et al., 1996, at 1055.

A few statutory definitions of medical necessity can be listed:

Medicare prohibits payment for services that "are not reasonable and necessary for the diagnosis or treatment of illness or injury or to improve the functioning of a malformed body member" 42 U.S.C. § 1395y(a)(1)(1988) (Section 1862(2)(1)(A) of the Social Security Act)

In the context of Medicaid, Minnesota specifies that covered services must "(A) be determined by prevailing community standards or customary practice and usage to: (1) be medically necessary; (2) be appropriate and effective for the medical needs of the recipient; (3) meet quality and timeliness standards; (4) be the most cost effective health service available for the medical needs of the recipient; (B) represent an effective and appropriate use of medical assistance funds." (Minn. R. 9505.0210)

From Florida's definition: "Covered outpatient services must be medically necessary, preventive, diagnostic, therapeutic or palliative services. . . . Requested service must be reasonably calculated to prevent, diagnose, correct, cure, alleviate, or prevent the worsening of conditions that threaten life, cause suffering or pain, result in illness or infirmity, or threaten to cause or aggravate a handicap, physical deformity, or malfunction, and there is no equally effectrive, more conservative or less costly course of treatment available." (Fla. Admin. Code Ann. r. 10C-7.040(1992))

South Dakota: "To be medically necessary, the covered service must meet the following conditions: (1) It is consistent with the recipient's symptoms, diagnosis, condition, or injury; (2) It is recognized as the prevailing standard and is consistent with generally accepted professional medical standards of the provider's peer group; (3) It is provided in response to a life-threatening condition; to treat pain, injury, illness or infection; to treat a condition that could result in physical or mental disability; or to achieve a level of physical or mental function consistent with prevailing communithy standards for diagnosis or condition; (4) It is not furnished primarily for the convenience of the recipient or the provider; and (5) There is no other equally effective courst of treatment available or suitable for the recipient requesting the service which is more conservative or substantially less costly." (S.D. Admin. R. 67: 16:01:06.02) California: "'A service is "medically necessary" or a "medical necessity" when it is reasonable and necessary to protect life, to prevent significant illness or significant disability, or to alleviate severe pain.'" (cited in Thie v. Davis, 688 N.E.2d 182, 187 [Ind.App. 1997].)

Health plans' corporate definitions can be somewhat more specific. The Travelers Insurance Company has used this definition:

"'The company determines, in its discretion, if a service or supply is medically necessary for the diagnosis or treatment of an accidental injury or sickness. This determination . . . [considers] the following:

- It is appropriate and required for the diagnosis or treatment of the accidental injury or sickness.
- It is safe and effective according to accepted clinical evidence reported by generally recognized medical professionals or publications.
- There is not a less intensive or more appropriate diagnostic or treatment alternative that could have been used in lieu of the service or supply given." *Doe* v. *Travelers Ins. Co.*, 971 F.Supp. 623, 629 (D.Mass. 1997).

In *McGraw* v. *Prudential Ins. Co. of America,* 137 F.3d 1253 (10th Cir. 1998), the Prudential Insurance criteria of medical necessity were identified:

"To be considered 'needed', a service or supply must be determined by Prudential to meet all of these tests:

(a) It is ordered by a Doctor.

(b) It is recognized throughout the Doctor's profession as safe and effective, is required for the diagnosis or treatment of the particular Sickness or Injury, and is employed appropriately in a manner and setting consistent with generally accepted United States medical standards.

(c) It is neither Educational nor Experimental or Investigational in nature." 137 F.3d 1256.

70. Mass. Eye and Ear Infirmary v. Com'r, 705 N.E.2d 592, 595 (Mass. 1999). The court quotes the Massachusetts statutory definition of medical necessity for Medicaid purposes, noting that a service is deemed to be necessary if: "'(1) it is reasonably calculated to prevent, diagnose, prevent the worsening of, alleviate, correct, or cure conditions in the recipient that endanger life, cause suffering or pain, cause physical deformity or malfunction, threaten to cause or to aggravate a handicap, or result in illness or infirmity; and (2) there is no comparable medical service or site of service available or suitable for the recipient requesting the service that is more conservative or less

costly. Medical services shall be a quality that meets professionally recognized standards of health care, and shall be sutstantiated by records including evidence of such medical necessity and quality. . . .'" 130 Cost Mass. Regs. § 450.204 (1997).

71. Havighurst, 1995.

72. In Bucci v. Blue Cross-Blue Shield of Connecticut, 764 F. Supp. 728 (D.Conn. 1991), Blue Cross/Blue Shield had implemented a 5-factor "Technical Evaluation Criteria" (TEC): "Summarized, the criteria are (1) government regulatory approval; (2) evidence which permits conclusions as to the effect on pateint health; (3) demonstrated improvement of the patient's health; (4) demonstration of medical benefit at least equal to that offered by established alternative treatment; and (5) improvement other than in investigational settings." 764 F. Supp. 731. In this case the court held the reliance on the TEC to be invalid on the ground that some portions were irrelevant, other portions subjective. 764 F. Supp. 732.

Daniels, Sabin, 1998; Morreim, 1997(b), at 8–16; Morreim, 2000(a); Hall, Anderson, 1992, at 1683–93; Bergthold, 1995, at 183; Mariner, 1994, at 1516; Bucci v. Blue Cross-Blue Shield of Connecticut, 764 F. Supp. 728 (D.Conn. 1991).

73. "Ambiguities in the plan should be resolved against the insurer." Bucci v. Blue Cross-Blue Shield of Connecticut, 764 F. Supp. 728, 730 (D.Conn. 1991). "If a court finds that an insurance policy is ambiguous, . . . an ambiguous policy will be construed in favor of the insured." Katskee v. Blue Cross/Blue Shield, 515 NW2d 645, 647 (Neb. 1994). See also Jerry, 1996, at 125–136.

74. Havighurst, 1995, at 182.

75. Van Vactor v. Blue Cross Ass'n, 365 N.E. 2d 638 (Ill. 1977).

76. McLaughlin v. Connecticut General Life Ins. Co., 565 F. Supp. 434 (Calif.1983).

77. Ex Parte Blue Cross-Blue Shield of Ala., 401 So.2d 783 (Ala. 1981). See also Haggard v. Blue Cross-Blue Shield of Ala., 401 So.2d 781 (Ala. App. 1980).

78. Group Hospitalization, Inc. v. Levin, 305 A.2d 248 (D.C.App. 1973).

79. A California appellate court held in Hughes v. Blue Cross of Northern Calif., 245 Cal. Rptr. 273 (Cal. App. 1 Dist. 1988), that when an insurer implemented a standard of medical necessity significantly different from prevailing community standards and did not properly investigate a claim, it stood to incur liability for bad faith.

In McGraw v. Prudential Ins. Co. of America, 137 F.3d 1253 (10th Cir. 1998), Prudential Insurance Company had denied physical therapy services for a patient with multiple sclerosis on the ground that it would not affect the course of the disease. Prudential's criteria of medical necessity required that the service be provided by a doctor, that it be recognized as safe and effective for the particular illness or injury, that it be employed in ways consistent with medical standards, and that it not be educational, experimental, or investigational (at 1256). The Tenth Circuit held that the denial of services was arbitrary and capricious on the ground that the insurer had covertly modified its definition of medical necessity to incorporate an additional requirement that the treatment provide a measurable, substantial increase in functional ability (at 1260).

On some occasions courts invoke government Medicare or Medicaid approaches to medical necessity in order to find for plaintiffs. See, e.g., Thie v. Davis, 688 N.E.2d 182 (Ind.App. 1997); Doe v. Travelers Ins. Co., 971 F.Supp. 623 (D.Mass. 1997).

Not every case goes against the health plan, of course. Sometimes a court is willing even to construe an interpretation of medical necessity as being plain enough to prevail. See, e.g., Lockshin v. Blue Cross of Northeast Ohio, 434 N.E. 2d 754 (Ohio App. 1980); Free v. Travelers Ins. Co., 551 F. Supp. 554 (D. Md.1982).

80. Judges' favor for injured plaintiffs sometimes goes further than invoking *contra proferentem.* In a pattern dubbed "judge-made insurance," courts have sometimes been quick to stretch contractual language to award benefits when desperate individuals seek treatment that may be their only hope for survival. Even when contractual language is quite clear, courts sometimes have gone out of their way to favor the needy individual over the large insurer. In Bailey v. Blue Cross/Blue Shield of Va., for instance, a woman with advanced breast cancer sought high-dose chemotherapy with peripheral stem cell rescue (a form of bone marrow transplant). The insurer's policy language stated: "Autologous bone marrow transplants and other forms of stem cell rescue . . . with high dose chemotherapy and/or radiation . . . are not covered." Bailey v. Blue Cross/Blue Shield of Va., 866 F.Supp. 277, 280 (E.D.Va. 1994). Although the policy listed some exceptions to this exclusion, it explicitly stated that breast cancer was not such an exception. Nevertheless, the court found for the plaintiff on the ground that the policy was ambiguous. Typically judges in these cases will argue on the grounds that the contract is ambiguous, that the ill patient may lose her life while the health plan loses only money, and that the patient will arguably prevail on the merits in any event.

For a more detailed discussion of judge-made insurance see, e.g., Abraham, 1981; Ferguson,

Dubinsky, Kirsch, 1993; Hall, Anderson, 1992; James, 1991; Havighurst, 1995; Kalb, 1990; Huber, 1988; Gottsegen, 1981; Great American Ins. Co. v. C.G. Tate Const., 279 S.E.2d 769 (N.C. 1981).

81. Morreim, 1995(a).

82. Often this occurs where the contract has an explicit exclusion.

83. "Ultimately, medical necessity can be thought of as a continuum, whereby services at one end of the continuum are clearly necessary for the diagnosis and treatment of an illness or injury, and services at the other end of the continuum are clearly unnecessary, and in between are services that have some degree of likelihood of benefitting a patient. As one moves along the continuum from clearly necessary to clearly unnecessary, the percentage of likelihood of a benefit from the provision of the health care involved decreases. The value judgment that must be made is how large the percentage of likelihood of a benefit should be for care to be provided. The closer that percentage is to 100%, the more likely it is that some individuals will be harmed by the withholding of care that could have benefitted them." Hirshfeld, Harris, 1996, at 24–25.

"Few medical problems respond to only one form of treatment; instead, a range of interventions, varying both in efficacy and cost, are usually available. Thus, a physician might attempt to treat a sore knee by prescribing rest, aspirin, a brace, or an artificial joint replacement. The optimal choice will vary from patient to patient, but in many cases the older, simpler, less costly treatments— treatments that alone might have constituted accepted medical practice a generation or two ago— will remain reasonably effective." Siliciano, 1991, at 463. See also Henderson, Siliciano, 1994, at 1390.

84. Eddy, 1996, at 654–55; Truog, Brett, Frader, 1992.

85. "Factors that influence the overuse of antibiotics for viral respiratory tract illnesses such as acute bronchitis include patient expectations for antibiotics, purulence of secretions, and physician workload." Gonzales, Steiner, Lum, et al., 1999, at 1518.

86. For further elaboration, see Morreim, 2000(a).

87. As Helvestine points out, health plans may even see an increased risk of liability if they permit their judgments of medical necessity to be influenced by economic considerations. Helvestine, 1989, at 174ff.

88. Pretzer, 1995, at 92–93. Data showed that for every 1000 services allowed:

*for office visit: Blue Shield of Northern Calif denied 12.1, while Wisconsin Physicians' Service denied 109.7;

*for real-time echocardiography: BCBS of Illinois denied zero, while Blue Shield of Calif. denied 2.2, while Transamerica Occidental denied 198.5;

*for myocardial perfusion imaging: BCBS of Ill. and Wisc. Physicians' Service denied zero, while Transamerica Occidental denied 252.3;

*for ambulance with basic life support: Blue Shield of Calif. denied 1.5, BCBS of So. Carolina denied 1.5, while Connecticut General denied 413.2.

Pretzer at 93.

See also Gleason, 1995, at 1483; Mariner, 1995.

This variability also has important implications for providers, since they can be accused of fraud if they provide and bill for "unnecessary" services. As pointed out by one commentator, "HCFA has elected . . . to allow each of its contractors to establish the medical necessity guidelines and parameters that will be applied in its service area. Thus, notwithstanding the national coverage 'speed limit,' HCFA allows—indeed, has encouraged—carriers and fiscal intermediaries to set up what are essentially 'speed traps' for the unwary by refusing to inform providers of local interpretations and parameters to be applied in processing their claims." Blanchard, 1999, at 102.

89. This discussion about quality of life issues is offered, in greater detail, in Morreim, 2000(b).

90. Goldzweig, Mittman, Carter, et al., 1997; Obstbaum, 1997.

91. Adelson v. GTE Corp., 790 F. Supp. 1265 (D.Md. 1992).

92. Retchin, Brown, Yeh, 1997; Webster, Feinglass, 1997.

In Bedrick v. Travelers Insur. Co. the insurer for a boy with cerebral palsy refused to continue most of the coverage for his physical therapy, occupational therapy, and speech therapy because these would not improve the boy's condition. Testimony that the services could preserve current function and prevent deterioration were to no avail until a federal court overturned the insurer's denial. Bedrick v. Travelers Insur. Co., 93 F.3d 149 (4th Cir, 1996).

93. Hirshfeld, 1994, at 93.

94. For further discussion see Morreim 2000(b). Goldzweig, Mittman, Carter, et al., 1997; SUPPORT Principal Investigators, 1995; Schreter, 1993; Borenstein, 1996; Stern, 1996; Lober, 1996; Russell, Kaplan, 1996.

95. Burnum, 1987; Wong, Lincoln, 1983; Hardison, 1979; Mold, Stein, 1986.

96. So long as health care remains so costly, and those costs are simply removed from workers' earnings before the workers ever realise it, people will have limited opportunity to spend their money on the things most important to them. Between 1970 and 1989, "employer expenditures . . . for wages and salaries increased only 1%. . . . In contrast, employer spending for employee health benefits increased 163%." Report to the Board of Trustees, 1995, at 1.

From another study: between 1980 and 1993, "private health insurance costs increased by 218 percent in inflation-adjusted dollars, while the inflation-adjusted gross domestic product per capita rose by just 17 percent." Kuttner, 1999, at 248.

97. Lockshin v. Blue Cross of Northeast Ohio, 434 N.E. 2d 754, 756 (Ohio App. 1980).

98. Eddy, 1996, at 654–55; Truog, Brett, Frader, 1992.

99. Canterbury v. Spence, 464 F.2d 772 (D.C. 1972); Cobbs v. Grant, 502 P.2d 1 (Cal. 1972).

For instance, removal of cataracts may be "necessary" for someone annoyed by an inability to do his favorite things, unimportant for someone who enjoys his life as is, and pointless for patients in a pemanent vegetative state. The key question is whether a particular medical risk or monetary cost is worth paying in order to achieve a desired goal such as possible prolongation of life, symptomatic relief, or functional improvement.

100. For further discussion of the ways in which health plans commonly require subscribers to purchase a level of care beyond what they might want, see Havighurst, 1995.

101. See Eddy, 1996; Bergthold, 1995; Mariner, 1994; Glassman, Model, Kahan, et al., 1997; Glassman, Jacobson, Asch, 1997; Daniels, Sabin, 1997; Enthoven, Singer, 1998, at 101.

102. Aston, 1999.

103. Ouellette v. Christ Hosp., 942 F.Supp. 1060 (S.D.Ohio 1996).

104. 942 F.Supp. 1162.

105. Klisch v. Meritcare Medical Group, Inc., 134 F.3d 1356 (8th Cir. 1998) (citing, with approval, Ouelette v. Subak, 391 NW2d 810, 816 (Minn. 1986)) See also Morlino v. Medical Center, 706 A.2D 721, 731 (N.J. 1998); Brannen v. Prince, 421 S.E.2d 76, 80 (Ga. App. 1992); Deyo v. Kinley, 565 A.2d 1286 (Vt. 1989); Jones v. Chidester, 610 A.2d 964 (Pa. 1992); Parris v. Sands, 25 Cal. Rptr. 2d 800 (Cal. App. 2 Dist. 1993); Riggins v. Mauriello, 603 A.2d 827 (Del. 1992); Tefft v. Wilcox, 6 Kan. 46 (1870); Aiello v. Muhlenberg R. Med. Ctr., 733 A.2d 433, 438 (N.J. 1999)(acknowledging the "exercise of judgment rule" but distinguishing this from poor exercise of skill and care).

106. Peregrine, Schwartz, 2000, at 459.

107. Peregrine, Schwartz, 2000, at 459. Four criteria for applying the rule are: "conscious exercise of judgment," "good faith and no interest," "the business decision must be an informed one," and "the director must rationally believe the decision is in the best interest of the corporation." Peregrine and Schwartz, 2000, at 465. As noted by Peregrine and Schwartz, these criteria apply likewise to not-for-profit entities.

108. Frahm v. Equitable Life Assur. Soc. of U.S., 137 F.3d 955 (7th Cir. 1998).

109. Frahm v. Equitable Life Assur. Soc. of U.S., 137 F.3d 955, 955 (7th Cir. 1998). The court went on to note the limits on accountability for corporate managers who commit errors of business administration.

> A corporate manager is the investors' fiduciary and must act loyally in their interests. But slipups in managing any complex enterprise are inevitable, and negligence—a violation of the duty of care—is not actionable. Quite the contrary, in corporate law managers rarely face liability even for gross negligence; if knowing how best to run a firm is a hard task for full-time managers, it is an impossible task for judges, who lack both the expertise and the incentives of managers.

Frahm v. Equitable Life Assur. Soc. of U.S., 137 F.3d 955, 959 (7th Cir. 1998). This book recommends that those who administer health plans should be liable in tort when their "slipups" are the product of inadequate knowledge, skill, judgment, or effort.

110. Jones v. Chicago HMO, 730 N.E.2d 1119, 1131 (Ill. 2000) (citing Advincula v. United Blood Services, 176 Ill. 2d 1, 32–34 (Ill. 1996)).

111. As noted in Chapter 5, instruments for profiling physicians can be seriously flawed. Hofer, Hayward, Greenfield, et al., 1999; Bindman, 1999; Kassirer, 1994; Salem-Schatz, Moore, Rucker, et al., 1994.

112. "Third party payors of health care services can be held legally accountable when medically inappropriate decisions result from defects in the design or implementation of cost containment mechanisms as, for example, when appeals made on a patient's behalf for medical or hospital care

are arbitrarily ignored or unreasonably disregarded or overridden." Wickline v. State of California, 192 Cal. App. 3d 1630, 1645 (1987).

113. Shannon v. McNulty, 718 A2d 828 (Pa Super 1998).

114. Shannon v. McNulty, 718 A2d 828, 835 (Pa Super 1998) (emphasis added).

115. Shannon v. McNulty, 718 A2d 828, 835 (Pa Super 1998) (emphasis added). See also Wilson v. Blue Cross of Southern Cal., 271 Cal. Rptr. 876, 883 (Cal. App. 2 Dist. 1990) (finding that a health plan or UR entity can be liable if its deficient performance is a "substantial factor" in causing the patient's injuries); and Thompson v. Nason Hosp., 591 A.2d 703, 707 (Pa. 1991) (holding that hospitals have a "duty to formulate, adopt and enforce *adequate* rules and policies to ensure quality care for patients.")

Other cases have likewise raised challenges when courts deem a health plan's guidelines to be medically unsound. In Bauman v. U.S. Healthcare, Inc., for instance, an infant was discharged 24 hours after birth, in accordance with her HMO's general policy. The next day, when the child seemed ill, the parents' repeated phone calls to their physician and to the health plan did not result in readmission to the hospital or even in the in-home nursing visit promised by the HMO. The infant died a day later from an undiagnosed, untreated Group B strep meningitis. Although part of the problem was the plan's failure even to do the things it had promised, a major claim was that its 24-hour postnatal discharge policy was inherently flawed. Bauman v. U.S. Healthcare, Inc., 1 F.Supp.2d 420 (D.N.J. 1998); aff'd, In re U.S. Healthcare, Inc. 193 F. 3d 151 (3rd Cir. 1999), cert. denied 120 SCt 2687 (2000).

116. 2000 Wash. Legis. Serv. 6199 (West) (Second Substitute Senate Bill 6199, as amended by the House; passed by Senate 3/6/200; passed by House of Representatives 3/3/2000). The applicable section reads, in part (new section 8, "Health Care Decisions," (amending RCW70.02.900 and 1991 c 335 s 901)): "Carriers that offer a health plan shall maintain a documented utilization review program description and written utilization review criteria based on reasonable medical evidence. The program must include a method for reviewing and updating criteria."

117. Crum v. Health Alliance Midwest, Inc., 47 F.Supp.2d 1013 (C.D.Ill. 1999).

118. A classic example of a dubious guideline came from the actuarial firm Milliman & Robertson. Their guides are used by such plans as Cigna, Prudential, and United Healthcare Corp, U.S. Healthcare Inc. The guideline regarding cataract surgery indicated that " 'After one lens has been removed, removal of the other lens is only indicated in a relatively young person who requires binocular vision for vocational function.' " The flaws of such a guideline are obvious: a frail, elderly person attempting to descend a staircase needs binocular vision at least as much as a younger working person. The guideline was eventually dropped. Anders, 1994.

119. Three recent Supreme Court cases have held that courts must undertake at least a limited screening of proposed expert testimony that should be anchored in "a reliable foundation," not just the vague "general acceptance" of the earlier *Frye* standard. See Daubert v. Merrell Dow Pharmaceuticals, Inc., 43 F. 3d 1311 (9th Cir. 1995); General Elec. Co. v. Joiner, 118 S.Ct. 512 (1997); Kumho Tire Co., LTD. v. Carmichael, 119 S.Ct. 1167 (1999).

120. For further discussion of *Daubert* in the context of health care, see Shuman, 2001; Jacobson, 2001.

121. Havighurst, 1992, at 1788.

122. Morreim, 2000(a); Morreim 1995(b); Morreim, 1997(b).

123. See Chapter 2, n. 125
Some of the early studies suggest that although patients receiving this treatment may have enjoyed a cancer-free state longer than those receiving conventional chemotherapy, in the final analysis they actually died sooner. ECRI, 1995, at 7.

124. See Meyer, Murr, 1994 (describing alleged inconsistencies in the way an HMO made decisions about ABMT for one patient versus for another).

125. For further discussion on causality issues, see Frankel, 1994, at 1328–31.

126. Cases in which plaintiff claims that the plan literally practiced medicine include Corcoran v. United Healthcare, Inc., 965 F2d 1321 (5th Cir 1992), cert denied 113 S.Ct. 812 (1992); Kuhl v. Lincoln Nat. Health Plan, 999 F.2d 298 (8th Cir. 1993) cert. denied 510 U.S. 1045, 114 S.Ct. 694 (1994); Williams v. Good Health Plus, Inc., 743 S.W.2d 373, 378 (Tex.App.–San Antonio 1988); Roessert v. Health Net, 929 F.Supp. 343 (N.D.Cal. 1996); Garrison v. Northeast Georgia Medical Center, Inc., 66 F.Supp2d 1336 (N.D.Ga. 1999); Williams v. California Physicians' Service, 85 Cal.Rptr.2d 497 (Cal.App. 3 Dist. 1999).

Some recent legislative actions authorize placing malpractice liability on health plans. See supra n. 55. This development is to be distinguished from earlier cases in which courts have considered whether physicians who, acting in their capacity as MCO medicial directors, have practiced medicine. Three such cases, already discussed, are relevant: Murphy v. Board of Medical Examiners, 949 P.2d 530 (Ariz.App.Dist.1 1997) (holding that an HMO's medical director did practice medicine in making UM decisions and was thus subject to supervision of the state medical board); Hand v. Tavera, 864 S.W.2d 678 (Tex.App.–San Antonio 1993) (holding that an HMO's on-call UM physician did have a physician–patient relationship with an enrollee, thus implicitly holding that the UM decisions constituted practicing medicine); Morris v. Dist. of Col. Bd. of Medicine, 701 A.2d 364 (D.C.App. 1997) (holding that a health plan's medical director's actions did not amount to practicing medicine). These cases do not place malpractice liability on MCOs; their reach extends solely to physicians and inquires whether UM activities fall within the ambit of medical practice.

127. In addition to these cases in which medical practice emerges through guideline implementation, it was also noted in Chapter 5 that health plans might practice medicine in any of their designated realms of control, including their business administration activities, construction of guidelines, or surveillance for patterns of poor care.

128. For some examples of guidelines, see the National Guidelines Clearinghouse at http://www.guideline.gov; "Clinical Evidence" guidelines, published by British Medical Journal, at www.clinicalevidence.org; Clinical Practice Guidelines Directory at http://www.ama-assn.org.

129. If such guides are adequately disseminated, as by computer links with physician offices, ideally there should be no need for physicians to contact health plans frequently. Open guidelines should thus, at least in principle, ameliorate a significant portion of the "hassle-factor" currently permeating many physicians' practices as they or their staffs must spend large amounts of time arguing with clerks about invisible edicts.

130. In another option for streamlining the process, health plans might leave the most routine decisions to physicians and patients and produce guidelines only for the costlier, more complex situations in which some measure of uniformity is more important. In such a don't-sweat-the-details arrangement, cost containment at these lower levels could be achieved by placing patients under medical savings accounts or similar financial incentives. Where patients and physicians have reasons to consider the economic as well as the medical wisdom of proposed interventions, there is little need for health plans to intervene. For a more detailed description of such approaches, see Morreim, 2000(a); Morreim 1995(b).

131. Morreim, 1992(b).

132. In Baer v. Regents of University of Cal., 972 P.2d 9, 13 (N.M.App. 1998), the New Mexico Supreme Court cites the Restatement (Third) of Torts (Proposed Final Draft 1998), Section 50(b)(1) and (2), which "addresses the apportionment of liability when damages can be divided by causation:

> '(b) Damages can be divided by causation when there is a reasonable basis for the factfinder to determine:
> (1) that any legally culpable conduct of a party or other relevant person to whom the factfinder assigns a percentage of responsibility was a legal cause of less than the entire damages for which the plaintiff has recovery and
> (2) the amount of damages separately caused by that conduct.'

As noted in that court's earlier decision in Scott v. Rizzo, 634 P.2d 1234, 1237 (N.M. 1981), by 1981 some 35 states had replaced old doctrines such as an all-or-none contributory negligence with comparative fault. "Regardless of the degrees of comparative fault of the parties, the principle of requiring wrongdoers to share the losses caused, at the ratio of their respective wrongdoing, more fairly distributes the burden of fault" (at 1241).

See also McIntyre v. Balentine, 833 S.W. 2d 52 (Tenn. 1992); Harlow v. Chin, 545 N.E. 2d 602, 608 (Mass. 1989); Smith v. Department of Ins., 507 So.2d 1080, 1090–92 (Fla. 1987); Lujan v. HealthSouth Rehabilitation Corp., 902 P.2d 1025 (N.M. 1995).

133. In Adnan Varol, M.D. v. Blue Cross & Blue Shield, 708 F. Supp. 826 (E.D. Mich. 1989), for instance, a district court found that psychiatrists who had agreed to a managed care arrangement and then found its terms intrusive were nevertheless contractually bound. The court noted that even when authorization for services was denied, the providers still received most of their fee. "[T]he Program in no way prevents providers from obtaining full payment even for rendering services that are not concurrently reviewed or preapproved. If the treating psychiatrist renders the service, that psychiatrist can still obtain 80 percent of his fee directly from BCBSM and collect the balance from the patient. So the denial of approval does not have the effect plaintiffs have urged; it merely changes from whom providers collect the 20 percent" (at 833). Although in this case the court's reasoning applied most directly to physicians, it also applied to patients, whom the physicians

would expect to pay the difference. In the eyes of the court, a reasonably affluent patient could make the copayment, while a reasonably affluent physician could absorb the defaults of those who cannot.

In Long v. Great West Life & Annuity Ins., 957 P.2d 823 (Wyo. 1998), a denial of payment authorization meant a far more substantial change in patients' cost-sharing and might be expected to have a considerably greater impact on decisions about the patient's care. "Under the contract, surgery performed without authorization would result in a payment penalty. Authorized surgery was paid at 80% up to $5000.00 less deductibles and then 100% over $5000, while unauthorized surgery would only be paid at 60% for all costs" (at 824). Nevertheless, it might be noted in this case and in a number of others that the patient actually received the treatment, paid out of pocket or from other sources, and then sued afterward for these expenses and other alleged damages.

See also Bast v. Prudential Ins. Co. of America, 150 F.3d 1003 (9th Cir. 1998) (patient paying for initial stages of autologous bone marrow transplant after payor denied coverage); Lenox v. Healthwise of Kentucky, Ltd, 149 F.3d 453, 455 (6th Cir. 1998) (patient eventually underwent successful heart transplant despite insurer's denial of coverage); Killian v. Healthsource Provident Administrators, 152 F.3d 514, 519 (6th Cir. 1998) (high-dose chemotherapy and peripheral stem cell rescue for breast cancer).

134. One major problem that many health plans encounter is attending physicians' failure to provide sufficient information, even after repeated requests. In Crocco v. Xerox Corp., 956 F.Supp. 129 (D.Conn. 1997), for instance, both the patient and the physician refused to provide detailed information about the patient's psychiatric condition. Sorting out problems surrounding inadequate factual information can pose interesting challenges. When a deficit is due to an attending physician's refusal to furnish the necessary information, then arguably the blame and liability for any resulting adverse outcomes should shift to the physician. But reciprocally, when a health plan places onerous administrative burdens or obstructions on its physician staff, the blame and liability can shift back toward the health plan. For further discussion, see Morreim, 1997(b), at 64–67.

135. In one poignant case, a young California girl diagnosed with Wilm's tumor could be cured with surgery. The operation is technically demanding, however, and can only be successful if performed by a highly experienced surgeon. TakeCare Health Plan, the family's HMO, insisted that the surgery be done by a general surgeon with no experience in this particular procedure, rather than by the highly experienced pediatric surgeon whom the family had requested. The child eventually received the surgery from the qualified surgeon, and the HMO was penalized by the California Department of Corporations. Hirshfeld, Harris, 1996, at 36–37.

136. Peregrine and Schwartz, 2000, at 465.

137. Peregrine and Schwartz, 2000.

Jacobson and Cahill offer another plausible description of this procedure-oriented evaluation, recommending that health plan administrators be judged according to traditional fiduciary law (Jacobson, Cahill, 2000). Fiduciaries, by definition, are empowered to act for the benefit of others, exercising discretion in making the kinds of decisions that cannot be determined in advance. Because these are the borderline cases that cannot be managed by simply reading a contract or by some other straightforward means, and because important needs and interests are at stake, administrators as fiduciaries are obligated by duties of loyalty and care. They should not labor under conflicts of interest that divert their focus from the beneficiaries' best interests, even if they cannot escape difficult conflicts of obligation to various individuals and constituencies within the enrollee population. And they should exercise reasonable care and skill in making their decisions (per *Varity Corp.* v. *Howe,* 516 U.S. 489, 504 (1996)).

In this mode, fiduciaries making a decision should first "gather and analyze sufficient information to make a reasoned judgment [and] . . . after the decision, . . . be able to articulate objectively the bases for that decision." Jacobson, Cahill, 2000, at 167. By the same token, judicial scrutiny of challenged decisions should require the fiduciary to demonstrate plausible reasons and show that those reasons actually motivated the decision. "Merely stating that the care should be denied or that providing care would adversely affect the patient population would not fulfill the fiduciary's obligations" (Jacobson, Cahill, 2000, at 169). See also Mehlman, 1990.

CHAPTER 9

1. "Ideally, then, the standard of care would be variable at the level of the individual health plan. This would require a legal regime that allowed beneficiaries and insurers to bargain over the duty of care in the insurance contract and that encouraged courts to defer to that bargain. Plan beneficiaries

could establish a more restrictive standard of care (or even a more generous one, should they be willing to pay for it) through contract language that either explicitly defined the decision rule to be applied in cases alleging negligent medical injury or made reference to a set of medical guidelines or practice protocols as a way of defining the procedures that a physician is obligated to provide to a given patient." Frankel, 1994, at 1327.

See also Havighurst, 1995; Morreim, 1995(a), at 256–57.

2. See Mehlman, 1990, at 374.

3. Morreim, 2000; 63–110; Morreim, 1997(b); Morreim, 1995(a).

4. Havighurst, for instance, has suggested a broad deregulation of health care. "Instead of visualizing a definitive set of guidelines that would be used to set the general tort-law standard for all care, [Havighurst] recommends encouraging the development of competing guidelines that might take different positions on specific issues. Such a strategy would be expressly designed to give health care providers, payors, and consumers new opportunities to choose a specific standard to govern their particular relationship. . . . Instead of defining the obligations of health professionals in universal terms, the law might contemplate that the physician's duty in a given malpractice case might be found in the contract between the physician and the patient. . . . If developed pluralistically, practice guidelines could facilitate both the rational exercise of consumer choice and the writing of contracts that specify just what health services insured groups of consumers do and do not wish to purchase on a prepaid basis. . . . Against this background, practice guidelines can be seen as a potential vehicle for finally enfranchising consumers to choose the style of medical care that best suits their preferences and pocketbooks." Havighurst, 1991, at 88, 108, 113. See also Havighurst, 1992; Havighurst, 1995.

Kalb proposes three tiers. His most basic level would encompass "those technologies demonstrated to be safe, effective, and cost-effective" (at 1119 [footnote omitted]). Thus, it might provide mainly generic medications except when a costlier drug is demonstrably safer or more effective. The next level would include "all those technologies covered by the basic insurance plan plus all technologies that are *not* cost effective" (at 1122). Subscribers at this level might have access to costlier medications that afford greater convenience and comfort than generic brands provide. Low-osmolar contrast media might be available to everyone on grounds of greater comfort. The top level might encompass innovative or "experimental" treatments that have not yet been proven effective. Autologous bone marrow transplant for breast cancer might exemplify treatments of this kind. The detailed content of each system could be spelled out by the particular guidelines or clinical protocols that indicate just what resources it would furnish for different kinds of conditions. See Kalb, 1990, at 1119–26.

Ellman and Hall propose to define health plans' contractual obligations in terms of budgets for specified pools of patients in an allocation model they call Budgeted Risk Preferences. In this system subscribers could choose a policy that would allocate a particular amount each year, e.g., for MRI or CT scans, and the actual expenditures would then be made on the basis of comparative need among subscribers. For instance, for MRI the plan might favor those people for whom MRI provided the best chance of yielding useful information. See Ellman, Hall, 1994. See also Hall, Anderson, 1992.

5. The following points are discussed further in Morreim, 2000.

6. Beauchamp, McCullough, 1984, at 37; Hanson, Callahan, 1998. See also Jonsen, Siegler, Winslade, 1992, at 17. These authors list the goals of medicine as (1) health promotion/disease prevention; (2) relieving symptoms, pain, suffering; (3) curing disease; (4) preventing untimely death; (5) improving functional status, maintaining compromised status; (6) educating, counseling patients; (7) avoiding harm to patients during care.

7. Hadorn, 1992(b), at 20.

8. Eddy, 1993(b).

9. Brandie Hinds, a three-year-old child with short bowel syndrome due to mid-gut volvulus with gangrene, had been nourished via total parenteral nutrition (TPN), a liquid nutrition usually administered by catheter into a large vein. Because this form of feeding ultimately destroys the liver, Hinds needed a liver transplant. However, because the continuing use of TPN would eventually destroy any transplanted liver, Hinds's physicians sought also to transplant bowel in hopes of returning her to normal nutrition. Hinds was a Medicaid patient, and the state's Medicaid office regarded the combined transplant procedure to be experimental and thus not covered by her health plan, which was one of the dozen MCOs in the state's TennCare managed competition plan. This type of surgery had been performed for only a few years at only a small number of institutions, and 58% of all patients had died. Hinds v. Blue Cross and Blue Shield of Tenn, No. 3:95–0508, M.D.TN, 12/28/95.

10. Cuttler, Silvers, Singh, et al., 1996; Bercu, 1996; Oberfield, 1999; Rose, 1995; Finkelstein, Silvers, Marrero, et al., 1998.

11. For further discussion of this issue, see Glazier, 1997; see also Katskee v. Blue Cross Blue Shield of Nebraska, 515 N.W.2d 645 (Neb. 1994).

12. Eddy, 1992; Jacobson, Rosenquist, 1988.

13. For further discussion about care oriented toward comfort, function, and quality of life, see Morreim, 2000(b)

14. Morreim, 2000.

15. Hibbard, Jewett, Legnini, et al., 1997, at 176; Farrell, 1997, at 287.

16. Note also that a relatively small number of tiers and guidelines would make intelligent resource decisions far easier for physicians, who currently must negotiate their way around a stunning diversity of rules and regulations in patients' widely varying health plans.

17. Many plans offer a "point-of-service" option that permits patients to see off-plan providers in exchange for higher payment, and many plans now have two- and three-tier drug formularies that permit patients to have costlier drugs by paying more for them.

18. "People can efficiently process and use only five or six variables or pieces of data in each decision. With more information, a person's ability to use that information declines." Hibbard, Jewett, Legnini, et al., 1997, at 176.

19. Pub. L. No. 101–508, § 4358, 104 Stat. 1388 (codified at 42 U.S.C. § 1395ss (1994)); see also Farrell, 1997, at 287. See also Fox, Snyder, Dallek, et al., 1999, at 41–42 (citing study showing that since the initiation of the MediGap changes, consumers' understanding of benefits "has been greatly enhanced" (at 42)); Hoffman , 1999, at 251 (citing 42 U.S.C. §§ 300e–300e-17 (1994)).

20. One major corporation creating such guidelines is Milliman and Robertson. See Healthcare management guidelines. New York: Milliman and Robertson, 1996–1998. See also Rosenbaum, Frankford, Moore, et al., 1999; Anders, 1994; Weiss v. CIGNA Healthcare Inc., 972 F.Supp. 748, 755 (S.D.N.Y. 1997).

21. These contributions might even come from MCOs, insurers, employers, and manufacturers of drugs and devices. MCOs, employers, and manufacturers are already spending enormous sums doing outcomes studies and pharmacoeconomics research—mostly under major conflicts of interest and too often with poor-quality science, as noted in Chapter 5. Instead, MCOs, corporations, and manufacturers might funnel their funds into such a private agency that could undertake or provide grants for careful, systematic outcomes and economics studies that could, in turn, be used to create guidelines at several levels, as proposed. Such guidelines would be more likely to have a guiding philosophy and conceptual integrity than most guidelines currently available and would be much easier to evaluate in terms of scientific quality. See Morreim, 2000.

Others have proposed a similar idea. Woosley proposes a dozen or so Centers for Education and Research in Therapeutics (CERTs) to study clinical outcomes of various drugs, to be funded collectively by pharmaceutical companies, governments, MCOs, and the like. Woosley, 1994. See also McGivney, 1992; Kong, Wertheimer, 1998; Neumann, Zinner, Paltiel, 1996, at 64.

Although such an entity(s) could be government-based, private agencies might be considerably less subject to the political pressures that recently closed the government's Office of Technology Assessment and precipitated major cutbacks in the scope of the Agency for Health Care Policy and Research. See Deyo, Psaty, Simon, et al., 1997; Kahn, 1998.

Encouragingly, some coordination of research is already beginning to occur. A large number of major corporations have pooled funds to create the Foundation for Accountability (FAcct), an organization that is conducting outcomes studies on a variety of conditions. The research looks not only at standard morbidity and mortality, as do many such studies, but also investigates quality of life, return to normal functions of living, and other matters important to a broader view of medical outcomes. See Keister, 1995, at 21; Terry, 1996.

In an analogous effort, the Managed Care Outcomes Study, funded by six MCOs and the National Pharmaceutical Council, recently led to publication of a study indicating that excessively stringent formulary limits tend perversely to increase patient visits to outpatient offices, emergency rooms, and hospitals, and to raise overall costs of care. See Horn, Sharkey, Tracy, et al., 1996, at 259. In the same vein, the HMO Research Network coordinates twelve research organizations located within integrated health care organizations. See Durham, 1998, at 114ff.

22. Havighurst recommends focusing litigation on the procedural aspects of implementing the contract in just this way. Havighurst, 1995, at 201.

23. See Chapter 8, n. 88 and accompanying text.

24. Blumstein, Sloan, 1981, at 865 (footnote omitted).

25. Siliciano, 1991, at 456–59.

26. Henderson, Siliciano, 1994, at 1398.

"Ideally, then, the standard of care would be variable at the level of the individual health plan. This would require a legal regime that allowed beneficiaries and insurers to bargain over the duty of care in the insurance contract and that encouraged courts to defer to that bargain. Plan beneficiaries could establish a more restrictive standard of care (or even a more generous one, should they be willing to pay for it) through contract language that either explicitly defined the decision rule to be applied in cases alleging negligent medical injury or made reference to a set of medical guidelines or practice protocols as a way of defining the procedures that a physician is obligated to provide to a given patient." Frankel, 1994, at 1327.

27. "An individual who purchases an economy car because of its price or low fuel consumption is unlikely, in a subsequent products liability action, to prevail on a theory that the car was not crashworthy because it was too small or too light. To hold otherwise would unduly impair consumer sovereignty, for if all cars must be as safe as Volvos, what will those who cannot pay the sticker price be able to drive?" Siliciano, 1991, at 439–40.

28. Morreim, 2000(b).

29. See Havighurst, 1995, at 179; Gawande, Blendon, Brodie, et al., 1998.

30. Blendon, Brodie, Benson, 1995, at 243; American College of Physicians, 1996, at 845.

31. Berenson, 1997, at 173.

Yet another study found that "[s]urveys have estimated that 44–58 percent of workers who have insurance are given no choice of plans. However, even persons who have options may be denied effective choice. For example, an employer may drop an employee's plan from the available list, forcing him or her to change." In this study, 42% of respondents said they had no choice of health plan when they enrolled in their current health plan. Of those with choices, 20% said they had too little choice; 31% said their employer forced them to change health plans in the past 5 years. Overall, 63% had no choice, inadequate variety, or a forced change of health plans. Gawande, Blendon, Brodie, 1998, at 186–88.

From a somewhat different vantage point, a study looking at workers rather than employers found that 48% of employees have only one health plan available, while 23% have only two plans to choose from, and 12% have three plans to choose from. Etheredge, Jones, Lewin, 1996 at 94.

32. Purchasing pools have been strongly endorsed by the American College of Physicians, which argues that "the mutual desire of physicians and patients for the maintenance of high-quality, accessible, affordable health care is clearly best served by the empowerment of individual persons in the marketplace. The College believes that this empowerment can be achieved through purchasing pools." American College of Physicians, 1996, at 847.

Such pools include Pacific Business Group on Health, a collaboration of 27 large West Coast firms that together spend some $3 billion to cover 25 million employees, dependents, and retirees; the Health Insurance Plan of California, a California consortium of small private employers covering some 100,000 lives; the Buyers' Health Care Action Group, a collection of 24 large firms in the Twin Cities area; and the Federal Employees Health Benefits Program. See Schauffler, Rodriguez, 1996; Robinson, 1995; Luft, 1995; Shewry, Hunt, Ramey, et al., 1996; Lipson, De Sa, 1996; Report to the Board of Trustees, AMA, 1995; Murata, 1996; O'Brien, 1996; Slomski, 1996; Wetzell, 1996; American College of Physicians, 1996; Butler, Moffit, 1995; Etheredge, Jones, Lewin, 1996; Cain, 1999.

See also Bodenheimer, Sullivan, 1998; Bodenheimer, Sullivan 1998(b); Long, Marquis, 1999.

33. See American College of Physicians, 1996, at 846.

Although there are various advantages and disadvantages to an employer-sponsored approach to providing health care, an additional advantage, aside from pooling for greater options, is that employers can use their purchasing clout to demand and monitor for quality. See Schauffler, Brown, Milstein, 1999; Reinhardt, 1992; Lave, Peele, Black, et al., 1999.

34. For example, rather than declaring a new drug to be either "necessary" or "unnecessary," a lower-cost health plan could offer a higher tier of more convenient or comfortable drugs as an "upgrade" available for purchase when they are not standard. Conversely, a higher-cost plan might include the newest drugs as a covered benefit for everyone, yet permit subscribers to share some savings if they opt to forego them in favor of more ordinary drugs.

35. See Morreim 1995(b). See also Goodman, Musgrave, 1992, at 439–62; Pauly, Goodman, 1995, at 129. For a variation on the MSA concept, see Morreim 1995(b).

36. See DeMott, 1988, at 903, noting some protections built into contract law: "the classical rules of offer and acceptance, by requiring that an acceptance precisely mirror the terms of the offer to which it responds, delay contract formation and thereby create opportunities for reflection and exit from improvident commitments" (footnotes omitted).

37. See Havighurst, 1995, at 181.

38. In this connection it is useful to think of "relational" contracts. These tend to be longer-term and guided more by a basic philosophy than by the crystal clear, highly transactional contract of the proverbial horse sale. See, e.g., Havighurst, 1992(b), at 126, stating that relational contracts, "instead of rigidly defining and anticipating every detail of the parties' future relationship, supply a basic structure that can accommodate unpredictable events and facilitate adaptations that further the parties' mutual long-term purposes." One can view these relational contracts as "frameworks for carrying on long-term, committed relationships, and parties routinely make major accommodations and suppress individual impulses in order to preserve harmonious relations." Havighurst, 1995, at 183; see also Farnsworth, 1990, at 28. For a particularly rich discussion of the concept, see Macneil, 1980, especially Chapter 3, "Relational Contract Law," at 71–117.

39. In addition to disclosing the guidelines' basic approach to care, it would seem appropriate for plans to provide information regarding how their guidelines were created. Those guidelines based on science may have more credibility than those created strictly by consensus of a few invited physicians.

For further discussion, see Havighurst, 1995, at 161–64.

40. Increasingly, a variety of Internet sites provide information for making choices among health plans. For example, the federal government has several sites for Medicare beneficiaries wishing to enroll in Medicare + Choice plans. At that site the Medicare Compare database provides info about each plan's premium costs, physician visit costs, prescription drug coverage, and the like. Similarly, the National Committee for Quality Assurance (NCQA) has several sites providing assessments of the various health plans it evaluates; some consumer organizations likewise have sites providing report card information, such as consumer satisfaction data and preventive care evaluations of various health plans. The state of New Jersey has a site permitting easy comparisons among various managed care plans within the state. And one HMO, Pacificare of California, has a site with information about the plan, including a "Quality Index" that rates the largest provider groups with which the HMO contracts. See Rai, 1999, at 397–400.

See also Weingarten, 1999, at 455: "The *Clinical Practice Guidelines Directory* (http://www.ama-assn.org) serves as a repository of guidelines on more than 2000 topics from more than 90 organizations. It is easy to use and can quickly point a reader toward the sources of guidelines on relevant topics. The *U.S. Preventive Services Task Force Guide to Clinical Preventive Services* (http://lww.com) is an evidence-based source of preventive care recommendations. . . . Another resource available on the Internet is the National Guideline Clearinghouse, which includes guidelines that meet specific criteria for being evidence-based. The Agency for Health Care Policy and Research, in partnership with the American Association of Health Plans and the American Medical Association, has invited developers of practice guidelines, including professional societies, to submit guidelines for possible inclusion in the National Guideline Clearinghouse. Guidelines must contain systematically developed statements that satisfy the Institute of Medicine's definition of a guideline; be developed under the auspices of a medical organization; be derived from a systematic review of the relevant literature and science; have been developed, reviewed, or revised in the past 5 years; and be available in English."

Furrow proposes putting a wide variety of guidelines on the Internet and lists a number of sites that already provide scientific research and guidelines. See Furrow, 1994, at 419–20. See also Hunt, Jaeschke, McKibbon, et al., 2000.

41. Interestingly, at least one court has held a health plan at fault for failing to reveal the guidelines as they related to the plaintiff-patient's situation. Doe v. Travelers Ins. Co, 971 F.Supp. 623 (D.Mass 1997). This ruling was overturned, however, in Doe v. Travelers Ins. Co., 167 F.3d 53 (1st Cir. 1999).

42. Interestingly, a recent study featuring interviews with a number of health plan executives showed that many were considering the possibility of shifting toward guidelines-based contracting. See Studdert, Sage, Gresenz, et al., 1999. As liability for health plans continues to expand, the authors noted, "contractors may be motivated to unbundle catchall terms such as *medical necessity* into a taxonomy of clinical scenarios or to develop detailed protocols for determining when treatments are experimental" (at 17).

> A majority espoused the view that heightened exposure would result in increased specificity and a greater tendency to clarify roles. One interviewee remarked on the possiblity of '900-page purchasing contracts,' with an accompanying 'incomprehensible road map' of benefits coverage. Another predicted that contractual expansion would likely be determined by 'problem' areas—those types of treatments that reveal themselves over time to be particularly

frequent or expensive targets of litigation. If plans chose not to allow wholesale coverage of such treatments, they might use the contract to carefully delineate them as excluded.

Id. at 18.

43. See, e.g., Rosenbaum, Frankford, Moore, et al., 1999, at 23.

44. Blumenthal points to 1993 as the first year of genuinely effective cost containment in health care. "Average annual rates of increase in per capita national health care expenditures ranged from 4 to 5 percent in the period from 1970 to 1993, but fell to 1.5 percent in the period from 1993 to 1996, and are estimated at 2.6 percent for the period from 1996 to 1998." Blumenthal, 1999, at 1916.

45. Robinson, 1999; Berwick, 1996; Robinson, Casalino, 1995; Robinson, Casalino, 1996.

46. See Chapter 10 § C.

47. See Herdrich v. Pegram, 154 F.3d 362 (7th Cir. 1998), reversed, Pegram v. Herdrich, 120 U.S. 2143 (2000); Shea v. Esensten, 107 F.3d 625 (8th Cir. 1997); Shea v. Esensten, 208 F3d 712, (8th Cir. 2000) ("Shea II"); Neade v. Portes, 710 N.E.2d 418 (Ill.App.2 Dist. 1999). But see Ehlmann v. Kaiser Foundation Health Plan, 20 F.Supp.2d 1008 (N.D.Tex. 1998), aff'd 198 F.3d 552 (5th Cir. 2000); Weiss v. CIGNA Healthcare Inc., 972 F.Supp. 748 (S.D.N.Y. 1997); D.A.B. v. Brown, 570 NW2d 168 (Minn.App. 1997); Spoor v. Serota, 852 P.2d 1292 (Colo.App. 1992); Awai v. Kotin, 872 P.2d 1332 (Colo. App. 1993). For further discussion see Chapter 10 §§ A and B-1.

Note, however, that the Supreme Court has ruled that the existence of incentive arrangements does not, in itself, constitute a breach of fiduciary duty in ERISA plans. Pegram v. Herdrich, 120 U.S. 2143 (2000).

48. The New Jersey statute was signed into law Aug. 7, 1997. Health Care Quality Act, ch. 192, 1997 N.J. Sess. Law Serv. 192 (West).

49. In new section 8, "Health Care Decisions," (amending RCW70.02.900 and 1991 c 335 s 901), the state's patient protection legislation mandates that "Carriers shall make clinical protocols, medical management standards, and other review criteria available upon request to participating providers."

In a somewhat related vein, plans have largely removed the infamous "gag clauses" that allegedly instructed physicians not to inform patients about limits on treatment or incentive structures. See Chapter 7, n. 7.

50. Freudenheim, 2001.

51. See Chapter 7 § B-1.

52. Courts uniformly discard such agreements. See, e.g., Tunkl v. Regents of Univ. Of Cal., 383 P.2d 441, 442 (Cal. 1963); Emory Univ. v. Porubiansky, 282 S.E.2d 903, 903–04 (Ga. 1981); Cudnik v. William Beaumont Hosp., 525 N.W.2d 891, 896 (Mich. Ct. App. 1994).

53. See Madden v. Kaiser Foundation Hospitals, 552 P.2d 1178 (Cal. 1976); Morris v. Metriyakool, 344 N.W. 2D 736, 753 (Mich. 1984); Sage, Jorling, 1994, at 1025 (noting that at the time of choosing among various health plans, people are "better able to make uncoerced decisions than they might be as patients seeking treatment."

54. See Schauffler, Rodriguez, 1996; Bodenheimer, Sullivan, 1998; Schauffler, Brown, Milstein, 1999; Terry, 1998.

55. See McGee v. Equicor-Equitable HCA Corp., 953 F.2d 1192, 1207 (10th Cir. 1992): "While it is readily apparent Mr. McGee sought the best possible care for his daughter, he was still obligated to work within the defined contractual borders of the HMO he *elected* to participate in" (emphasis added); see also Madden v. Kaiser Found. Hosps., 552 P.2d 1178, 1185–86 (Cal. 1976).

56. Madden v. Kaiser Found. Hosps., 552 P.2d 1178, 1185 (Cal. 1976).

57. As Havighurst notes, "[c]ourts are less likely to use these doctrines [e.g., adhesion] to invalidate a contract term, however, if they are satisfied by all the circumstances that the agreement was arrived at fairly. . . . Insurance law also supports the impression that contracts modifying tort rights will be judicially enforced if the bargaining circumstances seem fair." Havighurst 1986(a), at 166, 168. See also Morris v. Metriyakool, 344 N.W. 2D 736, 753 (Mich. 1984); Erickson v. Aetna Health Plans of Cal., 84 Cal.Rptr.2d 76 (Cal.App. 4 Dist. 1999); Hollister v. Benzl, 83 Cal.Rptr.2d 903, 906 (Cal.App.4 Dist. 1999).

58. In ERISA cases plaintiffs' claim in this scenario is that the administrator's denial of benefits was arbitrary and capricious or an abuse of discretion. Courts look mainly to the contract to resolve the question and additionally inquire whether the administrator's decision making process was reasonable. See, e.g. Vega v. Nat. Life Ins. Services, Inc., 188 F.3d 287 (5th Cir. 1999): the court's review "need not be particularly complex or technical; it need only assure that the administrator's decision fall somewhere on a continuum of reasonableness—even if on the low end" (188 F.3d

297). See also Kimber v. Thiokol Corp., 196 F.3d 1092 (10th Cir. 1999); Doe v. Travelers Ins. Co., 167 F.3d 53 (1st Cir. 1999); McGraw v. Prudential Ins. Co. of America, 137 F.3d 1253 (10th Cir. 1998); Hunt v. Hawthorne Associates, Inc., 119 F.3d 888 (11th Cir. 1997). For further discussion, see Chapter 11.

59. As further noted in Chapter 8, neither could an MCO have practiced medicine, as a special focus of tort, if it did not quite clearly owe the patient the particular care in question. This is because even if the MCO has made one or more medical judgments about the patient's care, it can not have actually *practiced* medicine if those judgments did not significantly affect the patient's actual course of care.

60. It is also possible, of course, for an MCO to commit a tort without any breach of contract. Chapter 6 pointed out that health plans can engage in sloppy business practices, poor-quality credentialing, and the like without necessarily violating any contractual provisions.

CHAPTER 10

1. For further discussion of these historical developments, see Starr, 1982; Morreim, 1991(a); Morreim, 2000(a).

2. Morreim, 1998.

3. In a number of recent cases, courts have based important rulings on serious misunderstandings about the financial structures of health plans and the implications that these structures do and do not have for the ways health care was delivered in that plan. For an extended discussion of three such cases, see Morreim, 2000(c).

4. As quoted in Chapter 7: "the physician who complies without protest with the limitations imposed by a third party payor, when his medical judgment dictates otherwise, cannot avoid his ultimate responsibility for his patient's care. He cannot point to the health care payor as the liability scapegoat when the consequences of his own determinative medical decisions go sour." A physician may be intimidated by a health plan's denial of coverage, but he is "not paralyzed . . . nor rendered powerless to act appropriately if other action was required under the circumstances." Wickline v. State of California, 192 Cal. App. 3d 1630, 1645 (1987) (dicta). Although subsequent decisions have held that physicians' obligations do not exempt health plans from their own liabilities (Wilson v. Blue Cross of Southern Cal., 271 Cal. Rptr. 876 (Cal. App. 2 Dist. 1990)), these do not negate the notion that physicians should make reasonable efforts to assist their patients to receive entitled resources. See also Chew v. Meyer, 527 A.2d 828 (Md. App. 1987); Tabor v. Doctors Memorial Hosp., 563 So.2d 233 (La. 1990). See also Chapter 7, n.9.

5. Neade v. Portes, 710 N.E.2d 418 (Ill.App. 1999); rev'd, 739 N.E.2d 496 (Ill. 2000).

6. Shea v. Esensten, 208 F3d 712, (8th Cir. 2000) ("Shea II"); see also Moore v. Regents of the University of California, 793 P.2d 479 (Cal. 1990), cert. denied 112 S. Ct. 2967 (1992).

7. Shea v. Esensten, 2001 WL 96192 (Minn. App. 2001).

8. See, e.g., D.A.B. v. Brown, 570 N.W. 2d 168 (Minn. App. 1997)(finding that nondisclosure of incentives does not create separate cause of action against physician for breach of fiduciary duty); Spoor v. Serota, 852 P.2d 1292 (Colo. App. 1992); Awai v. Kotin, 872 P.2d 1332 (Colo. App. 1993).

9. Morreim, 1991(c). These cases parallel recent litigation brought against health plans, e.g., for failing to disclose incentive arrangements. See Chapter 9 § C.

10. See Chapter 6 § B-2.

11. See particularly Chapter 8 § C-1–a, b.

12. For further discussion, see Chapters 3 and 8.

13. "A hospital has a duty to its patients to use reasonable care in formulating the policies, the procedures, the rules and the bylaws by which its medical staff and non-physician personnel are governed." Allred, Tottenham, 1996, at 467.

14. Wickline v. State of California, 192 Cal. App. 3d 1630, 1645 (1987) (dicta).

15. Wickline v. State of California, 192 Cal. App. 3d 1630, 1645 (1987).

16. Wilson v. Blue Cross of Southern Cal., 271 Cal. Rptr. 876, 883 (Cal. App. 2 Dist. 1990).

17. "The dicta in [*Raglin* and *Petrovich*] indicates [sic] there may be two kinds of HMO corporate negligence: one is the negligent selection or negligent control of the physician; the other consists of independent acts of negligence, for example, in the management of utilization control systems." Jones v. Chicago HMO Ltd. of Illinois, 703 N.E.2d 502, 508 (Ill. App. 1 Dist. 1998) (referring to Petrovich v. Share Health Plan of Illinois, 696 N.E.2d 356 (Ill. App. 1 Dist. 1998) and Raglin v. HMO Illinois, Inc., 595 N.E. 2d. 153 (Ill. App. 1. Dist. 1992)). See also Petrovich v.

Share Health Plan of Illinois, Inc., 7i9 NE 2d 756 (Ill. 1999). The *Jones* case was affirmed in part, reversed in part: Jones v. Chicago HMO, 730 N.E.2d 1119 (Ill. 2000).

18. See, e.g., Healthcare America Plans, Inc. v. Bossemeyer, 953 F.Supp. 1176 (D.Kan. 1996) affd w/o opin. 166 F.3d 347 (court emphasizing the importance of procedure by noting that despite some conflict of interest in an MCO's decision not to cover high-dose chemotherapy and peripheral stem-cell rescue for a patient with breast cancer, there was "no evidence that fiduciary did not conduct full and fair review or that those who reviewed claim were motivated by desire to enhance their personal or corporate financial position at beneficiary's expense") (at 1178).

19. See Chapter 8. See also, e.g., Weatherly v. Blue Cross Blue Shield Ins. Co., 513 N.W.2d 347, 354 (Neb. Ct. App. 1994).

For further discussion of bad faith doctrine, see Fletcher v. Western Nat'l Life Ins.Co., 89 Cal. Rptr. 78, 92–94 (Cal. Ct. App. 1970); Diamond, 1981, at 443–47 (1981); Louderback, 1982, at 192–96 (1982); Stern, 1983.

20. Petrovich v. Share Health Plan of Illinois, 696 N.E.2d 356, 362 (Ill. App. 1 Dist. 1998), aff'd 719 N.E.2d 756 (Ill. 1999). See also Kampmeier v. Sacred Heart Hospital, 1966 WL 220979 (E.D. Pa).

21. Herdrich v. Pegram, 154 F.3d 362 (7th Cir. 1998).

22. The court agreed with plaintiff Herdrich that a serious flaw inheres in the fact that the Carle Clinic's physician-owners "simultaneously control the care of their patients and reap the profits generated by the HMO through the limited use of tests and referrals. Under the terms of ERISA, Herdrich most certainly has raised the specter that the self-dealing physician/owners in this appeal were not acting 'solely in the interest of the participants' of the Plan." *Herdrich v. Pegram*, 154 F.3d 362, 373 (7th Cir. 1998). The court went on: "A doctor who is responsible for the real-life financial demands of providing for his or her family . . . might very well 'flinch' at the prospect of obtaining a relatively substantial bonus for himself or herself. *Here, the Carle physicians were intimately involved with the financial well-being of the enterprise in that the yearly 'kick-back' was paid to Carle physicians only if the annual expenditures made by physicians on benefits was less than total plan receipts. According to the complaint, Carle doctors stood to gain financially when they were able to limit treatments and referrals.* Due to the dual-loyalties at work, Carle doctors were faced with an incentive to limits costs so as to guarantee a greater kickback" (154 F.3d 379, emphasis in original).

Similarly, Illinois courts have opened the door to the possibility that a jury might take a capitation system into account in evaluating the quality of the patient's care. The HMO's "use of the capitation system could lead to the reasonable inference that Share's method of compensation to its participating physicians created a disincentive to order tests or make referrals and thus exerted control over its physicians' medical decisions. Here, plaintiff testified at her deposition that Dr. Kowalski told her that Share would not pay for more tests. This evidence was relevant to whether plaintiff was led to believe that Dr. Kowalski was controlled by [the HMO]." Petrovich v. Share Health Plan of Illinois, 696 N.E.2d 356, 362 (Ill. App. 1 Dist. 1998), aff'd 719 N.E.2d 756 (Ill. 1999).

See also Kampmeier v. Sacred Heart Hospital, 1966 WL 220979 (E.D. PA).

23. Pegram v. Herdrich, 120 U.S. 2143 (2000). The court's dicta seemed to accept the existence of incentives outside as well as within the ERISA context.

In Bush v. Dake, one of the earliest such cases, the plaintiff claimed that the delay in diagnosing her cervical cancer was due in part to her HMO's system of incentives and risk sharing. The court granted defendants' move for summary judgment on the ground that the legitimacy of such arrangements was a public policy matter for the legislature, not the courts, to determine. See File No. 86-25767 NM-2, State of Michigan, Circuit Court, County of Saginaw, 1989. Quoted and discussed in Furrow, Greaney, Johnson, et al., 1997.

Other early cases also downplayed the role of physician incentives. In Madsen v. Park Nicollet Medical Center, 419 N.W. 2d 511 (Minn. App. 1988), a Minnesota appellate court would not even permit information about the HMO physician's incentives to be introduced at trial:

we do not agree that the trial court abused its discretion in excluding evidence that Robin Madsen's status as an HMO member meant that her hospitalization could have adversely affected Dr. Solberg's profits. This evidence was only marginally relevant, and potentially very prejudicial. Even if evidence has probative value, [the trial court has] discretion to exclude it. . . . That discretion was not abused.

419 N.W. 2d 515.

In Pulvers v. Kaiser Foundation Health Plan, 160 Cal. Rptr. 392 (Cal. App. 1980), a California appellate court found that a nonprofit health plan's incentive arrangement to encourage conservative care did not constitute a fraudulent deception after plaintiffs alleged they had been induced to believe they would receive "the best" quality of care.

In Maltz v. Aetna Health Plans of New York, Inc., 114 F.3d 9 (2nd Cir. 1997), the Second Circuit held that a health plan's institution of capitation arrangements did not per se breach its ERISA fiduciary duty, even though the change prompted some physicians to quit the plan, so long as "enrollees are aware of the changes when they renew their contract with Aetna and Aetna provides them with competent, alternative physicians." 114 F.3d 12.

In Lancaster v. Kaiser Foundation Health Plan, 958 F.Supp. 1137 (E.D.Va. 1997), plaintiffs alleged that physicians' five-year delay in diagnosing brain tumor in an eleven-year-old girl was due to an incentive scheme that induced physicians to deny care. The case focused on ERISA preemption issues, and the court held that although the injuries to the child were quality matters that rightly belonged to state tort law, the legitimacy of incentive systems concerned the administrative structure of the plan and was therefore preempted by ERISA. The court noted that "Consistent with an HMO's goal of containing health care costs, the Incentive Program is ostensibly designed to encourage physicians to refrain from prescribing unnecessary and costly medical procedures and tests" (at 1140). Nevertheless, the court held that the physician's failure to order diagnostic tests was an issue of quality and not of quantity. Pointing to traditional views on the medical standard of care, the court held that financial incentives had no role in the plaintiff's malpractice claims because physicians are at fault for deviations from the standard of care no matter how they may be motivated. In other words, a physician's substandard care is ipso facto a quality problem, even if it involves a failure to provide resources and even if that deficiency was prompted by a financial incentive program (at 1146). ERISA will be discussed further in Chapter 11.

Ouelette v. Christ Hosp., 942 F.Supp. 1060 (S.D.Ohio 1996), was another ERISA case. The plaintiff claimed that her early hospital discharge was due to an incentive arrangement between her HMO and the hospital. The court concluded that the incentive arrangement did not present a reason to preempt the case from going to state courts.

24. Shea v. Esensten, 107 F.3d 625 (8th Cir. 1997). See also Drolet v. Healthsource, Inc., 968 F. Supp. 757 (D.N.H. 1997); Eddy v. Colonial Life Ins. Co. of America, 919 F.2d 747, 750–51 (D.C.Cir. 1990); Bixler v. Cent. Pa. Teamsters Health-Welfare Fund, 12 F.3d 1292 (3rd Cir. 1993); Lancaster v. Kaiser Foundation Health Plan, 958 F.Supp. 1137 (E.D. Va. 1997); Ouelette v. Christ Hosp. 942 F.Supp. 1060 (S.D.Ohio 1996) (identifying incentive issues but focusing on ERISA issues, holding that ERISA does not preempt other claims); Neade v. Portes, 710 N.E.2d 418 (Ill. App. 2 Dist. 1999)(holding that physician can breach fiduciary duty by failing to disclose incentives); rev'd, 739 N.E.2d 496 (Ill. 2000).

In Paul v. Humana Medical Plan, Inc., 682 So.2d 1119 (Fla. App. 4 Dist. 1996), (rev. denied, 695 So.2d 700 [Fla 1997]), it was noted that the defendant physician who failed to timely diagnose and adequately treat laryngeal cancer was paid via a monthly capitation fee. The plaintiff-appellant claimed that "financial considerations motivated the doctors who wanted to avoid incurring additional expenses for Mrs. Paul's hospitalization and treatment. Additionally, appellants claimed the doctors acted with extreme and outrageous conduct in failing to provide Mrs. Paul with adequate medical care and that they intentionally refused to render medical care and treatment with the knowledge that doing so would result in their increased profits and in Mrs. Paul's emotional distress." 682 So.2d 1121. The court ruled, with little discussion, that plaintiff had a cause of action against the physician for medical negligence.

25. The Fifth Circuit found that failure to disclose incentives does not specifically violate the duties of ERISA fiduciaries, basing its reasoning on the lack of any explicit statutory requirement for ERISA administrators to disclose incentives. See Ehlmann v. Kaiser Foundation Health Plan of Texas, 20 F.Supp.2d 1008 (N.D.Tex. 1998), aff'd 198 F.3d 552 (5th Cir. 2000). See also Weiss v. CIGNA Healthcare Inc., 972 F.Supp. 748 (S.D.N.Y. 1997) (holding there is not a fiduciary duty for ERISA plans to disclose incentive arrangements): "Weiss' contention that CIGNA's compensation package facially violates ERISA simply because it deprives her of her right to receive 'medical opinions and referrals unsullied by mixed motives,' . . . is tantamount to a claim that risk-sharing arrangements in managed care are inherently illegal, a position that is refuted by federal and New York law" (at 753). See also Anderson v. Humana, Inc. 24 F.3d 889 (7th Cir. 1994) (suit for failure to disclose HMO incentives held to be preempted by ERISA): Peterson v. Connecticut Gen. Life Ins. Co., 2000 WL 1708787 (E.D. Pa. 2000) (finding that to impose a duty on health plans to disclose financial incentives for physicians would be unduly burdensome). Note that these rulings would not preclude a finding that a failure to disclose incentives may violate other duties of insurers in the non-ERISA context, such as a breach of good faith and fair dealing.

26. See Chapter 8 § C-1-b.

27. Thompson v. Nason Hosp., 591 A.2d 703, 707 (Pa. 1991) (emphasis added); see also Welsh v. Bulger, 698 A.2d 581 (Pa. 1997).

28. Shannon v. McNulty, 718 A2d 828 (Pa Super 1998).

29. Shannon v. McNulty, 718 A2d 828, 835 (Pa Super 1998).

30. See Wickline v. State of California, 192 Cal. App. 3d 1630 (1987); Wilson v. Blue Cross of Southern Cal., 271 Cal. Rptr. 876 (Cal. App. 2 Dist. 1990); In re U.S. Healthcare, 193 F3d 151 (3d Cir. 1999), cert. denied 120 SCt 2687 (2000); Crum v. Health Alliance Midwest, Inc., 47 F.Supp.2d 1013 (C.D.Ill. 1999).

31. Creason v. Department of Health Services, 957 P.2d 1323 (Cal. 1998).

32. Creason v. Department of Health Services, 957 P.2d 1323, 1333 (Cal. 1998).

33. Doe v. Southeastern Penn. Transp. Auth. (SEPTA), 72 F.3d 1133 (3rd Cir. 1995).

34. Doe v. Southeastern Penn. Transp. Auth. (SEPTA), 72 F.3d 1133, 1141 (3rd Cir. 1995).

35. Barnett v. Kaiser Foundation Health Plan, Inc., 32 F.3d 413 (9th Cir. 1994).

36. The patient was e-antigen positive, meaning that the virus was rapidly replicating and not controllable. 32 F.3d 414. The criteria excluding patients with this type of hepatitis from transplant eligibility were taken largely from other medical centers, including University of California at San Francisco and Pittsburgh. 32 F.3d 417. As the court noted: "The doctors, as part of their professional responsibility, were legitimately concerned with distribution of livers to patients with the best chances of survival. Poor survival rate is an acceptable medical criterion." 32 F.3d 417.

37. The court explicitly noted that "[t]here is no evidence that the decision was motivated by financial concerns for cost savings to the Kaiser Health Plan" (Barnett v. Kaiser Foundation Health Plan, Inc., 32 F.3d 413, 417 (9th Cir. 1994)) and "that the decision was made . . . that the procedure was not medically appropriate for Barnett, rather than a cost savings to the Kaiser Plan" (at 416). However, although it thus noted that the decision was based on medical rather than financial criteria, the court did not actually reject financial considerations.

38. In Goepel v. Mail Handlers Benefit Plan, a New Jersey district court openly acknowledged financial resource constraints. Noting that new technologies save lives but unfortunately also drive the cost of medical care beyond some citizens' reach, the court pointed out that "rationing . . . already is, and may well remain, a reality until further technological, scientific, or social advances reduce, rather than escalate, health care costs." The court went on to uphold a denial of coverage for bone marrow transplant for breast cancer based on an unambiguous policy exclusion. Goepel v. Mail Handlers Benefit Plan (No. 93–3711, 1993 WL 384498 (D. N.J. 9/24/93)). The case was reversed and remanded on appeal, but for reasons of jurisdiction, not of substance. Goepel v. Mail Handlers Benefit Plan, 36 F.3d 306 (3rd Cir. 1994).

In New York Life Ins. Co. v. Johnson, the estate of a young man who died of AIDS was denied life insurance benefits because the man had lied about his smoking habits on the application form. Although it sympathized with the man's family, the Third Circuit court noted that if individuals who make such false statements are not denied benefits, as contractually stipulated, others will pay the price. "The victims will be the honest applicants who tell the truth and whose premiums will rise over the long run to pay for the excessive insurance proceeds paid out as a result of undetected misrepresentations in fraudulent applications." New York Life Ins. Co. v. Johnson, 923 F.2d 279, 284 (3rd Cir. 1991).

In a different sort of case that nevertheless raised the same concern, the First Circuit discarded a plaintiff's contention that a collagen anti-wrinkle treatment was a dangerous product, negligently designed and misrepresented in advertising. Noting that this device had been formally approved by the FDA, the court acknowledged the public's broader interests. If manufacturers' legal risks are

> too great, worthwhile medical devices may be left in the laboratory, to the public's loss. Public health is a valid federal purpose, and Congress can reasonably weigh possible loss to the idiosyncratic few against benefits to the public generally. . . . [the Medical Device Amendment] shows the principal emphasis to be on the protection of the individual user. But it also shows the intent to 'encourage . . . research and development' and 'permit new and improved devices to be marketed without delay.' Perfection is impossible and a few individuals may be denied full protection at the cost of benefitting the rest.

King v. Collagen Corp., 983 F.2d 1130, 1137–38 (1st Cir. 1993).

Along a similar line, a Maryland district court noted that "[b]ecause [these] cases frequently touch 'our human sympathies,' courts of appeal have cautioned judges 'to take care, for the general good of the community, that hard cases do not make bad law.'" Adelson v. GTE Corp., 790 F. Supp. 1265, 1274 (D.Md. 1992).

39. Johnson v. Dist. 2 Marine Eng. Beneficial Ass'n, 857 F.2d 514, 517 (9th Cir. 1988).

Likewise, the Fifth Circuit noted that "in any plan benefit determination, there is always some tension between the interest of the beneficiary in obtaining quality medical care and the interest of the plan in preserving the pool of funds available to compensate all beneficiaries. Corcoran v. United Healthcare, Inc., 965 F2d 1321, 1338 (5th Cir 1992), cert denied 113 S.Ct. 812 (1992).

Similarly, the Eleventh Circuit pointed out that although ERISA fiduciaries (particularly those in a conflict of interest) must ensure that their decisions benefit the individual beneficiary, an exception exists if "the fiduciary justifies the interpretation on the ground of its benefit to the class of *all* participants and beneficiaries." Brown v. Blue Cross & Blue Shield of Alabama, 898 F. 2d 1556, 1567 (11th Cir. 1990) (emphasis added).

40. Ricci v. Gooberman, 840 F.Supp. 316, 317 (D.N.J. 1993). Similarly, in Dukes v. U.S. Health Care Systems of Pennsylvania, the Eastern District of Pennsylvania voiced "a serious reservation about the policy implications of holding an HMO liable for state law claims arising from the negligence of physicians and hospitals. If an HMO such as USHC is obliged to act as a malpractice insurer for health care providers, higher costs will invariably be passed along to health care consumers. I do not comment on whether this spreading of risk and costs is desirable. Rather, I simply hesitate to approve such a potentially widesweeping policy. Congress spent considerable time and effort in debating and passing ERISA, and may soon put similar efforts into so-called health care 'reform.' If the legislature wishes to examine the scope of ERISA pre-emption so as to extend malpractice liability to health benefit plans, now may be an appropriate time for it to do so. It does not follow that I should do so." Dukes v. U.S. Health Care Systems of Pennsylvania, 848 F.Supp. 39, 43 (E.D.Pa. 1994), reversed, 57 F.3d 350 (3d. Cir. 1995), cert denied, 116 S.Ct. 564 (1995).

41. Mertens v. Hewitt Associates, 113 S.Ct. 2063, 2072 (1993).

42. "In sum, the detailed provisions of § 502(a) set forth a comprehensive civil enforcement scheme that represents a careful balancing of the need for prompt and fair claims settlement procedures against the public interest in encouraging the formation of employee benefit plans. The policy choices reflected in the inclusion of certain remedies and the exclusion of others under the federal scheme would be completely undermined if ERISA-plan participants and beneficiaries were free to obtain remedies under state law that Congress rejected in ERISA. . . . The deliberate care with which ERISA's civil enforcement remedies were drafted and the balancing of policies embodied in its choice of remedies argue strongly for the conclusion that ERISA's civil enforcement remedies were intended to be exclusive." Pilot Life Ins. Co. v. Dedeaux, 481 U.S. 41, 54 (1987).

In Holmes v. Pacific Mut. Life, a California district court saw a trade-off between the interests of particular aggrieved individuals and the needs of the wider group, as it explained that ERISA helps to ensure that employees can count on receiving their retirement and other benefits, partly by shielding plans from the unforeseen expenses that widespread litigation could cause. Holmes v. Pacific Mut. Life Ins. Co, 706 F.Supp. 733 (C.D.Cal. 1989), at 735.

43. Baptist Memorial Hosp. System v. Sampson, 969 S.W.2d 945 (Tex. 1998).

44. Sampson v. Baptist Memorial Hosp. System, 940 S.W. 2d 128 (Tex. App.-San Antonio, 1996).

45. Baptist Memorial Hosp. System v. Sampson, 969 S.W.2d 945, 948–49 (Tex. 1998).

46. Baptist Memorial Hosp. System v. Sampson, 969 S.W.2d 945, 949 (Tex. 1998). The Court held that a hospital can only be liable under ostensible agency if all three traditional criteria are met: "to establish a hospital's liability for an independent contractor's medical malpractice based on ostensible agency, a plaintiff must show that (1) he or she had a reasonable belief that the physician was the agent or employee of the hospital, (2) such belief was generated by the hospital affirmatively holding out the physician as its agent or employee or knowingly permitting the physician to hold herself out as the hospital's agent or employee, and (3) he or she justifiably relied on the representation of authority" (at 949).

47. James by James v. Ingalls Memorial Hosp., 701 N.E.2d 207 (Ill.App. 1 Dist. 1998); McClellan v. Health Maintenance Org., 660 A.2d 97 (Pa.Super. 1995).

In some other cases courts have been willing to find an ostensible agency relationship, based in part on the advertising practices of the MCO. See Jones v. Chicago HMO Ltd. of Illinois, 703 N.E.2d 502, 511 (Ill. App. 1 Dist. 1998), aff'd in part, rev'd in part, Jones v. Chicago HMO, 730 N.E.2d 1119 (Ill. 2000); Petrovich v. Share Health Plan of Illinois, 696 N.E.2d 356 (Ill. App. 1 Dist. 1998), aff'd, Petrovich v. Share Health Plan of Illinois, Inc., 719 NE 2d 756 (Ill. 1999).

48. Klisch v. Meritcare Medical Group, Inc., 134 F.3d 1356, 1360 (8th Cir. 1998)(citing Ouelette v. Subak, 391 N.W.2d 810, 816 (Minn. 1986)). See also Morlino v. Medical Center, 706 A.2D 721, 731 (N.J. 1998); Brannen v. Prince, 421 S.E.2d 76, 80 (Ga. App. 1992); Deyo v. Kinley, 565 A.2d 1286 (Vt. 1989); Jones v. Chidester, 610 A.2d 964 (Pa. 1992); Parris v. Sands, 25 Cal. Rptr. 2d 800

(Cal. App. 2 Dist. 1993); Riggins v. Mauriello, 603 A.2d 827 (Del. 1992); Tefft v. Wilcox, 6 Kan. 46 (1870); Aiello v. Muhlenberg R. Med. Ctr., 733 A.2d 433, 438 (N.J. 1999)(acknowledging the "exercise of judgment rule" but distinguishing this from poor exercise of skill and care).

49. See Jones v. Chicago HMO Ltd. of Illinois, 703 N.E.2d 502, 509 (Ill. App. 1 Dist. 1998), aff'd in part, rev'd in part, Jones v. Chicago HMO, 730 N.E.2d 1119 (Ill. 2000); Schleier v. Kaiser Found. Health Plan, 876 F.2d 174, 176 (D.C. Cir. 1989); Dearmas v. Av-Med, Inc., 865 F. Supp. 816, 818 (S.D. Fla. 1994); Kearney v. U.S. Healthcare, Inc., 859 F. Supp. 182, 184 (E.D. Pa. 1994); Ricci v. Gooberman, 840 F. Supp. 316, 316 (D.N.J. 1993); Elsesser v. Hospital of the Phila. College of Osteopathic Med., 802 F. Supp. 1286, 1289–1290 (E.D. Pa. 1992); Independence HMO, Inc. v. Smith, 733 F. Supp. 983, 986 (E.D. Pa. 1990); Raglin v. HMO Ill., Inc., 595 N.E.2d 153, 154–55 (Ill. App. Ct. 1992); Harrell v. Total Health Care, Inc., 781 S.W.2d 58, 59–60 (Mo. 1989); Dunn v. Praiss, 656 A.2d 413, 417 (N.J. 1995); Albain v. Flower Hosp., 553 N.E.2d 1038, 1041–42 (Ohio 1992); McClellan v. Health Maintenance Org., 604 A.2d 1053, 1057–59 (Pa. Super. Ct. 1992); Boyd v. Albert Einstein Med. Ctr., 547 A.2d 1229, 1231 (Pa. Super. Ct. 1988).

See also Chittenden, 1991, at 453–85; Conrad, Seiter, 1995, at 191, 194; Tiano, 1990, at 91–98; Wiehl, et al., 1993, at 12–15; Rice, 1996 , at 193, 193–94.

50. Baptist Memorial Hosp. System v. Sampson, 969 S.W.2d 945 (Tex. 1998).

51. Charter Peachford Behavioral v. Kohout, 504 SE2d 514 (Ga. App. 1998). The plaintiff alleged that it was erroneous to have assigned a diagnosis of multiple personality disorder and having been abused in satanic rituals

52. Charter Peachford Behavioral v. Kohout, 504 SE2d 514 (Ga. App. 1998).

53. As observed in Jones v. Chicago HMO Ltd. of Illinois, the duty to review and supervise medical treatment is "administrative and managerial in nature. . . . We have been especially cautious when treading through this new ground. While we believe there may be circumstances that establish the independent corporate negligence of an HMO, we also understand this territory is fraught with considerations of public interest, matters that courts are ill-equipped to determine." Jones v. Chicago HMO Ltd. of Illinois, 703 N.E.2d 502, 509 (Ill. App. 1 Dist. 1998).

The court went on to note that "two bills on managed care reform were considered, but not acted upon, by our legislature in 1998" (at 509). The court did find that the MCO could potentially be liable on grounds of apparent agency but declined to find a cause of action for direct negligence, noting that "corporate responsibility to patients has never been extended in this State to a duty to supervise an independent physician contractor in his private office outside the hospital" (703 N.E.2d 509).

As discussed in Chapter 6 §-A-2, on appeal the Illinois Supreme Court also held that a health plan can be liable on grounds of institutional negligence if it assigns too many patients to one physician. Jones v. Chicago HMO, 730 N.E.2d 1119 (Ill. 2000).

54. Chittenden, 1991, at 471–72. Chittenden goes on to note that "[a]s courts increasingly characterize MCOs as health care providers, and the collection of quality assurance data becomes more comprehensive, suits against MCOs for negligence in failing to use quality control data at their disposal are likely to surface. Again, determination of the appropriate standard of care will be the most difficult issue facing both the claimant and the MCO." Id., at 472–73.

55. See Chapter 3 § B-2, 3; Chapter 8 § A-4.

56. See, e.g., Brandon v. Aetna Services, Inc., 46 F.Supp.2d 110 (D.Conn. 1999); Corcoran v. United Healthcare, Inc., 965 F2d 1321 (5th Cir 1992), cert denied 113 SCt 812 (1992); Kuhl v. Lincoln Nat. Health Plan, 999 F.2d 298 (8th Cir. 1993) cert. denied 510 U.S. 1045, 114 S.Ct. 694 (1994); Williams v. Good Health Plus, Inc., 743 S.W.2d 373, 378 (Tex.App.–San Antonio 1988); Roessert v. Health Net, 929 F.Supp. 343 (N.D.Cal. 1996); Garrison v. Northeast Georgia Medical Center, Inc., 66 F.Supp2d 1336 (N.D.Ga. 1999); Williams v. California Physicians' Service, 85 Cal.Rptr.2d 497 (Cal.App. 3 Dist. 1999); Wilson V. Chestnut Hill Healthcare, 2000 WL 204368 (E.D.Pa., 2000).

57. Texas Civ. Prac & Rem. Code §§88.001(5).

58. Texas Civ. Prac & Rem. Code §§88.001–003, at §88.002(a). The statute continues: "(b) A health insurance carrier, health maintenance organization, or other managed care entity for a health care entity or a health care plan is *also* liable for damages for harm to an insured or enrollee proximately caused by the health care treatment deisions made by its:

(1) employees;

(2) agents;

(3) ostensible agents; or

(4) representatives who are acting on its behalf and over whom it has the right to exercise

influence or control or has actually exercised influence or control which result in the failure to exercise ordinary care." Texas Civ. Prac & Rem. Code §§88.001–003, at §88.002, emphasis added. Note that this second source of liability simply places a legislative endorsement on the vicarious liability health plans have already incurred for the misdeeds of their employees, agents, and ostensible agents.

59. The court found that ERISA preempted (1) the law's requirement for an independent appeals process for coverage denials, (2) its provision forbidding health plans to remove physicians because they had advocated for patients, and (3) its proscription of indemnification clauses.

60. Corporate Health Ins. Inc. v. Texas Dept. of Ins., 12 F.Supp.2d 597, 611–618 (S.D.Tex. 1998), aff'd in part, rev'd in part, 215 F.3d 526 (5th Cir. 2000).

61. It differed somewhat with the district court regarding the statute's other provisions, finding that ERISA does not preempt the statute's anti-retaliation or its anti-indemnity provisions. Only the requirement for independent review is preempted, the court said. Corporate Health Insurance, Inc. v. Texas Dept. of Insurance, 215 F.3d 526 (5th Cir. 2000). In contrast, the Seventh Circuit disagreed sharply about the independent review issue, holding that independent review requirements do not violate ERISA. *Moran* v. *Rush Prudential,* 230 F.3d 959 (7th Cir. 2000).

Interestingly, the Fifth Circuit seems to have misunderstood, or perhaps simply avoided, a central aspect of the controversy about health plans and medical decision making. Each time the court notes that ERISA does not preempt medical malpractice suits against health plans, it limits its discussion to instances in which a practicing physician, under the plan's auspices, has committed malpractice. That is, the court speaks only of instances in which the routine tort claim would allege ostensible agency. The court thus notes that "the Act would allow suit for claims that a treating physician was negligent in delivering medical services, and it imposes vicarious liability on managed care entities for that negligence" (at 534). Similarly: "A suit for medical malpractice against a doctor is not preempted by ERISA simply because those services were arranged by an HMO and paid for by an ERISA plan. Likewise, the vicarious liability of the entities for whom the doctor acted as an agent is rooted in general principles of state agency law. Seen in this light, the Act simply codifies Texas's already-existing standards regarding medical care" (at 535). The court seems to miss altogether the idea that the health plan itself may be practicing medicine when it makes benefits decisions based on medical necessity. This is the difficult question within this group of ERISA cases, and it remains untouched by this ruling.

62. See Chapter 8, n. 55.

63. See, eg., Tunkl v. Regents of Univ. of Cal., 383 P.2d 441, 441–42 (Cal. 1963); Emory Univ. v. Porubiansky, 282 S.E.2d 903, 906 (Ga. 1981); Cudnik v. William Beaumont Hosp., 525 N.W.2d 891, 896 (Mich. Ct. App. 1994); Olson v. Molzen, 558 S.W. 2D 429, 432 (Tenn. 1977); Ash v. New York University Dental Center, 564 N.Y.S.2d 308, 311 (A.D. 1 Dist. 1990); Mehlman, 1993, at 356.

However, courts have been willing to release providers from liability under the "assumption of risk" doctrine under certain conditions. When a person enters into an activity knowing about and agreeing to assume its risks, he exonerates in advance those who might otherwise be liable for the creation of those risks. In Schneider v. Revici a woman diagnosed with breast cancer rejected surgery and radiation in favor of unconventional nutrition therapy. The physician providing that alternative care clearly informed her that the therapy was not approved and also, once it had clearly proved ineffective for her, advised her several times to seek conventional treatment. When the woman finally did consult a surgeon, her disease had progressed too far for hope of cure. She sued the first physician over his worthless remedies, and the court held that in agreeing to opt for unapproved therapy despite its clearly stated risks, she had assumed the risk and could not hold the physician liable for her own choice. Schneider v. Revici, 817 F.2d 987 (2nd Cir. 1987). See also Massengill v. S.M.A.R.T., 996 P.2d 1132 (Wyo. 2000); Dowd v. New York O. & W. Ry. Co., 63 N.E. 541 (N.Y. 1902); Murphy v. Steeplechase Amusement Co., 166 N.E. 173 (N.Y. 1929); McEvoy v. City of New York, 42 N.Y.S.2d 746 (N.Y. App. 1943); aff'd 55 N.E.2d 517 (N.Y. 1944).

64. Wheeler v. St. Joseph Hosp., 133 Cal. Rptr. 775, 791 (Cal. Ct. App. 1976); Broughton v. CIGNA Healthplans of Cal., 65 Cal. Rptr 2d 558 (Cal. App. 2 Dist. 1997) (arbitration could not be compelled because arbitration clause could not provide injunctive relief); aff'd, 76 Cal.Rptr.2d 431 (Cal. App. 2 Dist. 1998); aff'd in part, rev'd in part, 90 Cal. Rptr.2d 334 (Cal. 1999). But see Madden v. Kaiser Found. Hosps., 552 P.2d 1178, 1184 (Cal. 1976); Morris v. Metriyakool, 344 N.W. 2D 736, 753 (Mich. 1984); Engalla v. Permanente Medical Center Group, 938 P.2d 903 (Cal. 1997) (arbitration clause was not unconscionable, although its implementation in instant case was problematic); Erickson v. Aetna Health Plans of Cal., 84 Cal.Rptr.2d 76 (Cal.App. 4 Dist. 1999)

(arbitration clause was not a contract of adhesion, and arbitration was mandatory rather than optional under HMO's contract); Hollister v. Benzl, 83 Cal. Rptr. 2d 903 (Cal. App. 4 Dist. 1999) (arbitration agreement not contractually void).

See Chapter 4, n. 27.

65. See Morreim, 1992(a), at 165–69.

66. See, e.g. Fuja v. Benefit Trust Life Ins. Co., 18 F.3d 1405, 1412 (7th Cir. 1994); Doe v. Group Hospitalization & Med. Servs., 3 F.3d. 80, 84 (4th Cir. 1993); Loyola Univ. v. Humana Ins. Co., 996 F.2d 895, 903 (7th Cir. 1993) Harris v. Mutual of Omaha Cos., 992 F.2d 706, 713 (7th Cir. 1993); McLeroy v. Blue Cross/Blue Shield, 825 F.Supp. 1064, 1071 (N.D. Ga. 1993); Arrington v. Group Hospitalization & Med. Serv., 806 F.Supp. 287, 290 (D.D.C. 1992); Gee v. Utah State Retirement Bd., 842, P.2d 919, 920–21 (Utah Ct. App. 1992).

67. Doe, 3 F.3d at 84.

68. Frahm v. Equitable Life Assur. Soc. of U.S., 137 F.3d 955, 962 (7th Cir. 1998). See also Pisciotta v. Teledyne Indus., Inc., 91 F.3d 1326, 1330 (9th Cir. Cir. 1996) (stating that "[I]n general, welfare benefits are not subject to vesting requirements under ERISA, 29 U.S.C.§ 1501 (1). Employers may adopt, modify or terminate welfare benefit plans").

69. See Morreim, 1992(a), at 165–66.

70. See Pretzer, 1995, at 92–93; Gleason, 1995, at 1483; Mariner, 1995. See also Morreim, 1992(a), at 165–66.

71. See Chapter 8 § B-3; see also United States General Accounting Office, Mar. 1, 1994; United States General Accounting Office, Dec. 19, 1994.

72. See Alexander v. Choate, 469 U.S. 287, 306 (1985).

73. See Alexander v. Choate, 469 U.S. 287, 303 (1985).

74. Ross v. Moffitt, 417 U.S. 600 (1974), discussed in Siliciano, 1991, at 470–71.

In a similar vein, "few courts would seriously entertain a claim that an economy car should have exactly the same level of safety features as a luxury car." Thus, the Supreme Court of Washington found that the purchaser of a Volkswagen cannot reasonably expect the same degree of safety as would the buyer of the much more expensive Cadillac" (Seattle-First Nat'l Bank v. Tabert, 542 P.2d 774, 779 (Wash. 1975), discussed in Henderson, Siliciano, 1994, at 1395).

75. See generally Morreim, 1992(a); Morreim, 1987.

76. See Hall v. Hilbun, 466 So.2d 856, 866 (Miss. 1985).

77. See, e.g., George v. Jefferson Hosp. Ass'n, Inc., 987 S.W.2d 710 (Ark. 1999); Fulton-DeKalb Hosp. Auth. v. Fanning, 396 S.E.2d 534 (Ga. Ct. App. 1990); Lazerson v. Hilton Head Hosp., Inc., 439 S.E.2d 836 (S.C. 1994) (upholding validity of damage limits for charitable organizations); Cutts v. Fulton-DeKalb Hosp. Auth., 385 S.E.2d 436, 437 (Ga. Ct. App. 1989); Clark v. Maine Med. Ctr., 559 A.2d 358, 360 (Me. 1989); Johnson v. Mountainside Hosp., 571 A.2d 318 (N.J. Super. Ct. App. Div. 1990). See also English v. New Eng. Med. Ctr., 541 N.E.2d 329, 331 (Mass. 1989) (providing a cap on damages for charitable institutions); Creason v. Department of Health Services, 957 P.2d 1323 (Cal. 1998) (finding that plaintiffs' action was not covered by sovereign immunity statute, but accepting statute as valid); Helton v. Phelps County Regional Medical Center, 817 F.Supp. 789 (E.D. Mo. 1993) (finding that in instant case, sovereign immunity was preempted by EMTALA, but not challenging overall validity of statute); Thompson v. Regional Medical Center at Memphis, 748 F. Supp. 575 (W.D. Tenn. 1990) (finding defendants absolutely immune from liability, pursuant to sovereign immunity statute); Wynn v. Fulton-DeKalb Hosp. Authority, 395 S.E.2d 343 (Ga. App. 1990) (finding that hospital enjoyed charitable immunity under statute).

78. See Brown, 1996, at 437–38.

79. See OR. Rev. Stat. § 414.745 (1987).

80. See Nazay v. Miller, 949 F.2d 1323, 1338 (3d Cir. 1991).

81. Nazay v. Miller, 949 F.2d 1323, 1326 (3d Cir. 1991).

82. Nazay v. Miller, 949 F.2d 1323, 1336 (3rd Cir. 1991). The court went on to note that it is legitimate for those who pay for health care to attempt to contain their rising costs (at 1328). In this case, a corporation gave teeth to its precertification requirement by imposing a thirty percent penalty on those who failed to comply. If this requirement were overruled, the corporation "and its employees would be deprived of an important weapon in their joint battle against rising healthcare costs" (at 1338).

83. Loyola University of Chicago v. Humana Ins. Co., 996 F.2d 895 (7th Cir. 1993).

84. Loyola University of Chicago v. Humana Ins. Co., 996 F.2d 903.

85. Loyola University of Chicago v. Humana Ins. Co., 996 F.2d 903.

86. McGee v. Equicor-Equitable HCA Corp., 953 F.2d 1192 (10th Cir. 1992) (citing Firestone

Tire & Rubber Co. v. Bruch, 489 U.S. 101 [1989]). The Tenth Circuit did require the HMO to pay for some benefits that did, in fact, meet their utilization requirements.

87. McGee v. Equicor-Equitable HCA Corp., 953 F.2d 1192, 1207 (10th Cir. 1992).

88. McGee v. Equicor-Equitable HCA Corp., 953 F.2d 1192, 1207 (10th Cir. 1992).

89. The same Seventh Circuit that ruled in *Loyola* came to a similar result in Fuja v. Benefit Trust Life Ins. Co., 18 F.3d 1405 (7th Cir. 1994), in which a woman sought autologous bone marrow transplant (ABMT) for advanced breast cancer. The insurance contract excluded research treatments, and the court found that ABMT for her disease was research. "Under the present state of the law, we are bound to interpret the language of the specific contract before us and cannot amend or expand the coverage contained therein." 18 F.3d 1412 The court went on to observe "Although we fully realize the heartache Mrs. Fuja's family has endured, as judges we are called upon to resolve the legal question presented in this appeal, i.e., interpreting the Benefit Trust insurance contract." 18 F.3d 1407.

Analogously, a district court in Georgia pointed out in McLeroy v. Blue Cross/Blue Shield of Oregon that it was "well within the bargaining rights of the parties" to determine the conditions under which special alternative services might be provided. McLeroy v. Blue Cross/Blue Shield of Oregon, Inc., 825 F.Supp. 1064, 1071 (N.D. Ga. 1993).

In Goepel v. Mail Handlers Benefit Plan a New Jersey district court held that the plaintiffs' policy was clearly written, with adequate notice of policy changes, and enabled the plaintiffs to make an informed purchase. Significantly, the court also expressed an interest in the responsibilities of subscribers. "This Court is also troubled by the invitation to recognize a cause of action, not based on the fact that the policy was unclear, but rather, as plaintiffs suggest, on the premises that insureds (1) do not read the full brochure detailing policy coverage and (2) do not heed the admonotion in the secion on 'How the Plan Changes' to review the entire policy." Goepel v. Mail Handlers Benefit Plan (No. 93–3711, 1993 WL 384498 (D. N.J. 9/24/93)). This decision was subsequently overturned by the Third Circuit, but not on grounds of its substance. Rather, the issue was jurisdictional: the preemption from state to federal court should not have been done automatically. The preemption question required further adjudication. Goepel v. National Postal Mail Handlers Union, 36 F.3d 306 (3rd. Cir. 1994).

In the same vein, a federal district court in Maryland held that an insurer was not obligated to pay for the patient's laetrile expenses. See Free v. Travelers Ins. Co., 551 F.Supp. 554, 560 (D.Md. 1982):

> [T]he plaintiff's unfettered right to select a physician and follow his advice does not create a corresponding responsibility in the [health care plan] to pay for every treatment so chosen. As one court noted, "it is simply not enough to show that some people, even experts, have a belief in [the] safety and effectiveness [of a particular drug]. A reasonable number of Americans will sincerely attest to the worth of almost any product or even idea." . . . Finally, the Court notes that the plaitiff, by his own admission, was well aware that laetrile and nutritional therapy are disapproved of by the majority of cancer specialists. He was equally well informed of the accepted alternative chemotherapy.

Id. (citations omitted) (some alterations in original).

90. Andrews-Clarke v. Travelers Ins., Co., 984 F.Supp. 49, 52–53 (D. Mass. 1997).

91. Bechtold v. Physicians Health Plan, 19 F.3d 322 (7th Cir. 1994).

92. Bechtold v. Physicians Health Plan, 19 F.3d 322, 327 (7th Cir. 1994) citing Senn v. United Donimion Indust., Inc., 951 F.2d 806, 818 (7th Cir. 1992).

93. Bechtold v. Physicians Health Plan, 19 F.3d 322, 327 (7th Cir. 1994) citing Heller v. Equitable Life Assur. Soc. of U.S., 833 F.2d 1253, 1257 (7th Cir. 1987).

94. "Courts may not, under cloak of construction of insurance policy, make new contract for parties by adopting preferred interpretation contrary to language of the policy." O'Rourke v. Access Health, Inc., 668 N.E.2d 214, 215 (Ill. App. 1 Dist. 1996).

In Gee v. Utah State Retirement Bd, the Utah Court of Appeals upheld an insurer's denial of coverage for removal of breast implants, holding that the policy was not ambiguous. "Insurance policies are contracts, and are interpreted under the same rules governing ordinary contracts. . . . [A] policy term is not ambiguous simply because one party ascribes a different meaning to it to suit his or her own interests" (842 P.2d 919, 920–21 (Utah App. 1992)).

Other courts have expressed similar views. "Moreover, because of the plain language of the contract, we would have no choice but to affirm the denial of coverage even if, *arguendo,* we were to review that decision *de novo.*" Harris v. Mutual of Omaha Companies, 992 F.2d 706, 713 (7th Cir. 1993).

"The plan is clear and not ambiguous. . . . The contract is clear. HDC-ABMT is not covered under the 1992 Plan. Accordingly, Blue Cross/Blue Shield's decision denying coverage and OPM's review and affirmance of that decision are rational. Denial of coverage is clearly not an arbitrary and capricious decision; indeed, because of the plain language of the contract, the Court would affirm denial of coverage even if that decision were reviewed *de novo.*" Arrington v. Group Hospitalization & Med. Serv., 806 F.Supp. 287, 290 (D.D.C. 1992).

In Richards v. Engelberger, 868 F.Supp. 117 (D.Md. 1994), a physician sued to receive payment for breast reduction surgery. The court ruled in favor of the insurer on the gound that the contract clearly, explicitly excluded coverage for breast reductions—this, despite the fact that the breast reduction was arguably "medically necessary" because large breasts were causing the patient shoulder, upper back, and neck pain.

In Adnan Varol, M.D. v. Blue Cross & Blue Shield, 708 F. Supp. 826 (E.D. Mich. 1989), a district court informed a group of psychiatrists that they were expected to adhere to their contract with an insurer, even though they now disagreed with its cost containment provisions. In Williams v. HealthAmerica, 535 N.E.2d 717 (Ohio App. 1987) an Ohio appellate court ruled that although a malpractice action against an HMO physician should go to arbitration, the patient also could pursue separately a breach of contract action against that physician.

See also Madden v. Kaiser Foundation Hospitals, 552 P.2d 1178 (Cal. 1976) (holding that an employee who had chosen his HMO from among several options negotiated on his behalf by a state agency was bound by the arbitration clause to which he had agreed and noting that "[o]ne who assents to a contract is bound by its provisions and cannot complain of unfamiliarity with the language"); Erickson v. Aetna Health Plans of Cal., 84 Cal.Rptr.2d 76 (Cal.App. 4 Dist. 1999) (following *Madden*'s willingness to uphold clause mandating arbitration); Sarchett v. Blue Shield of California, 729 P. 2d 267 (Cal. 1987) (upholding insurer's right to deny payment based on its own judgment of medical necessity).

See also Barnett v. Kaiser Foundation Health Plan, Inc., 32 F.3d 413 (9th Cir. 1994); Goepel v. Mail Handlers Benefit Plan (No. 93–3711, 1993 WL 384498 (D. N.J. 9/24/93)); Nesseim v. Mail Handlers Ben. Plan, 995 F.2d 804 (8th Cir., 1993); Farley v. Benefit Trust Life Ins. Co., 979 F.2d 653 (8th Cir. 1992); Harris v. Blue Cross Blue Shield of Missouri, 995 F.2d 877 (8th Cir. 1993); McLeroy v. Blue Cross/Blue Shield of Oregon, Inc., 825 F.Supp. 1064 (N.D. Ga. 1993); Thomas v. Gulf Health Plan, Inc., 688 F. Supp. 590 (S.D. Ala. 1988); Doe v. Group Hospitalization & Medical Services, 3 F.3d 80 (4th Cir. 1993); Mire v. Blue Cross/Blue Shield of Florida, 43 F.3d 567 (11th Cir 1994); Healthcare America Plans, Inc. v. Bossemeyer, 953 F.Supp. 1176 (D.Kan. 1996) affd w/o opin. 166 F.3d 347; England v. John Alden Life Ins. Co., 846 F.Supp. 798 (W.D.Mo. 1994); O'Rourke v. Access Health, Inc., 668 N.E.2d 214 (Ill.App. 1 Dist. 1996); Hollister v. Benzl, 83 Cal.Rptr.2d 903 (Cal.App.4 Dist. 1999); Massengill v. S.M.A.R.T., 996 P.2d 1132 (Wyo. 2000); Morton v. Smith, 91 F.3d 867 (7th Cir. 1996).

95. See Farnsworth, 1990, § 12.2, at 845–48, 860.

96. See Farnsworth, 1990, § 12.6, at 845–48, 860.

97. See Farnsworth, 1990, § 12.3, at 845–48, 860. But see Friedmann, 1989, at 2 (concluding that "the simple entitlement approach which provides that a party is generally bound to perform his contractual promises unless he obtains a release from the promisee, fares better on both [entitlement and economic efficiency] scores").

98. See Farnsworth, 1990, § 12.6, at 856, 860.

99. See Florence Nightingale Nursing Serv., Inc. v. Blue Cross/Blue Shield, 41 F.3d 1476, 1483–84 (11th Cir. 1995); Bailey v. Blue Cross/Blue Shield, 866 F. Supp. 277, 280–82 (E.D. Va. 1994), aff'd, 67 F.3d 53 (4th Cir. 1995); Calhoun v. Complete Health Care, Inc., 860 F. Supp. 1494, 1501 (S.D. Ala. 1994), aff'd, 61 F.3d 31 (11th Cir. 1995); Leonhardt v. Holden Business Forms Co., 828 F. Supp. 657, 667–72 (D. Minn.1993); Wilson v. Group Hospitalization & Med. Servs., Inc., 791 F. Supp. 309, 313–14 (D.D.C. 1992), appeal dismissed, 995 F.2d 306 (D.C. Cir. 1993); Pirozzi v. Blue Cross-Blue Shield, 741 F. Supp. 586, 594 (E.D. Va. 1990).

100. Dearmas v. Av-Med, Inc., 814 F. Supp. 1103 (S.D. Fla. 1993).

101. Dearmas v. Av-Med, Inc., 814 F. Supp. 1103, 1105 (S.D. Fla. 1993). Because his HMO was an employment benefit, all of the plaintiff's tort claims, including negligence, dumping, and loss of consortium, were preempted by ERISA. The district court in this case preempted claims based on a theory that the HMO had violated federal "anti-dumping" laws. In a subsequent suit the same district court also preempted claims regarding negligent administration of the plan but did not rule out a claim for vicarious liability. See Dearmas v. Av-Med, Inc., 865 F. Supp. 816, 818 (S.D. Fla. 1994).

See also Nealy v. U.S. Healthcare HMO, 844 F. Supp. 966, 969 (S.D.N.Y. 1994) (describing a series of authorization denials for a patient's access to specialists and prescriptions causing delays that allegedly led to the patient's death from massive myocardial infarction).

102. See Schaber, Rohwer, 1984, § 172, at 326.

That is, courts seek to protect "the expectation that the injured party had when making the contract by attempting to put the injured party in as good a position as that party would have been in had the contract been performed, that is, had there been no breach." Farnsworth, 1990, § 12.8, at 840.

Cooter and Friedman define perfect compensation as "damages that restore the victim to the same position that she would have been in but for the wrong. Perfect compensation thus leaves the victim no better or worse off than if the injurer had done no wrong." Cooter, Freedman, 1991, at 1059.

See also DeMott, 1988, at 900–01: "Contract remedies . . . are less exotic, and the plaintiff typically receives only money damages equal to the value of his lost expectation."

103. Farnsworth, 1990, at 42, 840. Similarly, Schaber and Rohwer point out that "expectancy of the bargain damages" are "calculated to place the innocent party, to the extent that money can do so, in the position he would have been in had the contract been performed." Schaber, Rohwer, 1984, at 326.

104. When a person has changed his position to his detriment by relying on a promise (e.g., by making expenditures to prepare land for a house to be built), courts might measure his *reliance interest* "in an attempt to put the *promisee back in the position in which the promisee would have been had the promise not been made.*" In still other cases recovery is based on the fact that the promisee might actually confer a benefit on the promisor and is "measured by the promisee's *restitution interest,* in an attempt to put the *promisor back in the position in which the promisor would have been had the promise not been made.*" Farnsworth, at 42, 843.

"Reliance damages consist of the amount necessary to reimburse the innocent party for the loss caused by his reliance on the contract. Reliance damages are designed to take the innocent party back to the position he would have been in had the contract never been made (status quo ante). This is distinctly different from expectancy damages." Schaber, Rohwer, 1984, § 173, at 327. "Restitution damages consist of returning or restoring to the innocent party the dollar value of any benefit he has conferred upon the other party." Schaber, Rohwer, 1984, § 173, at 327.

105. Farnsworth, 1990, § 12.9, at 879. Farnsworth also states that "since the court is attempting to measure the expectation of the injured party itself, the *loss in value* should be the loss to that party, not to some hypothetical reasonable person or on some market. It will depend on the circumstances of the injured party or those of that party's enterprise." *Id.*

106. Farnsworth, 1990, § 12.9, at 880–91 (footnote omitted); see also 907. There are other factors that can be involved in calculating damages. Because courts will not grant recovery for losses that could reasonably have been avoided, injured parties sometimes incur costs and losses that occur when the injured party tries to minimize his loss. See *id.* § 12.12, at 882–93. In health care, perhaps there is some room for expecting patients to make reasonable efforts to minimize losses by cooperating with treatment—much as contributory negligence can diminish or negate tort remedies. However, the patient's imminent need for help often renders him sufficiently vulnerable that it is not reasonable to expect him to shop for other care. Further, patients have the autonomous right to refuse treatments they consider unacceptable. Hence, avoiding costs and losses will not often be relevant in calculating contract damages, which leaves loss in value and consequential damages as the primary focus.

107. See Corcoran v. United Healthcare, Inc., 965 F.2d 1321, 1324 (5th Cir. 1992), cert denied 113 S.Ct. 812 (1992) (death of fetus alleged to be due to defendants's decision to authorize only part-time home nursing care, rather than permitting hospitalization or full-time nursing care in high-risk pregnancy). All common law claims in this case, however, were preempted by ERISA. See *id.* at 1331.

108. See Farnsworth, 1990, § 12.5, at 856 ("Along with any equitable relief by specific performance or injunction, a court may also award damages and grant other relief."). "Because an order granting equitable relief seldom results in performance within the time required by the contract, damages for delay are often appropriate." *Id.* § 12.5, at 857.

109. Cases invoking the tort/contract doctrine of "bad faith breach of contract" can involve punitive damages, but such suits reach beyond ordinary contract and must satisfy a demanding list of criteria. See, e.g., Abraham, 1994; Allen, 1982; Crespi, 1994; Diamond, 1981; Jerry, 1986; Kornblum, 1988; Louderback, 1982; Stern, 1983.

110. See Farnsworth, 1990, § 12.8, at 874–75: "[N]o matter how reprehensible the breach, damages that are punitive, in the sense of being in excess of those required to compensate the injured party for lost expectation, are not ordinarily awarded for breach of contract. It is a funda-

mental tenet of the law of contract remedies that, regardless of the character of the breach, an injured party should not be put in a better position than had the contract been performed" (footnote omitted).

"The basic rule is that damages for pain and suffering, emotional distress and other types of harm to the person are only available where there is a tort cause of action. In some jurisdictions, an action for personal injuries can be treated as a breach of contract." Schaber, Rohwer, 1984, at 342. See also Farnsworth at 934.

111. Schaber, Rohwer, 1984, § 176, at 342.

112. See Gergen, 1994, at 1254, 1257.

113. Jerry, 1994, at 1341 (footnote omitted); see also Jerry, 1986, at 298. When promises to "be there" are broken, adverse consequences are foreseeable:

> Given the real promise of the insurance relationship, [it is consistent with existing law] to award an insured compensation for the emotional and financial consequences of the insurance company's absence.
>
> Contract law is replete with exceptions to the traditional rule against damages for emotional distress. Such damages are permitted for breaches of burial contracts, contracts for long-term care, contracts for repair of family heirlooms, contracts for the construction or improvement of family homes, contracts related to memorable events like weddings and vacations, and other contracts in which emotional distress is a foreseeable consequence of breach.

Baker, 1994, at 1426 (footnotes omitted). "[E]motional distress is at least a foreseeable, if not inevitable, result of an insurance company's failure to 'be there' in time of need. . . . As the sales stories make clear, a primary reason for buying insurance is to avoid emotional distress." *Id.,* at 1428.

114. Farnsworth, 1990, § 12.9, at 881. See also Baker, 1994, at 1424 ("[C]ommon-law contract damage limitations appear to rest on a surprisingly narrow foundation. Peeling away the onion of precedent reveals a final core of nineteenth-century books that simply recite the classical contract damages 'rules' without analysis.") (footnote omitted).

115. Jerry, 1986, at 299–300 (footnotes omitted).

116. See Jerry, 1986, at 312; Jerry, 1994, at 1341–42.

117. See, e.g., Farnsworth, 1990, § 12.8, at 873; Schaber, Rohwer, 1984, § 174, at 338.

Reasonableness of the promisee's efforts is an important element. "The injured party is not, however, expected to guard against unforeseeable risks nor to take steps that involve undue burden, risk, or humiliation." Farnsworth, 1990, § 12.12, at 897–98.

118. See, e.g., Farnsworth, 1990, § 12.8, at 842, 874; Schaber, Rohwer, 1984, § 174, at 331.

119. See, e.g., Farnsworth, 1990, § 12.14, at 912; Schaber, Rohwer, 1984, § 174, at 337. Farnsworth notes:

> In spite of the vagueness of the concept of foreseeability, a few general propositions can be asserted with some assurance. First, foreseeability is to be determined as of the time of the making of the contract and is unaffected by events subsequent to that time. The question is not what was foreseeable at the time of the breach, but what was foreseeable at the time of contracting. Second, what must be foreseeable is only that the loss would result if the breach occurred. There is no requirement that the breach itself or the particular way that the loss came about be foreseeable. Third, it is foreseeability only by the party in breach that is determinative. . . . Fourth, foreseeability has an objective character. When one makes a contract one takes the risk not only of those consequences that one actually did foresee, but also of those that one ought reasonably to have foreseen. Fifth, the loss need only have been foreseeable as a probable, as opposed to a necessary or certain, result of the breach. The mere circumstance that some loss was foreseeable, however, may not suffice to impose liability for a type of loss that was so unusual as not to be foreseeable.

Farnsworth, 1990, § 12.14, at 915.

120. Schaber, Rohwer, 1984, § 174, at 331–32.

121. See, e.g., Mimbs v. Commercial Life Ins. Co., 832 F. Supp. 354, 358 (S.D. Ga. 1993); Conrad, Seiter, 1995, at 191: "Because lack of coverage frequently translates, at least as a practical matter, to lack of access to care, prospective and concurrent utilization review can expose a health plan to liability claims of a kind from which indemnity plans are largely insulated".

122. See, e.g., Farnsworth, 1990, § 12.8, at 842, 859, 874; Schaber, Rohwer, 1984, § 174, at 333 ("Restatement, Second, [of Contracts] Section 35 provides: 'Damages are not recoverable for loss

beyond an amount that the evidence permits to be established with reasonable certainty.' Two problems are involved: proof with certainty that some damages were caused by the breach, and proof with certainty of the amount of the damages in dollars and cents.").

123. See generally Farnsworth, 1990, § 12.15, at 924.

124. See Farnsworth, 1990, § 12.15, at 922.

125. See generally Grumet, 1989, at 609; Light, 1994, at 499.

126. See, e.g., Farnsworth, 1990, § 12.1, at 42, 841; Schaber, Rohwer, 1984, § 174, at 333.

127. Quite possibly, such a minimum benefits standard might deter some litigation. If all subscribers are assured of at least some modicum of care, and if government further has specified that this level is satisfactory, then courts may be much less inclined to second-guess these and other health plans' limits.

128. See, e.g., *In re* Baby K, 16 F.3d 590, 592 (4th Cir. 1994).

129. See generally Morreim, 1995(c), at 883; Morreim 1995(a), at 247.

130. See Havighurst, 1995, at 181 (arguing that the legitimacy of the contract should depend on the legitimacy of the procedures under which it was chosen). Hall and Anderson offer a detailed description of the ways in which health plans' procedures for determining benefits might be assessed and why such procedural fairness should be the chief focus of litigation in this area. See Hall, Anderson, 1992, at 1684; see also Anderson, Hall, Steinberg, 1993, at 1637.

131. This scenario is based on, but not perfectly faithful to, Schwartz v. FHP International Corp.,947 F.Supp. 1354, 1357 (D. Ariz. 1996). In this case the court held that ERISA preempted tort claims, such as for vicarious liability, breach of contract, fraud, and emotional distress.

132. See Schwartz v. FHP International Corp.,947 F.Supp. 1354 (D. Ariz. 1996). A federal district court preempted this plaintiff's claims on the ground that the HMO's failure to administer benefits properly was a "quantity" issue preempted by ERISA. See *id.* at 1359.

133. The plaintiff alleged such an arrangement in Schwartz v. FHP International Corp.,947 F.Supp. 1359 (D. Ariz. 1996).

134. See also Pappas v. Asbel, 675 A.2d 711 (Pa. Super. Ct. 1996), aff'd, 724 A.2d 889 (Pa. 1998), vacated, 120 S.Ct. 2686. A man appeared at a community hospital with a cervical epidural abscess, a neurologic emergency requiring immediate surgery. The emergency room (ER) physician phoned for immediate admission to a nearby hospital with facilities for the necessary care, but the ambulance transport service informed the ER physician that this facility was not among the providers authorized by the patient's HMO. The ER physician tried to obtain permission from the HMO to send him to the original hospital but was told to send the patient to one of two alternate hospitals. Instead of sending the patient to one of the two authorized alternatives, the ER physician continued to try to secure authorization for the hospital of his first choice. Ultimately, the delays resulted in permanent quadriplegia for the patient. The case raises numerous questions: whether someone on either side might have been misinformed and, if so, why the person was not better informed; whether someone may have been stubborn; and so forth.

In some cases, court opinions provide too little factual detail even to speculate whether the real issues were mainly expertise, resources, or a mixture of both. See, e.g., Santitoro v. Evans, 935 F. Supp. 733 (E.D.N.C. 1996) (alleging without further examination that medical malpractice and misconduct occurred during the delivery of medical services); Prihoda v. Shpritz, 914 F. Supp. 113, 115 (D. Md. 1996) (stating that a kidney tumor was not diagnosed but now showing how the failure occurred); Frappier v. Wishnov (*In re* Estate of Frappier), 678 So. 2D 884, 885 (Fla. Dist. Ct. App. 1996) (alleging that physicians were incompetent but failing to explain the basis of the charge).

CHAPTER 11

1. Employee Retirement Income Security Act, 29 U.S.C. §§ 1001–1461 (1994).

2. For further discussion of ERISA, see Jacobson, Pomfret, 1998; Pomfret, 1998; Wethly, 1996; Cantor, 1997; Shah, 1996; Cerminara, 1999; Flint, 1994; Rossbacher, Cahill, Griffis, 1997; American Bar Asociation, 1991; Fox, Schaffer, 1989; Muir, 1995; Rouco, 1994; Koutoulogenis, 1998.

3 Holmes v. Pacific Mut. Life Ins. Co., 706 F.Supp. 733, 735 (C.D. Cal. 1989); see also Mertens v. Hewitt Assocs., 508 U.S. 248, 264 (1993) (White, J., dissenting):

Concerned that many pension plans were being corruptly or ineptly mismanaged and that American workers were losing their financial security in retirement as a result, Congress in 1974 enacted ERISA, "declar[ing] [it] to be the policy of [the statute] to protect . . . the interests of participants in employee benefit plans and their beneficiaries, by requiring the disclosure and reporting to participants and beneficiaries of financial and other information with respect [to the plans], by establishing standards of conduct, responsibility, and obligation for fiduciaries of employee benefit plans, and by providing for appropiate remedies, sanctions, and ready access to the Federal courts." Id. (alterations in original).

4. See, e.g., Ingersoll-Rand Co. v. McClendon, 498 U.S. 133, 137 (1990); Pilot Life Ins. Co. v. Dedeaux, 481 U.S. 41, 44 (1987).

It might also be noted that during the same period, many large corporations were interested in expanding their businesses into the Southern states, where labor laws were often quite different than in the North. These discrepancies created a further impetus for unifying employee benefits under a single set of federal laws.

5. "Congress' avowed purposes in enacting ERISA was to 'protect interstate commerce . . . and the interests of participants in employee benefit plans' by initiating reporting and disclosure requirements and by establishing federal standards of conduct for those running such benefit plans. Congress further sought to establish uniform minimum standards regarding requirements of the vesting of plan benefits, fiscal responsibility of plan administrators and disclosure of plan specifics. Concerned that a full one-half of all non-agricultural private employees remained without coverage of any sort of retirement plan, Congress hoped that ERISA's clear and uniformly regulated statutory scheme would encourage employers to further expand their use of employee benefit plans." Wethly, 1996, at 826.

6. "Congress has distinguished between 'employee pension benefit plans' and 'employee welfare benefit plans,' exempting the latter from much of ERISA's panoply of requirements including its vesting provisions. Welfare benefits such as medical insurance . . . are not subject to the rather strict vesting, accrual, participation, and minimum funding requirements that ERISA imposes on pension plans." Pittman v. Blue Cross & Blue Shield, 24 F.3d 118, 121 (10th Cir. 1994) (quoting Wise v. El Paso Natural Gas Co., 986 F.2d 929, 935 (5th Cir. 1993) (omission in original). See also 29 U.S.C. § 1001 (1994).

"In general, welfare benefits are not subject to vesting requirements under ERISA. Employers may adopt, modify or terminate welfare benefit plans." Curtiss-Wright Corp v. Schoonejongen, 514 U.S. 73, 78 (1995). In the context of this article, however, the distinction will not play a role.

7. "ERISA does not mandate that employers provide any particular benefits . . ." Shaw v. Delta Air Lines, Inc., 103 S.Ct. 2890, 2897 (1983).

"In general, welfare benefits are not subject to vesting requirements under ERISA, 29 U.S.C. § 1501 (1). Employers may adopt, modify or terminate welfare benefit plans." Pisciotta v. Teledyne Indus., Inc., 91 F.3d 1326, 1330 (9th Cir. 1996)(citing Curtiss-Wright Corp v. Schoonejongen, 514 U.S. 73, 78 (1995)).

See also Pitman v. Blue Cross & Blue Shield, 24 F. 3D 118, 121–122 (10th Cir. 1994) ("'[T]he employer may modify or withdraw these benefits at any time, provided the changes are made in compliance with ERISA and the terms of the plan.'") (alteration in originial) (quoting Doe v. Group Hospitlization & Medical Servs., 3 F.3d 80, 84 (4th Cir. 1993)); McGann v. H&H Music Co., 946 F.2d 401, (5th Cir. 1991) cert. denied 113 S.Ct. 482 (1992) (holding that employers can change benefits at will, so long as the change does not intentionally discriminate against any particular group); Doe v. Group Hospitalization & Medical Services, 3 F.3d 80, 84 (4th Cir. 1993); Nazay v. Miller, 949 F.2d 1323, 1324, 1329 (3rd Cir. 1991); Maltz v. Aetna Health Plans, Inc., 114 F.3d 9, 12 (2nd Cir. 1997); Senn v. United Dominion Industries, Inc., 951 F.2d 806, 816–17 (7th Cir. 1992); Frahm v. Equitable Life Assur. Soc. of U.S., 137 F.3d 955, 962 (7th Cir. 1998); American Medical Security, Inc. v. Bartlett, 111 F.3d 358 (4th Cir. 1997).

8. "ERISA applies only to benefit plans offered by employers engaged in interstate commerce." Settles v. Golden Rule Ins. Col, 927 F.2d 505, 507–8 (10th Cir. 1991) (citing 29 U.S.C. § 1003(a)(1)).

9. "The 'pre-emption clause' (§514(a)) [of ERISA] provides that ERISA supersedes all state laws insofar as they 'relate to any employee benefit plan.'" Pilot Life Ins. Co. v. Dedeaux, 481 U.S. 41, 41 (1987).

10. See 29 U.S.C. § 1001 (1994).

11. See, e.g., 29 U.S.C.§ 1114(a) (1994); Pilot Life Ins. Co., 481 U.S. at 45; Corcoran v. United Healthcare, Inc., 965 F.2d 1321, 1339 (5th Cir. 1992); see also Pomeroy v. Johns Hopkins Med. Servs., Inc., 868 F. Supp. 110, 116 (D.Md. 1994) (preempting claim against HMO for failure to cover treatment for diplopia, chronic back pain, facial tic, severe depression, and addiction to prescription pain medications); Hemphill v. Unisys Corp., 855 F.Supp. 1225, 1229, 1232 (D. Uah 1994) (preempting various tort claims related to insurer's failure to cover certain benefits after auto accident); Rollo v. Maxicare, 695 F.Supp. 245, 246–47 (E.D. La. 1988) (preempting claim against HMO for poor care after an auto accident).

12. Note also that preemption of state-based causes of action also entails preemption of state-based remedies, such as punitive damages.

13. "ERISA preemption, which shields ERISA employee benefit plans from unforeseen liabilities . . . is critical to the entire statutory scheme." Holmes v. Pacific Mut. Life Ins. Co., 706 F. Supp. 733, 735 (C.D. Cal. 1989). See also Johnson v. Dist. 2 Marine Eng. Beneficial Ass'n: "Plan trustees are reqired to discharge their duties 'solely in the interest of the participants and beneficiaries.' . . . At the same time, however, they have a duty to keep the Fund financially stable. '[T]he purpose of a Fund is to provide benefits to as many intended beneficiaries as is economically possible while protecting the financial stability of the Fund'" (Johnson v. Dist. 2 Marine Eng. Beneficial Ass'n, 857 F.2d 514, 517 [9th Cir. 1988]). See also Chittenden, 1991, at 489.

Thus, ERISA is designed to protect employee-beneficiaries, partly by protecting the various plans on which they depend.

14. These instances primarily occur when claims against the health plan are ERISA-preempted and there is also no separate cause of action against the physician. In Corcoran v. United Healthcare, Inc., for instance, the health plan denied a pregnancy treatment the physician recommended. Since no physician malpractice was alleged, there was no claim against a physician. And all claims against the health plan were preempted, leaving the plaintiff with no remedy at all. Corcoran v. United Healthcare, Inc., 965 F2d 1321 (5th Cir 1992), cert denied 113 SCt 812 (1992). See also Cannon v. Group Health Service of Oklahoma, Inc., 77 F.3d 1270 (10th Cir. 1996); Turner v. Fallon Community Health Plan Inc., 953 F.Supp 419 (D.Mass 1997); Tolton v. American Biodyne, Inc., 48 F.3d 937 (6th Cir. 1995); Nealy v. U.S. Healthcare HMO., 844 F.Supp. 966 (S.D.N.Y. 1994) (in *Nealy,* the New York Court of Appeal subsequently held that causes against the primary care physician were not preempted: Nealy v. US HealthCare HMO, 711 N.E.2d 621 (N.Y. 1999)).

15. "The 'pre-emption clause' (§ 514(a)) [of ERISA] provides that ERISA supersedes all state laws insofar as they 'relate to any employee benefit plan,' but ERISA's 'saving clause' (§ 514(b)(2)(A)) exempts from the pre-emption clause any state law that 'regulates insurance.' ERISA's 'deemer clause' (§ 514(b)(2)(B)) provides that no employee benefit plan shall be deemed to be an insurance company for purposes of any state law 'purporting to regulate insurance.'" Pilot Life Ins. Co. v. Dedeaux, 481 U.S. 41, 41 (1987).

16. Metropolitan Life Ins. Co. v. Massachusetts, 471 U.S. 724 (1984).

17. In 1992 one estimate found that there were at least one thousand such state mandates. Pitsenberger, 1999, at 308.

Another study found that with respect to states' assorted mandates requiring health plans to cover various specified services, from 59% to 90% of the costs of these mandates are translated into wage reductions. Blumberg, 1999, at 58. See also Butler, 1991, at 2543; Goodman, Musgrave, 1992, at 197–98, 340–50.

18. In American Medical Security, Inc. v. Bartlett, 111 F.3d 358 (4th Cir. 1997), the state of Maryland had required all benefit plans, including self-funded ones, to carry stop-loss coverage. The Fourth Circuit overturned this statute as a violation of ERISA.

One exception is Hawaii, which enacted legislation mandating employers to provide health insurance in 1974; this program has an exemption from ERISA. See Law, 2000; Lewin, Sybinsk, 1993.

The U.S. Supreme Court has permitted states to collect money for uninsured health care by imposing levies on institutions such as for-profit health insurers so long as there are no specific dictates regarding the amount or type of benefits these plans must provide. New York State Conference of Blue Cross v. Travelers Ins., 115 S.Ct. 1671 (1995). See also Cal. Labor Stds. Enforcement v. Dillingham Const., 117 S.Ct. 832 (1997); De Buono v. NYSA-ILA Medical and Clinical Services, 117 S.Ct. 1747 (1997).

19. Mertens v. Hewitt Associates, 113 S.Ct. 2063 (1993); Massachusetts Mutual Life Ins. Co. v. Russell, 473 U.S. 134 (1985); Novak v. Andersen Corp., 962 F.2d 757, 760 (8th Cir. 1992). See also Younger, Conner, Cartwright, 1994, at 6.

For instance, in Juliano v. Health Maint. Organ. of New Jersey, 221 F.3d 279 (2nd Cir. 2000), an HMO denied coverage for home nursing care to a beneficiary suffering from multiple sclerosis. The Second Circuit determined after examining the contract that the beneficiary (or more precisely, her estate, since the plaintiff was deceased by the time of the ruling) would be entitled to the monetary value of the treatment in a skilled nursing facility, as offered earlier by the HMO. Although this amount was greater than the amount the HMO would have spent for home nursing, it was the amount that the HMO would have been obligated to spend under the terms of the plan.

20. Dearmass v. Av-Med, Inc., 814 F. Supp. 1103 (S.D. Fla. 1993).

21. Dearmass v. Av-Med, Inc., 814 F. Supp. 1103 (S.D. Fla. 1993). The district court in this case preempted claims based on a theory that the HMO had violated federal "anti-dumping" laws. In a

subsequent suit the same district court also prerempted claims regarding negligent administration of the plan but did not rule out a claim for vicarious liability. Dearmass v. Av-Med, Inc., 865 F.Supp. 816 (S.D.Fla. 1994).

22. Kuhl v. Lincoln Nat. Health Plan, 999 F.2d 298 (8th Cir. 1993).

23. See, e.g., Spain v. Aetna Life Ins. Co., 11 F.3d 129 (9th Cir. 1993), cert. denied 511 U.S. 1052, 114 S.Ct. 1612 (1994); Sweeney v. Gerber Products Co. Med. Benefits Plan, 728 F.Supp. 594, (D.Neb. 1989); Exbom v. Central States Health and Welfare Fund, 900 F.2d 1138 (7th Cir. 1990)(preempting claim of morbidly obese patient protesting denial of coverage for gastroplasty); Rollo v. Maxicare of Louisiana, Inc., 695 F. Supp. 245 (E.D.La. 1988) (preempting claim against HMO for poor care after an auto accident); Pomeroy v. Johns Hopkins Medical Services, Inc., 868 F.Supp. 110 (D.Md. 1994)(preempting claim against HMO for failure to cover treatment for diplopia, chronic back pain, facial tic, severe depression, and addiction to prescription pain medications); Hemphill v. Unisys Corp., 855 F.Supp. 1225 (D.Utah 1994) (preempting various tort claims related to insurer's failure to cover certain benefits after auto accident); Holmes v. Pacific Mut. Life Ins. Co, 706 F.Supp. 733 (C.D.Cal. 1989); Corcoran v. United Healthcare, Inc., 965 F2d 1321 (5th Cir 1992), cert denied 113 SCt 812 (1992); Ricci v. Gooberman, 840 F.Supp. 316 (D.N.J. 1993); Cannon v. Group Health Service of Oklahoma, Inc., 77 F.3d 1270 (10th Cir. 1996); Andrews-Clarke v. Travelers Ins. Co., 984 F. Supp 49 (D.Mass. 1997); Nealy v. U.S. Healthcare HMO., 844 F.Supp. 966 (S.D.N.Y. 1994); Tolton v. American Biodyne, Inc., 48 F.3d 937 (6th Cir. 1995); Jass v. Prudential Health Care Plan, Inc., 88 F.3d 1482 (7th Cir. 1996); Bast v. Prudential Ins. Co. of America, 150 F.3d 1003 (9th Cir. 1998); Foster v. Blue Cross Blue Shield of Michigan, 969 F.Supp. 1020 (E.D.Mich. 1997); Huss v. Green Spring Health Services, Inc., 18 F.Supp.2d 400 (D.Del. 1998); Pryzbowski v. U.S. Healthcare, Inc., 64 F.Supp.2d 361 (D.N.J. 1999).

24. Corcoran v. United Healthcare, Inc., 965 F2d 1321, 1338 (5th Cir 1992), cert denied 113 SCt 812 (1992)

"This case, thus, becomes yet another illustration of the glaring need for Congress to amend ERISA to account for the changing realities of the modern health care system." Andrews-Clarke v. Travelers Ins. Col, 984 F.Supp. 49, 53 (D.Mass. 1997).

"The Court is not unmindful this holding leaves plaintiff with no remedy under ERISA for the needless and tragic loss she has suffered. . . . Nevertheless, the Court must respect Congress' intent to have the civil enforcement mechanism of ERISA be the exclusive remedy for such claims. . . . "There is sound reason to alter ERISA in order to provide relief to plaintiffs who present claims like this one; however, amending ERISA to accommodate those causes of action is for Congress, not the courts." Huss v. Green Spring Health Services, Inc., 18 F.Supp.2d 400, 408 (D.Del. 1998).

"Although ERISA provides a remedy for the improper denial of benefits—it is not the remedy that plaintiffs desire. Plaintiffs misconstrue the nature of ERISA preemption. That ERISA does not provide the full range of remedies available under state law in no way undermines ERISA preemption. The policy choices reflected in the inclusion of certain remedies and the exclusion of others under the federal scheme would be completely undermined if ERISA-plan participants and beneficiaries were free to obtain remedies under state law that Congress rejected in ERISA." Tolton v. American Biodyne, Inc., 48 F.3d 937, 943 (6th Cir. 1995).

"Although forcing the Basts to assert their claims only under ERISA may leave them without a viable remedy, this is an unfortunate consequence of the compromise Congress made in drafting ERISA" Bast v. Prudential Ins. Co. of America, 150 F.3d 1003, 1010 (9th Cir. 1998).

"ERISA preempts all causes of actions that attempt to recover for a denial of benefits. This may seem harsh result in this case, but it is an unfortunate consequence of the breadth of ERISA's preemption clause." Foster v. Blue Cross Blue Shield of Michigan, 969 F.Supp. 1020, 1024 (E.D.Mich. 1997)

See also Jass v. Prudential Health Care Plan, Inc., 88 F.3d 1482 (7th Cir. 1996); Turner v. Fallon Community Health Plan Inc., 953 F.Supp 419, 424 (D.Mass 1997); aff'd, Turner v. Fallon Community Health Plan, Inc., 127 F.3d 196 (1st Cir. 1997); Cannon v. Group Health Serv., 77 F.3d 1270, 1274 (10th Cir.) cert denied, 117 S. Ct. 66 (1996); Nealy v. U.S. Healthcare HMO, 844 F. Supp. 966, 974 (S.D.N.Y. 1994); Olson v. General Dynamics Corp., 960 F.2d 1418, 1423–25 (Judge Reinhardt, concurring) (9th Cir. 1991).

25. Haas v. Group Health Plan, Inc., 875 F. Supp. 544 (S.D. Ill. 1994).

26. Haas v. Group Health Plan, Inc., 875 F. Supp. 544, 548–49 (S.D. Ill. 1994). "This Court concludes that when an HMO plan elected to directly provide medical services or leads a participant to reasonably believe that it has, rather than simply arranging and paying for treatment, a

vicarious liability medical practice claim based on substandard treatment by an agent of the HMO plan is not preempted."
Id., at 548.

27. Kearney v. U.S. Healthcare, Inc., 859 F.Supp. 182 (E.D. Pa. 1994).

28. Kearney v. U.S. Healthcare, Inc., 859 F.Supp. 182, 186 (E.D. Pa. 1994) (emphasis added).

29. Similar reasoning can be found in Schachter v. Pacificare, Inc., 923 F.Supp. 1448, 1451 (N.D. Okla.), mandamus denied sub nom. Pacificare, Inc. v. Burrage, 59 F.3d 151 (10th Cir. 1995), and Jackson v. Roseman, 878 F.Supp. 820, 826 (D.Md. 1995).

30. Dukes v. U.S. Healthcare, 57 F.3d 350 (3d. Cir. 1995).

31. Dukes v. U.S. Healthcare, 57 F.3d 350, 354 n.2 (3d. Cir. 1995); citing ERISA § 502(a)(1)(B), 29 U.S.C. § 1132(a)(1)(B).

32. Dukes v. U.S. Healthcare, 57 F.3d 350, 356 (3d. Cir. 1995). "Instead of claiming that the welfare plans in any way withheld some quantum of plan benefits due, the plaintiffs . . . complain about the low quality of the medical treatment that they actually received." *Id.*, at 357. The court went on to note that "[q]uality control of benefits, such as the health care benefits provided here, is a field traditionally occupied by state regulation and we interpret the silence of Congress as reflecting an intent that it remain such." *Id.*

33. Dukes v. U.S. Healthcare, 57 F.3d 350, 361 (3d. Cir. 1995). The court did not go on to note that a state court might nevertheless rule that ERISA preempted the ostensible agency claim. See *id.*, at 355. In *Dukes* and in the Seventh Circuit's ensuing decision in Rice v. Panchal, 65 F.3d 637 (7th Cir. 1995), the courts distinguished carefully between complete preemption, which will only occur if the provisions of 502(a)(1)(B) are invoked (i.e., If the suit's question concerns withholding of benefits due, enforcement of rights under the terms of the plan, or clarification of rights to future benefits), and conflict preemption, which can be adjudicated in state or federal courts according to the plaintiff's well-pleaded complaint. See Id.at 355; Rice, 65 F.3d at 637, 639–40.

34. Herrera v. Lovelace Health Systems, Inc., 35 F.Supp.2d 1327 (D.N.M . 1999).

35. Herrera, 35 F.Supp.2d 1330, citing Pacificare of Oklahoma, Inc. v. Burrage, 59 F.3d 151, 154 (10th Cir. 1995).

36. Crum v. Health Alliance-Midwest, Inc., 47 F.Supp.2d 1013 (C.D.Ill. 1999).

37. Tufino v. N.Y. Hotel & Motel Trades Council, 646 N.Y.S.2d 799 (A.D. 1 Dept. 1996).

38. In Prihoda v. Shpritz, 914 F.Supp. 113 (D.Md. 1966), the plaintiff sued his HMO on grounds of vicarious liability when its physicians failed to diagnose his kidney cancer. "Prihoda does not claim that the HMO Defendants withheld benefits due Leisher. Prihoda does not ask the courts to enforce rights created under the terms of the plan. Nor does she ask the court to clarify future benefits. Her complaint is concerned solely with the quality of the benefits provided." 914 F.Supp. 118.

Similarly, In Re Estate of Frappier, 678 So.2d 884 (Fla.App. 4 Dist. 1996), agreed with the *Dukes* dichotomy and held that when the plaintiff's complaint concerns "failing to provide, arrange for, or supervise qualified doctors to provide the actual medical treatment for the plan participants, federal preemption is inappropriate."

39. Tolton v. American Biodyne, Inc.,48 F.3d 937 (6th Cir. 1995).

40. Tolton v. American Biodyne, Inc.,48 F.3d 937, 941(6th Cir. 1995).

41. Turner v. Fallon Community Health Plan Inc., 953 F.Supp. 419 (D.Mass.), aff'd, 127 F.3d 196 (1st Cir. 1997).

42. Turner v. Fallon Community Health Plan Inc., 127 F.3d 196 (1st Cir. 1997).

43. Cannon v. Group Health Service, 77 F.3d 1270 (10th Cir.) cert denied, 117 S.Ct. 66 (1996).

44. See Cannon v. Group Health Service, 77 F.3d 1270, 1273–74 (10th Cir.) cert denied, 117 S.Ct. 66 (1996). See also Jass v. Prudential Health Care Plan, Inc., 88 F.3d 1482 (7th Cir. 1996); Parrino v. FHP, Inc., 146 F.3d 699 (9th Cir. 1998); Schmid v. Kaiser Foundation Health Plan, 963 F.Supp 942 (D.Or. 1997); Foster v. Blue Cross Blue Shield of Michigan, 969 F.Supp. 1020 (E.D.Mich. 1997); Huss v. Green Spring Health Services, Inc., 18 F.Supp.2d 400 (D.Del. 1998); Healthcare America Plans, Inc. v. Bossemeyer, 953 F.Supp. 1176 (D.Kan. 1996) affd w/o opin. 166 F.3d 347; Garrison v. Northeast Georgia Medical Center, Inc., 66 F.Supp2d 1336 (N.D.Ga. 1999); Danca v. Private Health Care Sys., Inc., 185 F.3d 1 (1st Cir. 1999).

45. See Cannon v. Group Health Service, 77 F.3d 1270,1274–75 (10th Cir.) cert denied, 117 S.Ct. 66 (1996).

In Maltz v. Aetna Health Plans, Inc., 114 F.3d 9 (2nd Cir. 1997), the Second Circuit preempted any challenge to an HMO's decision to pay its physicians by capitation rather than by the more traditional fee-for-service. See *id.*, at 11–12. "Nothing in the contract between Aetna and its enrollees . . . limits Aetna's ability to make significant changes in its relationship with its doctors as long as the enrollees are aware of the changes when they renew their contract with Aetna and Aetna provides them with competent, alternative physicians." *Id.*, at 12 (footnote omitted).

In Hull v. Fallon, 188 F.3d 939 (8th Cir. 1999), claims that the health plan's medical director had practiced medicine and done so negligently in denying a request for a thallium stress test, were preempted on the ground that the claims concerned the administration of benefits.

In Pryzbowski v. U.S. Healthcare, Inc., 64 F.Supp.2d 361 (D.N.J. 1999), seven months of delays in processing requests for a patient's back surgery allegedly led to complications in her condition. The federal district court held that negligence claims against the plan were preempted because they concerned the administration of benefits rather than the quality of the actual care delivered.

46. See, e.g., Rice v. Panchal, 65 F.3d 637, 645 (7th Cir. 1995); Newton v. Tavani, 962 F.Supp. 45, 47–48 (D.N.J. 1997); Lancaster v. Kaiser Foundation Health Plan, 958 F.Supp. 1137 (E.D.Va. 1997); Turner v. Fallon Community Health Plan Inc., 953 F.Supp. 419, 424 (D.Mass.), aff'd, 127 F.3d 196 (1st Cir. 1997); Schwartz v. FHP Int'l Corp., 947 F.Supp. 1354, 1360 (D. Ariz. 1996); Ouellette v. Christ Hosp., 942 F.Supp. 1160, 1164–65 (S.D. Ohio 1996); Santitoro v. Evans, 935 F.Supp. 733, 736 (E.D.N.C. 1996); Prihoda v. Shpritz, 914 F.Supp. 113, 118 (D.Md. 1996); Roessert v. Health Net, 929 F.Supp. 343, 349–50 (N.D. Cal. 1996); Kampmeier v. Sacred Heart Hosp., No. CIV. A. 95–7816, 1996 WL 220979, *2–3 (E.D. Pa. May 2, 1996); Frappier v. Wishnov (*In re* Estate of Frappier), 678 So. 2D 884, 889 (Fla. Dist. Ct. App. 1996); Pappas v. Asbel, 675 A.2d 711, 716 (Pa. Super. Ct. 1996); affirmed, 724 A.2d 889 (Pa. 1998), vacated, 120 S.Ct. 2686; Negron v. Patel, 6 F.Supp.2d 366 (E.D.Pa. 1998) (case concerned federal employees' health benefits plans (FEHBP) rather than ERISA); Wartenberg v. Aetna U.S. Healthcare, Inc., 2 F.Supp.2d 273 (E.D.N.Y. 1998); Bauman v. U.S. Healthcare, Inc., 1 F.Supp.2d 420 (D.N.J. 1998), aff'd, *In re* U.S. Healthcare, 193 F3d 151 (3d Cir. 1999), cert. denied 120 SCt 2687 (2000); Moreno v. Health Partners Health Plan, 4 F.Supp.2d 888 (D.Ariz. 1998); Moscovitch v. Danbury Hosp., 25 F.Supp.2d 74 (D.Conn. 1998); Corporate Health Ins. Inc. v. Texas Dept. of Ins., 12 F.Supp.2d 597 (S.D.Tex. 1998), aff'd in part, rev'd in part, 215 F.3d 526 (5th Cir. 2000); Chaghervand v. CareFirst, 909 F.Supp 304 (D.Md. 1995); Schmid v. Kaiser Foundation Health Plan, 963 F.Supp 942 (D.Or. 1997); Brandon v. Aetna Services, Inc., 46 F.Supp.2d 110 (D.Conn. 1999); Plocica v. NYLCare of Texas, Inc., 43 F.Supp.2d 658 (N.D.Tex. 1999); Fritts v. Khoury, 933 F.Supp. 668 (E.D. Mich. 1996); Bast v. Prudential Ins. Co. of America, 150 F.3d 1003 (9th Cir. 1998); Newton v. Tavani, 962 F.Supp. 45 (D.N.J. 1997); Negron v. Patel, 6 F.Supp.2d 366 (E.D.Pa. 1998); Wartenberg v. Aetna U.S. Health-care, Inc., 2 F.Supp.2d 273 (E.D.N.Y. 1998); Dykema v. King, 959 F.Supp. 736 (D.S.C. 1997); Brewer v. Geisinger Clinic Inc., 2000 WL 114270 (Pa. Com. Pl. 2000); Howard v. Sasson, 1995 WL 581960 (E.D.Pa. 1995); Morton v. Mylan Pharmaceuticals, 2000 WL 340196 (E.D.Pa. 2000); Whelan v. Keystone Health Plan East, 1995 WL 394153 (E.D.Pa. 1995).

47. Both these scenarios are envisioned by the Third Circuit in the Dukes case.

> We recognize that the distinction between the quantity of benefits due under a welfare plan and the quality of those benefits will not always be clear in situations like this where the benefit contracted for is health care services rather than money to pay for such services. There well may be cases in which the quality of a patient's medical care or the skills of the personnel provided to administer that care will be so low that the treatment received simply will not qualify as health care at all. In such a case, it well may be appropriate to conclude that the plan participant or beneficiary has been denied benefits due under the plan. . . .
>
> We also recognize the possibility that an ERISA plan may describe a benefit in terms that can accurately be described as related to the quality of the service. Thus, for example, a plan might promise that all X-rays would be analyzed by radiologists with prescribed level of advanced training.

Dukes v. U.S. Healthcare, 57 F.3d 350, 357, 358 (3d. Cir. 1995), cert denied, 116 S.Ct. 564 (1995).

48. Dukes v. U.S. Healthcare, 57 F.3d 350, 357 (3d. Cir. 1995), cert denied, 116 S.Ct. 564 (1995).

49. Metropolitan Life Ins. Co. v. Massachusetts, 471 U.S. 724 (1984); American Medical Security, Inc. v. Bartlett, 111 F.3d 358 (4th Cir. 1997) (overturning state law requiring self-insured ERISA plans to carry stop-loss insurance).

50. See supra n. 7.

51. Ouellette v. Christ Hospital, 942 F.Supp. 1160 (S.D. Ohio 1996).

52. Bauman v. U.S. Healthcare, Inc., 1 F.Supp.2d 420 (D.N.J. 1998); aff'd as *In re* U.S. Health-care, Inc., 193 F. 3d 151 (3rd Cir. 1999), cert. denied 120 SCt 2687 (2000).

53. The district court did call the denial of a home visit a benefits denial, preempting that question to federal court under ERISA. However, even this concession to identifying resource issues was put aside by the Third Circuit. "The mere fact that the Baumans referred in their complaint to a benefit promised by their health care plan does not automatically convert their state-law negligence claim into a claim for benefits under section 502. If, as the Baumans contend, U.S. Healthcare failed to meet the standard of care required of health care providers by failing to arrange for a pediatric nurse in a timely manner, Count Six sets forth an ordinary state-law tort claim for medical malpractice." *In re* U.S. Healthcare, Inc., 193 F. 3d 151, 164 (3rd Cir. 1999), cert. denied 120 SCt 2687 (2000).

54. Beebe, Britton, Britton, et al., 1996; Chin, 1997; Edmonson, Stoddard, Owens, 1997; Liu, Clemens, Shay, et al., 1997; Gazmarian, Koplan, Cogswell, et al., 1997; Lane, Kauls, Ickovics, et al., 1999.

55. See supra n. 7.

56. Kampmeier v. Sacred Heart Hospital, No. CIV. A. 95–7816, 1996 WL 220979 (E.D. Pa. May 2, 1996).

57. In this case, any administrative slip-ups that led to the initial denial of the test could, of course, constitute breaches of expertise duties on the part of the health plan.

58. Plocica v. NYLCare of Texas, Inc., 43 F.Supp.2d 658 (N.D.Tex. 1999).

59. Moscovitch v. Danbury Hosp., 25 F.Supp.2d 74 (D.Conn. 1998).

60. Plocica v. NYLCare of Texas, Inc., 43 F.Supp.2d 663.

61. Plocica v. NYLCare of Texas, Inc., 43 F.Supp.2d 663.

62. Similarly, in Lancaster v. Kaiser Foundation Health Plan, 958 F.Supp. 1137 (E.D.Va. 1997), the court found that the plaintiffs' claims fell outside ERISA § 502(a)(1)(B), "because they focused on the 'quality' of the medical benefits received, as opposed to the 'quantity' of the medical benefits delivered." 958 F.Supp. 1145.

63. Moreno v. Health Partners Health Plan, 4 F.Supp.2d 888, 889 (D.Ariz. 1998).

64. Rice v. Panchal, 65 F3d 637, 639, 646 (7th Cir. 1995). This principle is also called the "well-pleaded complaint" rule. The court went on: "This court, like a defendant, cannot recharacterize a plaintiff's claim in order to create federal question jurisdiction, for if we did so, then 'the plaintiff would be master of nothing'" (at 646).

65. Jass v. Prudential Health Care Plan, Inc., 88 F.3d 1482 (7th Cir. 1996).

66. Jass v. Prudential Health Care Plan, Inc., 88 F.3d 1482, 1489 (7th Cir. 1996) (citing Oglesby v. RCA Corp., 752 F.2d 272, 277–78 (7th Cir. 1985), quoting Salveson v. Western States Bankcard Assoc., 525 F.Supp. 566, 572 (N.D.Cal. 1981)).

67. Huss v. Green Spring Health Services, Inc., 18 F.Supp.2d 400, 404 (D.Del. 1998); citing Kuhl v. Lincoln Nat. Health Plan, 999 F.2d 298, 303–4 (8th Cir. 1993). See also Parrino v. FHP, Inc., 146 F.3d 699, 704 (9th Cir. 1998); Danca v. Private Health Care Sys., Inc., 185 F.3d 1 (1st Cir. 1999); Pryzbowski v. U.S. Healthcare, Inc., 64 F.Supp.2d 361, 369 (D.N.J. 1999); Hull v. Fallon, 188 F.3d 939, 943 (8th Cir. 1999) (citing Kuhl v. Lincoln Nat. Health Plan, 999 F.2d 298, 303 (8th Cir. 1993).

See also Maio v. Aetna, Inc., 221 F.3d 472, 485 n.12 (3rd Cir. 2000): "Moreover, while our standard of review requires us to accept as true all factual allegations in the complaint, 'we need not accept as true "unsupported conclusions and unwarranted inferences.'" West Penn Power Co., 147 F.3d at 263 n. 13 (quoting Schuylkill Energy Resources . . .) '[C]ourts have an obligation in matters before them to view the complaint as a whole and to base rulings not upon the presence of mere words but, rather, upon the presence of a factual situation which is not justiciable. We do not draw on the allegations of the complaint, but in a realistic, rather than a slavish, manner.' *Id.*, at 263"

68. In one case in which ERISA preemption was reluctantly imposed, a federal district judge nevertheless issued strong criticism of the law. "This case, thus, becomes yet another illustration of the glaring need for Congress to amend ERISA to account for the changing realities of the modern health care system. Enacted to safeguard the interests of employees and their beneficiaries, ERISA has evolved into a shield of immunity that protects health insurers, utilization review providers, and other managed care entities from potential liability for the consequences of their wrongful denial of health benefits." Andrews-Clarke v. Travelers Ins. Col, 984 F.Supp. 49, 53 (D.Mass. 1997). The court went on to say: "Under any criterion, however, the shield of near absolute immunity now provided by ERISA simply cannot be justified. . . . [E]ven more disturbing to this Court is the failure of Congress to amend a statute that, due to the changing realities of the modern health care system, has gone conspicuously awry from its original intent. Does anyone care? Do you?" (984 F.Supp. 63, 65).

69. Pappas v. Asbel, 675 A.2d 711 (Pa.Super. 1996); aff'd, Pappas v. Asbel, 724 A.2d 889 (Pa. 1998), vacated, 120 S.Ct. 2686. In this case a patient presented to a community hospital with a cervical epidural abscess, which is a neurological emergency requiring immediate surgery. Wrangling between the ER physician and HMO representatives over which hospital he should be sent to resulted in delays that left the patient quadriplegic. For further detail see Chapter 10, n. 134.

70. As the court suggested:

> The type of recovery sought is based on negligence attributable to the delay occasioned by a cost containment protocol set by a for-profit organization, and which is aimed at conserving and increasing its profits, an intention diametrically opposed to ERISA's general purpose of protecting the rights of a plan's beneficiaries. Decisions such as that made by USHC concerning where Mr. Pappas might receive treatment are propelled by dollar savings, not the protection of worker's [sic] rights, in this case the right to the most effective medical care, which was the original focus of ERISA. . . . Considerations of cost containment of the type which drive the decision making process in HMO's did not exist for employee welfare plans when ERISA was enacted. It cannot therefore be argued that the type of recovery sought here was deliberately excluded from the Congressional schema in order to protect ERISA plans from conflicting directives which would, in attempting to control expenses, affect medical judgments. . . . To find that such claims are preempted because they may interfere with what is in essence a business decision made in the financial interests of a commercial entity is inconsistent with the intention of ERISA and should not "suffice to trigger preemption."

Pappas v. Asbel, 675 A.2d 711, 716 (Pa.Super. 1996) aff'd, Pappas v. Asbel, 724 A.2d 889 (Pa. 1998), vacated, 120 S.Ct. 2686. The court continued: "The negligence claims at issue here . . . have, in fact, no connection to the benefit scheme which Congress sought to protect by preempting laws tending to produce conflicting systemic demand; ERISA is in no way implicated by the claim that USHC negligently caused Mr. Pappas' injuries by its delay in authorizing his transfer." *Id.*, at 717. "We, too, do not believe that Congress can have intended, prior even to invention of the cost containment system which inheres in USHC's review process, to foreclose recovery to plan beneficiaries injured by negligent medical decisions. We therefore conclude that the negligence claims against appellee are not preempted by ERISA." *Id.*, at 718. Other commentators have noticed this oddity in the emerging application of the *Dukes* distinction.

> The most glaring failure of this distinction arises in cases when a physician fails to detect (and therefore to treat) a medical problem. In this case, the complaint could be characterized as one of quantity of benefits, yet no direct cause of action may be leveled at the MCO if the failure to detect a medical problem did not result from the MCO's negligence. In this situation, a vicarious liability complaint would be proper. Even deeming failure-to-detect cases as quality-oriented does not solve the issue. It merely encourages the astute plaintiff's counsel, in a state forum, to plead the case as a failure-to-detect case (i.e., vicarious liability, not preempted) rather than as an improper UR case (i.e., direct liability, preempted). . . . Because they are not tethered to the reality of managed care, these distinctions are easily manipulated. Some courts, for example, have achieved a result contrary to *Dukes* by tinkering with and collapsing these distinctions. Other courts see the provision of substandard care as a constructive denial of benefits, or have determined that medical decisions are benefit determinations.

Jacobson, Pomfret, 1998, at 1028–30 (citations omitted).

71. Lancaster v. Kaiser Foundation Health Plan, 958 F.Supp. 1137 (E.D. Va. 1997).

72. Lancaster v. Kaiser Foundation Health Plan, 958 F.Supp. 1137, 1145 (E.D. Va. 1997) (emphasis added).

73. Lancaster v. Kaiser Foundation Health Plan, 958 F.Supp. 1137, 1146 (E.D. Va. 1997) (emphasis added). It is interesting to note the court's ambivalence about the role of the incentives. On one hand, the court acknowledged that Kaiser's incentive system was designed to influence resource use. "[T]he gravamen of these claims is that Kaiser purposefully established and implemented an administrative policy that had the effect of inducing [Drs.] Campbell and Pauls to deny benefits to Lancaster, thereby causing her injuries" (958 F.Supp. 1146). However, the court found that the plaintiff's claims against the plan were preempted be because they

> attack an administrative decision, not a medical one. Properly construed, these claims focus on Kaiser's administrative decision to curb rising health care costs by employing a system of financial incentives that rewarded physicians for not ordering tests or treatments. In other

words, [they] challenge an administrative decision that had the effect of denying benefits to Lancaster as a plan participant because it inappropriately influenced Campbell and Pauls to take non-medical factors, most notably, their incomes, into account when prescribing treatment. These claims for direct negligence and fraud against Kaiser trigger § 502(a)(1)(B) and support complete preemption since they challenge an administrative decision that has the effect of denying benefits.

958 F.Supp. 1147.

On the other hand, when the incentives actually showed signs of effectiveness—when, as the court says just above, they "had the effect of denying benefits to Lancaster as a plan participant because it inappropriately influenced Campbell and Pauls to take non-medical factors . . . into account"—the court insisted that the physicians' conduct was limited to quality issues, not benefit denial. 958 F.Supp. 1146.

74. Other courts share *Lancaster's* assumption that ERISA preemption applies essentially to "administration" of the plan, with the implicit assumption that only administrators do the administrating and make the benefits decisions. "[T]his court concludes that the claims at issue here do not clearly involve 'utilization review' and instead are more accurately considered claims based on the 'quality' of medical care received rather than an administrative decision." Crum v. Health Alliance-Midwest, Inc., 47 F.Supp.2d 1013, 1021 (C.D.Ill. 1999). Although such references to "administrative" decisions do not absolutely entail that such decisions can only be made by a plan administrator, the distinction, as drawn between administration and "medical care," does seem fairly clearly to separate according to persons' job titles as well as their functions.

"Despite plaintiff's attempts to craft defendants' actions as medical malpractice, the wrong committed in this case relates to the administration of the plan, not to the provision or supervision of medical services. In fact, the overarching problem was that no medical treatment was ever initiated let alone provided." Huss v. Green Spring Health Services, Inc., 18 F.Supp.2d 400, 405 (D.Del. 1998).

See also In Re Estate of Frappier, 678 So.2d 884, 887 (Fla.App. 4 Dist. 1996); Roessert v. Health Net, 929 F.Supp. 343, 350 (N.D.Cal. 1996); Santitoro v. Evans, 935 F.Supp. 733, 736 (E.D.N.C. 1996); Haas v. Group Health Plan, Inc., 875 F.Supp. 544, 548 (S.D.Ill. 1994); Schachter v. Pacificare of Oklahoma, Inc., 923 F.Supp. 1448, 1452 (N.D.Okl. 1995); Dearmass v. Av-Med, Inc., 865 F.Supp. 816, 818 (S.D. Fla. 1994); Turner v. Fallon Community Health Plan Inc., 953 F.Supp 419, 423 (D.Mass 1997); Turner v. Fallon Community Health Plan, Inc., 127 F.3d 196, 198, 199 (1st Cir. 1997).

75. "In Virginia as elsewhere, medical malpractice plaintiffs need only show that a deviation from the standard of medical care occurred; they are not required to show why it occurred. A health care provider's deviation from the standard of care is actionable whether it was occasioned by inadvertence, ignorance, mistake, superstition, or indeed for any reason at all." Lancaster v. Kaiser Foundation Health Plan, 958 F.Supp. 1137, 1140 (E.D. Va. 1997).

76. Schachter v. Pacificare, Inc., 923 F.Supp. 1448, 1452 (N.D. Okla. 1995), mandamus denied sub nom. Pacificare, Inc. v. Burrage, 59 F.3d 151 (10th Cir. 1995).

A Florida court, similarly, held that although claims for ostensible agency were not preempted, direct negligence and corporate liability claims against the health plan were preempted. "[W]e concur with the lower court's decision that these allegations would be completely preempted because they present issues unequivocally related to the administration of the plan and are within the scope of section 502(a)(1)(B)." Frappier v. Wishnow (*In re* Estate of Frappier), 678 So. 2d 884, 887 (Fla. Dist. Ct. App. 1996). See also Dearmas v. Av-Med., Inc., 865 F.Supp. 816, 818 (S.D. Fla. 1994); Stroker v. Rubin, 1994 WL 719694 (E.D.Pa. 1994).

77. For a discussion of the difference between "complete preemption" and "conflict preemption," see Rice v. Panchal, 65 F3d 637, 640–41 (7th Cir. 1995); Dukes v. U.S. Health Care, Inc., 57 F.3d 350, 355 ff. (3rd Cir. 1995).

78. ERISA preemption applies to claims "to recover benefits due . . . under the terms of [the] plan, to enforce . . . rights under the terms of the plan, or to clarify . . . rights to future benefits under the terms of the plan."Dukes v. U.S. Health Care, Inc., 57 F.3d 350, 356 (3rd Cir. 1995), citing ERISA § 502(a)(1)(B), 29 U.S.C. § 1132(a)(1)(B).

79. See supra n. 7.

80. Interestingly, the *Dukes* court entertained the possibility that quality of care issues might be preempted if the plan made explicit promises regarding quality or if the quality was so low that it did not constitute health care at all. Dukes v. U.S. Health Care, Inc., 57 F.3d 350, 358 (3rd Cir. 1995).

81. Other observers have likewise noticed the oddity of supposing that claims for direct liability must invariably be preempted, even while claims for indirect liability such as ostensible agency

may be permitted. "[T]o deny preemption in vicarious liability cliams while allowing preemption in direct negligence cliams will lead to the anomalous result of decreasing HMO liability in correlation with the extent of its involvement in providing care." Ricci v. Gooberman, 840 F.Supp. 316, 317–18 (D.N.J. 1993).

In any given case, careless credentialing could stem from a deficiency of knowledge, skill, or diligence on the part of a health plan. Perhaps administrators were hasty in assembling the plan's provider network, signing up anyone who would agree to their fee scale rather than scrutinizing the quality of each prospective provider; or perhaps they didn't take the time to verify that each physician is indeed licensed. These issues do not directly implicate benefits or rights under the terms of the health plan and can be remanded to state courts.

82. *In re* U.S. Healthcare, 193 F3d 151 (3d Cir. 1999), cert. denied 120 SCt 2687 (2000); see discussion just above, in §B-1 of this chapter.

83. *In re* U.S. Healthcare, 193 F3d 151, 163 (3d Cir. 1999).

84. Danca v. Private Health Care Sys., Inc., 185 F.3d 1 (1st Cir. 1999).

85. Danca v. Private Health Care Sys., Inc., 185 F.3d 1, 6 n.6 (1st Cir. 1999).

86. See Dukes v. U.S. Health Care, Inc., 57 F.3d 350, 360–61 (3rd Cir. 1995): "The difference between the 'utilization review' and the 'arranging for medical treatment' roles is crucial for the purposes of § 502(a)(1)(B) because *only in a utilization-review role is an entity in a position to deny benefits due* under an ERISA welfare plan" (emphasis added). Kampmeier v. Sacred Heart Hospital, 1996 WL 220979, 220981 (E.D. PA) (favorably citing *Dukes* position above).

87. At most, such plans may receive a formal request for reimbursement in unusual situations, such as when a member has received care out of network while traveling; or when someone seeks explicit authorization for an unusual or costly procedure; or when someone, following a denial of such authorization, purchases the services out-of-pocket and demands reimbursement. Shy of these uncommon situations, "denials of benefits" in capitated plans are simply a failure to provide services or resources that patients were promised by the plan.

88. For further discussion of this point, see Morreim, 2000(c).

89. See Chapter 10 § D. The case of Jass v. Prudential Health Care Plan, Inc., 88 F.3d 1482 (7th Cir. 1996), is interesting and on point. As recounted by Jacobson and Pomfret,

> a physician and UR nurse allegedly acted negligently by discharging a patient without needed rehabilitation and the patient suffered permanent injury. After conceding that the UR nurse's decision was medical and that she was a registered nurse, the court nevertheless held that the nurse's job title was UR *administrator* and, pursuant to that position, was determining benefits within the meaning of ERISA. The court also pointed out that the nurse had no contact with the plaintiff, perhaps concluding that this lack of contact transformed the medical nature of the nurse's determination into an administrative decision. In framing the issue in this manner, the court was clearly thinking in terms of a paradigm in which medical decision making is only pursued by treating physicians in direct contact with patients. Jacobson, Pomfret, 1998, at 1028.

Although the *Jass* court was confused in its apparent presumption that the bare fact that an administrator made the decision rendered the issue a benefits issue, arguably the court was nevertheless correct in concluding that denial of physical therapy services involved a resource issue. What is not clear from the facts provided is whether there were additionally any expertise issues. On the one hand, if the MCO's contract placed clear, explicit limits and criteria on the use of physical therapy, then resources are the only issue. On the other hand, if the contract asks its UR personnel to make judgments about the medical necessity of the therapy, and if those judgments were characterized by expertise deficiencies, then there may indeed be room for state-based tort litigation.

90. For further discussion about the importance of understanding the precise financial structures operating in a given health plan, see Morreim, 2000(c).

91. See Chapter 6, § B-2. Recall that physician-level capitation (e.g., an individual physician is capitated just to provide his professional services to his own patients) is distinguished from group-level capitation (e.g. a physician group receives a fixed sum to provide primary care services for a large panel of patients), and distinguished further from global capitation (e.g. a provider group that accepts the entire premium in exchange for providing all care).

92. Although physicians are often fiduciaries in the common law sense, as described in Chapter 7, ERISA has a very specialized concept. The statute and the Supreme Court define the ERISA fiduciary functionally as "one who 'exercises any discretionary authority or discretionary control respecting management of [a] plan or exercises any authority or control respecting management or disposition of its assets.'" Firestone Tire & Rubber Co. v. Bruch, 489 U.S. 101, 113 (1989); see

also Mertens v. Hewitt Associates, 113 S.Ct. 2063, 2071 (1993). More particularly, "a person is a fiduciary with respect to a plan to the extent (i) he exercises any discretionary authority or discretionary control respecting management of such plan . . . [or (ii)] he has any discretionary authority or discretionary responsibility in the administration of such plan." 20 U.S.C.A. § 1002(21)(A) (West Supp. 1996).

An ERISA fiduciary might be the person or people who make claims decisions within a commercial insurer or MCO, as when an employer has purchased a policy in the marketplace; or the fiduciary could be an individual person or group within the benefits department of a self-insured employer-corporation; or it might be an outside organization, as when a self-insured employer hires an outside agency such as an insurance company to administer claims and make benefits decisions (called TPAs, or third-party administrators). Arrangements vary widely. For the courts, however, the central question is which person, group, or entity actually had the authority to make the particular benefit decision in question and whether that decision maker was permitted to exercise discretion in making this specific benefit determination. If the answer to the latter is yes, then there is an ERISA fiduciary. For further discussion, see Morreim 1998(b), at 518–19.

The question of whether financially incentivized physicians can be fiduciaries was directly considered in the case of Pegram v. Herdrich, 120 U.S. 2143 (2000). The court held that so-called "mixed" decisions, which combine medical decisions and benefit eligibility decisions, are not fiduciary decisions under ERISA. Accordingly, incentive arrangements that might influence the care physicians provide do not inherently constitute a breach of fiduciary duty. The Court's decision does not necessarily mean that a fully capitated physician cannot be an ERISA fiduciary, however, because the incentive arrangement in this particular case featured only an indirect, limited relationship between the physicians' incentives and their medical decisions. In cases in which physicians are fully at financial risk, so that they and no one else are responsible to administer the health plan's funds and make discretionary decisions, the court might well take a different stand.

93. The case of the male impotence drug, Viagra, illustrates the point. See McGarvey, 2000; Smith, Roberts, 2000.

94. See § C-1.

95. " 'Where discretion is conferred upon the trustee with respect to the exercise of a power, its exercise is not subject to control by the court except to prevent an abuse by the trustee of his discretion.' " Firestone Tire & Rubber Co. v. Bruch, 489 U.S. 101, 111 (1989). The fiduciary has the difficult task of balancing the interests of all the beneficiaries who depend on him to administer the plan in their interests. And when he errs, he is "personally liable for damages . . . for restitution . . . and for . . . equitable relief." Mertens v. Hewitt Associates, 113 S.Ct. 2063, 2066 (1993). See also Varity Corp. v. Howe, 116 S.Ct. 1065, 1080 (1996).

As noted in Adelson v. GTE Corp., 790 F. Supp. 1265, 1270 (D.Md. 1992): "It must be remembered that the decisions of plan administrators are entitled to deference because the plan administrators are *fiduciaries* charged with the responsibility to make decisions critical to the lives of individual citizens. To a very real degree they are on the front line in determining the extent and the quality of health care being delivered in this country. They have the duty to assure that the financial integrity of health plans is preserved by denying improper claims, however difficult such decisions may be. In so doing they assist in placing restraints upon health care providers who, if left to their own devices, might well permit health care costs to continue to spiral upward. However, that said, plan administrators have a duty to assure that valid claims of beneficiaries who are in need of medical care are not denied simply because of the cost of such care."

96. As noted by the Eleventh Circuit in Brown v. Blue Cross & Blue Shield of Alabama, 898 F. 2d 1556, 1564–65 (11th Cir. 1990): "The disinterested, impartial decision maker deserves the greatest deference. 'Where . . . the claimant does not argue or is unable to show that the trustees had a significant conflict of interest, we reverse the denial of benefits only if the denial is completely unreasonable.' "

From the Tenth Circuit: " 'The Administrator['s] decision need not be the only logical one nor even the best one. It need only be sufficiently supported by facts within [his] knowledge to counter a claim that it was arbitrary or capricious. *Woolsey,* 934 F.2d at 1460. The decision will be upheld unless it is 'not grounded on any reasonable basis.' *Id.* (citation omitted). The reviewing court 'need only assure that the administrator's decision fall[s] somewhere on a continuum of reasonableness-even if on the low end." Kimber v Thiokol Corp., 196 F.3d 1092, 1098 (10th Cir. 1999)

In Doe v. Group Hospitalization & Medical Services, 3 F.3d 80, 85 (4th Cir. 1993) the Fourth Circuit pointed out: "where a fiduciary with authorized discretion construes a disputed or doubtful term, we will not disturb the interpretation if it is reasonable, even if we come to a different conclusion."

From the Ninth Circuit, in Johnson v. Dist. 2 Marine Eng. Beneficial Ass'n, 857 F.2d 514, 516 (9th Cir. 1988): "A decision is not arbitrary or capricious if it is based on a reasonable interpretation of the plan's terms and was made in good faith."

The Eighth Circuit finds that courts should uphold a denial if the decision is reasonable, meaning that it is "supported by reasoned explanation, even if another reasonable, but different, interpretation may be made." Birdsell v United Parcel Service, 94 F.3d 1130, 1131 (8th Cir. 1996).

From Doe v. Travelers Ins. Co., 971 F.Supp. 623, 630 (D.Mass. 1997): " '[i]f the administrator makes an informed judgment and articulates an explanation for it that is satisfactory in light of the relevant facts, then the administrator's decision is final.' "

97. For further discussion of this predicament, see Morreim, 1998(b).

98. For further discussion, see Morreim 1998(b).

99. From Chapter 4, three scenarios are to be distinguished. In the prospective scenario, a patient who has been denied a particular treatment but who can nevertheless still benefit from it seeks to mandate coverage or treatment. In the second scenario the patient has secured treatment, but the health plan refuses reimbursement. In the third, needed treatment has been delayed or denied, and the patient has been harmed.

In at least some instances, the patient claims harm even though the treatment has been received and the claim paid. In Redmond v. Secure Horizons, Pacificare, Inc., 60 Cal. App.4th 96 (Cal. App. 1997), for instance, the HMO of a Medicare enrollee denied a claim, then eventually paid it. Because of the delays, the patient wanted to bring various actions in state courts for bad faith breach of contract, emotional distress, etc. However, the court ruled that only federal remedies were available. The case was not ERISA, but raises pertinent issues since federal remedies govern in both situations.

100. ERISA § 502(a)(1)(B), 29 U.S.C. § 1132(a)(1)(B).

101. Although ERISA's fiduciaries are modeled in many respects after traditional trustees, the Supreme Court recognizes that the analogy is limited. The ordinary trustee is obligated, for example, to avoid conflicts of interest, but under ERISA that is not always possible. The very same employer that establishes the benefit plan might also (depending on how the plan is set up) function as the fiduciary for that plan. Hence, the employer could incur significant conflicts of interest, since every decision it makes about what to include or exclude from that benefit plan can have significant financial implications for its business. Congress did not wish for ERISA to constrain businesses in this way, and so it resolved the tension by creating its highly functional definition of the ERISA fiduciary: only when specifically acting in the capacity of making discretionary decisions over the assets belonging to the benefit plan will that individual or group be regarded as an ERISA fiduciary. See, e.g., Varity Corp. v. Howe, 116 S.Ct. 1065, 1085–86 (1996); Pegram v. Herdrich, 120 S.Ct. 2143, 2151–52 (2000).

102. 29 USC §1104(a)(1)(A).

103. " 'Any person who is a fiduciary with respect to a plan who breaches any of the responsibilities . . . imposed upon fiduciaries by [ERISA] shall be personally liable to make good to such plan any losses to the plan resulting from each such breach . . .' " 29 U.S.C. § 1109(a), discussed in Herdrich v. Pegram, 154 F.3d 362, 380 (7th Cir. 1998), reversed, Pegram v. Herdrich, 120 U.S. 2143 (2000). See also Massachusetts Mut. Life Ins. Co. v. Russell, 473 U.S. 134, 139 (1985); Reid v. Gruntal & Co., Inc., 763 F.Supp. 672, 673 (D.Me. 1991); Doe v. Travelers Ins. Co, 971 F.Supp. 623, 639 (D.Mass 1997).

104. Firestone Tire & Rubber Co. v. Bruch, 489 U.S. 101 (1989). See also Wiehl JG, et al. Legal Issues Related to Systems Integration. In: Integrated Health Care Delivery Systems, Fine A, ed. New York: Thompson Publishing Group, Inc., 1993; 9–38, at 23; Younger, Conner, Cartwright, 1994, at 11; Johnson v. Dist. 2 Marine Eng. Beneficial Ass'n, 857 F.2d 514, 517 (9th Cir. 1988)

105. The deference accorded to fiduciary administrators is reduced if those administrators are in a conflict of interest, as when they represent both the interests of the individual beneficiaries and the profitability interests of the plan. See Firestone Tire & Rubber Co. v. Bruch, 489 U.S. 101 (1989); Brown v. Blue Cross & Blue Shield of Alabama, 898 F. 2d 1556 (11th Cir. 1990); Pitman v. Blue Cross & Blue Shield, 24 F.3d 118 (10th Cir. 1994); Doe v. Group Hospitalization & Medical Services, 3 F.3d 80 (4th Cir. 1993).

106. Bailey v. Blue Cross/Blue Shield, 866 F. Supp. 277 (E.D. Va. 1994), aff'd, 67 F.3d 53 (4th Cir. 1995).

107. Bailey v. Blue Cross/Blue Shield, 866 F. Supp. 277, 280 (E.D. Va. 1994), aff'd, 67 F.3d 53 (4th Cir. 1995).

108. Bailey v. Blue Cross/Blue Shield, 866 F. Supp. 277, 283 (E.D. Va. 1994), aff'd, 67 F.3d 53 (4th Cir. 1995). In part, the court found the ambiguity by separating the high-dose chemotherapy

part of treatment from the bone marrow rescue part. The chemotherapy was already covered by the policy, the court opined, so there must be uncertainty about whether the bone marrow rescue was also covered. Such reasoning is dramatically at odds with medical realities. Given current medical technology, high-dose chemotherapy (as distinct from standard chemotherapy) cannot be undertaken without a reinfusion of healthy bone marrow to restore the patient's ability to produce the vital blood cells that carry oxygen and fight infection. To regard the two as somehow separable is rather like regarding the sutures that close a surgical incision as separable from the surgery and potentially optional—as though the surgery is to fix the problem, while the sutures are simply to prevent potential later problems.

109. DiDomenico v. Employers Co-op. Industry Trust, 676 F.Supp. 903 (N.D. Ind. 1987); Leonhardt v. Holden Business Forms Co., 828 F. Supp. 657 (D. Minn. 1993); Nesseim v. Mail Handlers Ben. Plan, 792 F. Supp. 674, 675 (D.S.D. 1992); Pirozzi v. Blue Cross-Blue Shield of Virginia, 741 F.Supp. 586 (E.D. Va. 1990); Wilson v. Group Hospitalization , 791 F.Supp. 309 (D.D.C. 1992); Weaver v. Phoenix Home Life Mut. Ins. Co., 990 F.2d 154 (4th Cir. 1993); Calhoun v. Complete Health Care, Inc., 860 F.Supp. 1494 (S.C.Ala. 1994); Wilson v. CHAMPUS, 65 F.3d 361 (4th Cir. 1995)(applied to CHAMPUS plan rather than ERISA); Doe v. Travelers Ins. Co, 971 F.Supp. 623 (D.Mass 1997); Heasley v. Belden & Blake Corp., 2 F.3d 1249 (3rd Cir. 1993).

But see Johnson v. Dist. 2 Marine Eng. Beneficial Ass'n, 857 F.2d 514 (9th Cir. 1988); McLeroy v. Blue Cross/Blue Shield of Oregon, Inc., 825 F.Supp. 1064 (N.D. Ga. 1993); Sweeney v. Gerber Products Co. Med. Benefits Plan, 728 F.Supp. 594 (D.Neb. 1989); Thomas v. Gulf Health Plan, Inc., 688 F. Supp. 590 (S.D. Ala. 1988); Martin v. Blue Cross & Blue Shield of Va., Inc., 115 F3d 1201 (4th Cir. 1997); Turner v. Fallon Community Health Plan, Inc., 127 F.3d 196 (1st Cir. 1997); Jones v. Kodak Medical Assistance Plan, 169 F.3d 1287 (10th Cir. 1999); Healthcare America Plans, Inc. v. Bossemeyer, 953 F.Supp. 1176 (D.Kan. 1996) affd w/o opin. 166 F.3d 347; Bechtold v. Physicians Health Plan, 19 F.3d 322 (7th Cir. 1994); Martin v. Blue Cross & Blue Shield of Va., Inc., 115 F3d 1201 (4th Cir. 1997)

110. Brown v. Blue Cross & Blue Shield of Alabama, 898 F. 2d 1556, 1561–62 (11th Cir. 1990). See also Firestone Tire & Rubber Co. v. Bruch, 489 U.S. 101 (1989).

111. Morreim 1998(b). See also Firestone Tire & Rubber Co. v. Bruch, 489 U.S. 101 (1989); Brown v. Blue Cross & Blue Shield of Alabama, 898 F. 2d 1556 (11th Cir. 1990); Doe v. Group Hospitalization & Medical Services, 3 F.3d 80 (4th Cir. 1993); Pitman v. Blue Cross & Blue Shield, 24 F.3d 118 (10th Cir. 1994); Nightingale v. Blue Cross, 41 F.3d 1476 (11th Cir 1995); Bedrick v. Travelers Insur. Co., 93 F.3d 149 (4th Cir, 1996); Bucci v. Blue Cross-Blue Shield of Connecticut, 764 F. Supp. 728 (D.Conn. 1991); Wilson v. Group Hospitalization 791 F.Supp. 309 (D.D.C. 1992); Adelson v. GTE Corp., 790 F. Supp. 1265 (D.Md. 1992); Mattive v. Healthsource of Savannah, Inc., 893 F.Supp. 1559 (S.D.Ga. 1995); McKinnon v. Blue Cros-Blue Shield of Alabama, 691 F.Supp. 1314 (N.D.Ala. 1988); Lee v. Blue Cross/Blue Shield of Alabama, 10 F.3d 1547 (11th Cir. 1994); McGraw v. Prudential Ins. Co. of America, 137 F.3d 1253 (10th Cir. 1998).

Although many recent court decisions have shown very little deference to fiduciaries in a conflict of interest, the rule is far from dead. See Jones v. Kodak Medical Assistance Plan, 169 F.3d 1287 (10th Cir. 1999) (explicitly affirming a 'sliding scale' approach to evaluating a fiduciary's conflict of interest); Healthcare America Plans, Inc. v. Bossemeyer, 953 F.Supp. 1176 (D.Kan. 1996) affd w/o opin. 166 F.3d 347; Anderson v. Blue Cross/Blue Shield of Alabama, 907 F.2d 1072 (11th Cir. 1990).

112. In Hunt v. Hawthorne Associates, Inc., 119 F.3d 888 (11th Cir. 1997), the Eleventh Circuit emphasized that ERISA plan fiduciaries have duties to all the beneficiaries of that plan, not just to a complaining individual. "[T]he terms of the Plan make clear that the administrator owes an equal fiduciary duty to all Plan participants. . . . The administrator is required to treat all participants equally at all times in running the Plan." An ERISA administrator has the power to determine questions regarding the application of the plan . . . " '*provided that each Participant shall be granted the same treatment under similar conditions*' " Id., at 913, emphasis added by Hunt court.

113. "By one estimate, for every 1% increase in premiums that occurs due to mandated benefits, 400,000 Americans lose insurance coverage. Other studies peg the cost of mandated benefits at amounts ranging up to 15.5% of total premium costs." Pitsenberger, 1999, at 323.

Various studies have found that, depending on the type and size of the corporation, somewhere between 56% and 85% of the costs of health care are directly shifted back to workers through reduced wages. Another study found that, with respect to states' assorted mandates for health plans to cover various specified services, from 59% to 90% of the costs of these mandates are translated into wage reductions. Blumberg, 1999, at 58.

114. Huss v. Green Spring Health Services, Inc., 18 F.Supp.2d 400, 408 (D.Del. 1998).

See also Andrews-Clarke v. Travelers Ins. Col, 984 F.Supp. 49, 52–53 (D.Mass. 1997): "this Court had no choice but to pluck Diane Andrews-Clarke's case out of the state court in which she sought redress (and where relief to other litigants is available) and then, at the the behest of Travelers and Greenspring, to slam the courthouse doors in her face and leave her without any remedy." See also Corcoran v. United Healthcare, Inc., 965 F2d 1321, 1338 (5th Cir 1992), cert denied 113 SCt 812 (1992); Tolton v. American Biodyne, Inc., 48 F.3d 937, 943 (6th Cir. 1995); Bast v. Prudential Ins. Co. of America, 150 F.3d 1003, 1010 (9th Cir. 1998); Foster v. Blue Cross Blue Shield of Michigan, 969 F.Supp. 1020, 1024 (E.D.Mich. 1997); Jass v. Prudential Health Care Plan, Inc., 88 F.3d 1482 (7th Cir. 1996); Turner v. Fallon Community Health Plan Inc., 953 F.Supp 419, 424 (D.Mass 1997); aff'd, Turner v. Fallon Community Health Plan, Inc., 127 F.3d 196 (1st Cir. 1997); Cannon v. Group Health Serv., 77 F.3d 1270, 1'274 (10th Cir.) cert denied, 117 S. Ct. 66 (1996); Nealy v. U.S. Healthcare HMO, 844 F. Supp. 966, 974 (S.D.N.Y. 1994).

115. Massachusetts Mutual Life Ins. Co. v. Russell, 473 U.S. 134, 147 (1985) (cited with approval in Pilot Life Ins. Co. v. Dedeaux, 481 U.S. 41, 54 (1987)).

116. Mertens v. Hewitt Associates, 113 S.Ct. 2063 (1993). See also Harsch v. Eisenberg, 956 F.2d 651 (7th Cir. 1992); Novak v. Andersen Corp., 962 F.2d 757 (8th Cir. 1992).

117. Haywood v. Russell Corp., 584 So. 2d 1291, 1297 (Ala. 1991) (citing House Education and Labor Committee regarding ERISA's intent).

118. Haywood v. Russell Corp., 584 So. 2d 1291, 1297 (Ala. 1991).

119. "The majority candidly acknowledges that it is plausible to interpret the phrase 'appropriate equitable relief' . . . as meaning that relief which was available in the courts of equity for a breach of trust . . . The majority also acknowledges that the relief petitioners seek here—a compensatory monetary award—*was* available in the equity courts under the common law of trusts, not only against trustees for breach of duty but also against nonfiducaiaries knowingly participating in a breach of trust. . . . Finally, there can be no dispute that ERISA was grounded in this common-law experience and that 'we are [to be] guided by principles of trust law' in construing the terms of the statute. . . . Nevertheless, the majority today holds that in enacting ERISA Congress strippped ERISA trust beneficiaries of a remedy against trustees and third parties that they enjoyed in the equity courts under common law." Mertens v. Hewitt Associates, 113 S.Ct. 2063, 2072 (1993).

120. "Moreover, while the majority of courts adhere to the view that equity courts, even in trust cases, cannot award punitive damages, . . . a number of courts in more recent decades have drawn upon their 'legal' powers to award punitive damages even in cases that historically could have been brought only in equity. While acknowledging the traditional bar against such relief in equity, these courts have concluded that the merger of law and equity authorizes modern courts to draw upon both legal and equitable powers in crafting an appropriate remedy for a breach of trust." Mertens v. Hewitt Associates, 113 S.Ct. 2063, 2076 (1993).

The dissenters go on the cite a number of cases supporting the conclusion that the "present day Chancery Division can 'afford the full range of equitable and legal remedies for breach of trust,' including punitive damages." *Id.*, at 2076. The dissenters then conclude: "Because some forms of 'legal' relief in trust cases were thus not avilable at equity, limiting the scope of relief under § 502(a)(3) to the sort of relief historically provided by the equity courts for a breach of trust provides a meaningful limitation and, *if one is needed,* a basis for distinguishing 'equitable' from 'legal' relief. Accordingly, the statutory text does not compel the majority's rejection of the reading of 'appropriate equitable relief' advanced by petitioners and the Solicitor General—a reading that the majority acknowledges is otherwise plausible. . . ." Mertens v. Hewitt Associates, 113 S.Ct. 2063, 2077 (1993) (emphasis added)

In an earlier case, Massachusetts Mut. Life Ins. Co. v. Russell, 473 U.S. 134 (1985), four justices (Brennan, White, Marshall, Blackmun) argued in a concurring opinion that, as Congress intended to base ERISA on traditional trust law, there is good reason to think that remedies under ERISA can expand to encompass " 'such remedies as are necessary for the protection of their interests' " (at 156).

121. Reid v. Gruntal & Co., Inc., 763 F.Supp. 672 (D.Me. 1991).

122. The court continued: "The remedy for a common law claim of promissory estoppel may include both expectation damages and reliance damages, but 'reliance damages would appear to be the minimum remedy appropriate in order to avoid the injustice from lack of any enforcement at all.' . . . Reliance damages 'put the plaintiff back in the position the plaintiff would have occupied had the reliance not taken place.' " Reid v. Gruntal & Co., Inc., 763 F.Supp. 672, 678–79 (D.Me. 1991) (omitting references).

123. Russell v. Northrop Grumman Corp., 921 F.Supp. 143 (E.D.N.Y. 1996) (pension benefits case concerning employee who was fired just 7 months before his 20-year vesting in the retirement plan).

124. Russell v. Northrop Grumman Corp., 921 F.Supp. 143, 152 (E.D.N.Y. 1996).

125. Weems v. Jefferson-Pilot Life Ins. Co., Inc., 663 So.2d 905 (Ala. 1995).

126. Ingersoll-Rand concerned an employee who had been fired just four months before his pension would have been vested. The employee complained that he was fired so that the employer would not have to pay his pension benefits and requested damages for future lost wages and emotional distress in addition to punitive damages. The Court pointed out that unlawful termination in order to avoid paying pension benefits is already illegal under ERISA, so there was no need to go to state courts for enforcement of this provision. The Court then noted that, while ERISA remedies were carefully crafted, "[i]t is clear that the relief requested here is well within the power of federal courts to provide. Consequently, it is no answer to a pre-emption argument that a particular plaintiff is not seeking recovery of pension benefits." Ingersoll-Rand Co. v. McClendon, 111 S.Ct. 478, 485–86 (1990).

127. In 1997, for instance, the First Circuit noted that "the Supreme Court has stressed that ERISA does not create compensatory or punitive damage remedies where an administrator of a plan fails to provide the benefits due under that plan. . . . This is not a minor technicality: damage awards may increase effective coverage but may also add significantly to the costs of coverage. . . . [T]he Supreme Court has adamantly ruled that ERISA's express remedies are a signal to courts not to create additional remedies of their own." Turner v. Fallon Community Health Plan, Inc., 127 F.3d 196, 198 (1st Cir. 1997).

Similarly, the Seventh Circuit held that Congress excluded compensatory damages against health plans when they have wrongly denied benefits. As the court noted, permitting such a recovery would "conflict with Congress' intent that a plan not be subject to a myriad of [sic] state laws applying to employee benefit plans." Jass v. Prudential Health Care Plan, Inc., 88 F.3d 1482, 1493 (7th Cir. 1996).

The Ninth Circuit emphasized that punitive damages are not available under ERISA, even though plaintiffs may be left without alternative or adequate remedy. Bast v. Prudential Ins. Co. of America, 150 F.3d 1003, 1009 (9th Cir. 1998). And from Olson v. General Dynamics Corp., 960 F.2d 1418, 1424 (9th Cir. 1991): "the federal courts have consistently ruled that ERISA plaintiffs may not recover extracontractual damages."

128. 2000 Wash. Legis. Serv. 6199 (West) (Second Substitute Senate Bill 6199, as amended by the House; passed by Senate 3/6/200; passed by House of Representatives 3/3/2000). New section 17, "Carrier Liability" (amending chapter 41.05 RCW) provides:

"(7) (a) A person may not maintain a cause of action under this section against a health carrier unless:

(i) The affected enrollee has suffered substantial harm. As used in this subsection, 'substantial harm' means loss of life, loss or significant impairment of limb, bodily or cognitive function, significant disfigurement, or severe or chronic physical pain; and

(ii) The affected enrollee or the enrollee's representative has exercised the opportunity established in section 11 of this act to seek independent review of the health care treatment decision."

129. Jacobson, Pomfret, 1998, at 993–94.

130. Jacobson, Pomfret, 1998, at 994, 1048. For other commentators favoring a limited ERISA, see also Wethly, 1996; Pomfret, 1998; Koutoulogenis, 1998; Cerminara, 1999.

131. New York State Conference of Blue Cross v. Travelers Ins., 115 S.Ct. 1671 (1995).

132. Cerminara, 1999, at 353 (references omitted).

133. New York State Conference of Blue Cross v. Travelers Ins., 115 S.Ct. 1671, 1680 (1995). "Cost uniformity almost certainly is not an object of preemption" (at 1673).

134. New York State Conference of Blue Cross v. Travelers Ins., 115 S.Ct. 1671, 1672 (1995).

135. Parrino v. FHP, Inc., 146 F.3d 699 (9th Cir. 1998).

136. Foster v. Blue Cross Blue Shield of Michigan, 969 F.Supp. 1020, 1020 (E.D.Mich. 1997). "Congress intended ERISA to preempt at least three categories of state law that can be said to have a connection with an ERISA plan: (1) laws that mandate employee benefit structures or their administration, (2) laws that bind employers or plan administrators to particular choices or preclude uniform administrative practice, thereby functioning as a regulation of an ERISA plan itself, and (3) laws providing alternative enforcement mechanisms for employees to obtain ERISA plan benefits." Moreno v. Health Partners Health Plan, 4 F.Supp.2d 888, 891–92 (D.Ariz. 1998).

See also Corporate Health Ins. Inc. v. Texas Dept. of Ins., 12 F.Supp.2d 597, 611 (S.D.Tex. 1998), aff'd in part, rev'd in part, 215 F.3d 526 (5th Cir. 2000); Roessert v. Health Net, 929 F.Supp. 343, 351 (N.D.Cal. 1996); Pappas v. Asbel, 675 A.2d 711, 714–15 (Pa.Super. 1996); Pappas v. Asbel, 724 A.2d 889, 892 (Pa. 1998), vacated, 120 S.Ct. 2686; Shea v. Esensten, 107 F.3d 625, 627 (8th Cir. 1997); Tolton v. American Biodyne, Inc., 48 F.3d 937, 941 (6th Cir. 1995); Chaghervand v. CareFirst, 909 F.Supp 304, 310–11 (D.Md. 1995); Negron v. Patel, 6 F.Supp.2d 366, 370 (E.D.Pa.

1998); Huss v. Green Spring Health Services, Inc., 18 F.Supp.2d 400, 406 (D.Del. 1998). See also Jacobson, Pomfret, 1998.

137. "Concerned that a full one-half of all non-agricultural private employees remained without coverage of any sort of retirement plan, Congress hoped that ERISA's clear and uniformly regulated statutory scheme would encourage employers to further expand their use of employee benefit plans." Wethly, 1996, at 826.

138. Holmes v. Pacific Mut. Life Ins. Co., 706 F.Supp. 733, 735 (C.D. Cal. 1989)

139. Holmes v. Pacific Mut. Life Ins. Co., 706 F.Supp. 733, 735 (C.D. Cal. 1989).

140. Holmes v. Pacific Mut. Life Ins. Co., 706 F.Supp. 733, 735 (C.D. Cal. 1989) (emphasis added).

141. Pilot Life Ins. Co v. Dedeaux, 481 U.S. 41 (1987).

142. Pilot Life Ins. Co v. Dedeaux, 481 U.S. 41, 54 (1987) (emphasis added).

143. Varity Corp. v. Howe, 116 S.Ct. 1065, 1070 (1996) (emphasis added).

144. Frahm v. Equitable Life Assur. Soc. of U.S., 137 F.3d 955, 962 (7th Cir. 1998).

145. Gable v. Sweetheart Cup Co., Inc., 35 F.3d 851, 859–60 (4th Cir. 1994).

146. See supra n. 7.

147. Inter-modal Rail v. Atchison, Topeka & Santa Fe Ry., 117 S.Ct.1513, 1516 (1997) (emphasis added) (citing Heath v. Varity Corp., 71 F.3d 256, 258 (CA 7, 1995)).

148. New York State Conference of Blue Cross v. Travelers Ins., 115 S.Ct. 1671, 1683 (1995).

In a similar vein, dissenting judges in the Seventh Circuit's refusal to rehear Herdrich v. Pegram en banc pointed out that if employers are precluded from selecting managed care plans for their employees on the ground that they carry unpalatable conflicts of interest, then fewer employers will offer the costlier fee-for-service benefit plans. "If alternatives such as fee-for-service medicine are more expensive, then plan sponsors will be inclined to offer less medical coverage, and participants may be worse off. . . . The panel's opinion thus implies that the principal organizational forms through which medical care is delivered today are unlawful. If this conclusion is correct, then the cost-saving achieved by managed care must be abandoned, and the cost of medical care will rise perhaps substantially." Herdrich v. Pegram, 170 F.3d 683, 685, 686 (7th Cir. 1999)(dissent).

"Congress enacted ERISA to protect participants and beneficiaries of employee benefit plans by creating a statutory system that would encourage employers to offer benefit plans, establish 'standards of conduct, responsibility, and obligation for fiduciaries,' and provide plan participants and beneficiaries with 'appropriate remedies. . . . and ready access to the Federal courts.' " Bins v. Exxon Co. U.S.A., 189 F.3d 929, 933–34 (9th Cir. 1999) (citing Varity v. Howe, 516 U.S. 489, 497, 513).

"In enacting ERISA, Congress found that 'the soundness and stability of plans with respect to adequate funds to pay promised benefits may be endangered (19 U.S.C. § 1101(a) (1994)) due to a lack of uniformity in the regulations of such plans. . . . Congress's intent in engrafting section 514(a) on ERISA was to establish regulation of the *administration* of employee benefit plans as an exclusviely federal concern [citing *Travelers*]. . . . In *Travelers,* the Court noted that the purpose of section 514(a) is to ensure that benefit plans are subjected to a uniform body of law that minimizes the administrative and financial burden of complying with conflicting directives among states or between states and the federal government." Hinterlong v. Baldwin, 720 N.E.2d 315, 321–22 (Ill.App. 2 Dist. 1999).

"Purpose of ERISA is to ensure that plans and plan sponsors are subject to a uniform body of benefits law, to minimize administrative and financial burden of complying with conflicting directives among states or between states and federal govt, and to prevent potential for conflict in substantive law requiring tailoring of plans and employer conduct to peculiarities of each jurisdiction." Foster v. Blue Cross Blue Shield of Michigan, 969 F.Supp. 1020, 1020 (E.D.Mich. 1997).

149. See Chapter 10.

CHAPTER 12

1. They were Martin Luther King, Jr., Robert F. Kennedy, and George Wallace.

2. It is probably no accident that contemporary bioethics began to flower during that turbulent decade from the mid-1960s to the mid-1970s. In picking through those days' piles of upended values we can find several major candidates: research scandals proving that abuses were not limited to Nazis; incredible new life-prolonging technologies prompting physicians and society to wonder whether everything that can be done should be done; and a flurry of lawsuits demanding informed consent, rejecting traditional physician paternalism in favor of patient autonomy. In the last decade

we added an even greater impetus for contemporary bioethics: the economic upheaval that now causes such profound consternation yet also opens such important opportunities to reconsider what is important and what is dispensible in this enormous field we call health care. See Beecher, 1966; Caplan, 1992; Matter of Quinlan, 355 A.2d 647 (N.J. 1976); Salgo v. Leland Stanford Jr. University Bd. of Trust., 317 P.2d 170 (Cal. 1957); Natanson v. Kline, 350 P.2d 1093 (Kan. 1960), 354 P.2d 670 (Kan. 1960); Canterbury v. Spence, 464 F.2d 772 (D.C. 1972); Cobbs v. Grant, 502 P.2d 1 (Cal. 1972).

3. Morreim 1994(a).

4. Hume, 1973; Book III: Of Morals; Part II: Of justice and injustice; II: Of the origin of justice and property.

5. Mount Isa Mines, Ltd. v. Pusey (1970) 125 C.L.R. 383, 395.

REFERENCES

Abraham KS. The natural history of the insurer's liability for bad faith. Texas Law Review 1994; 72: 1295–1315.

Abraham KS. Judge-made law and judge-made insurance: Honoring the reasonable expectations of the insured. Virginia Law Review 1981; 67:1151–1191.

Abraham KS, Weiler PC. Enterprise medical liability and the evolution of the American health care system. Harvard Law Review 1994; 108: 381–486.

Abraham KS, Weiler PC. Enterprise medical liability and the choice of the responsible enterprise. Am J Law & Medicine 1994(b); 20: 29–36.

Abrams FR. Patient advocate or secret agent? Journal of the American Medical Association 1986; 256: 1784–1785.

Allen GL. Insurance bad faith law: the need for legislative intervention. Pacific Law Journal 1982; 13: 833–857.

Allen MC, Donohue PK, Dusman AE. The limit of viability—neonatal outcome of infants born at 22 to 25 weeks' gestation. New Engl J Med 1993; 329: 1597–1601.

Allred AD, Tottenham TO. Liability and indemnity issues for integrated delivery systems. St. Louis University LJ 1996; 40: 457–542.

American Bar Asociation. Developments in common law remedies under ERISA. American Bar Association 1991; 1–21.

American College of Physicians. The oversight of medical care: a proposal for reform. Ann Intern Med 1994; 120: 423–431.

American College of Physicians. Magnetic resonance imaging of the brain and spine: a revised statement. Ann Intern Med 1994(b); 120: 872–75.

American College of Physicians. Voluntary purchasing pools: a market model for improving access, quality, and cost in health care. Ann Intern Med 1996; 124: 845–53.

Anders G. More insurers pay for care that's in trials. Wall St J, February 15, 1994; B-1.

Anders G. Limits on second-eye cataract surgery are lifted by major actuarial firm. Wall St J December 15, 1994; B-6.

Anderson EG. Why some patients sue: learning from a plaintiffs' lawyer. Physician's Management 1995; 35(4): 39–45.

Anderson GF, Hall MA, Steinberg EP. Medical technology assessment and practice guidelines: their day in court. American Journal of Public Health 1993; 83: 1635–1639.

Anderson GF, Weller WE. Methods of reducing the financial risk of physicians under capitation. Arch Fam Med 1999; 8: 149–155.

Anderson RE. Billions for defense: the pervasive nature of defensive medicine. Arch Intern Med 1999; 159: 2399–2402.

Andreson JS. Is utilization review the practice of medicine? implications for managed care administrators. J Legal Med 1998; 19: 431–54.

Antman KH, Heitjan DF, Hortobagyi GN. High-dose chemotherapy for breast cancer. JAMA 1999; 282: 1701–1703.

Asch SM, Sloss EM, Hogan CH, et al. Measuring underuse of necessary care among elderly Medicare beneficiaries using inpatient and outpatient claims. JAMA 2000; 284: 2325–33.

Ashton CM, Petersen NJ, Souchek J, Menke TJ, Yu HJ, Pietz K, Eigenbrodt ML, Barbour G, Kizer KW, Wray NP. Geographic variations in utilization rates in Veterans Affairs hospitals and clinics. New Engl J Med 1999; 340: 32–39.

Aston G. No consensus on medical necessity. Amer Med News May 10, 1999; 28.

Avanian JZ, Landrum MB, Normand ST, Guadagnoli E, McNeil B. Rating the appropriateness of coronary angiography—do practicing physicians agree with an expert panel and with each other? New Engl J Med 1998; 338: 1896–1904.

Avorn J, Soumerai SB, Taylor W, Wessels MR, Janousek J, Weiner M. Reduction of incorrect antibiotic dosing through a structured educational order form. Arch Intern Med 1988; 148: 1720–1724.

Avorn J. Putting adverse drug events into perspective. JAMA 1997; 277: 341–42.

Avorn J, Solomon DH. Cultural and economic factors that (mis)shape antibiotic use: the nonpharmacologic basis of therapeutics. Ann Intern Med 2000; 133: 128–35.

Avorn J, Chen M, Hartley R. Scientific versus commercial sources of influence on the prescribing behavior of physicians. Am J Med 1982; 73: 4–8.

Ayres WH. Dilemmas and challenges: a clinician's perspective. J Am Acad Child Adolesc Psychiatry 1994; 33: 153–157.

Azevedo D. Taking back health care: doctors must work together. Medical Economics 1996; 73(12): 156–67.

Azevedo D. Did an HMO doctor's greed kill Joyce Ching? Medical Economics 1996(b); 73(4): 43–56.

Azevedo D. New owners drive this group to unionize. Medical Economics 1997; 74(6): 196, 199–200, 202, 204–207.

Baker SE. The nurse practitioner in malpractice actions: standard of care and theory of liability. Health Matrix 1992; 2: 325–55.

Baker T. Constructing the insurance relationship: sales stories, claims stories, and insurance contract damages. Texas Law Review 1994; 72: 1395–1433.

Balas EA, Kretschmer RAC, Gnann W, et al. Interpreting cost analyses of clinical interventions. JAMA 1998; 279: 54–57.

Balas EA, Weingarten S, Garb CT et al. Improving preventive care by prompting physicians. Arch. Intern. Med. 2000; 160: 301–8.

Barber J. Experimental treatment exclusions from medical insurance coverage: who should decide? Widener Law Symposium Journal 1996; 1(1): 389–424.

Barrett BJ, Parfrey PS, McDonald JR, Hefferton DM, Reddy ER, McManamon PJ. Nonionic low-osmolality versus ionic high-osmolality contrast material for intravenous use in patients perceived to be at high risk: randomized trial. Radiology 1992; 183:105–110.

Barrett BJ, Parfrey PS, Vavasour HM, O'Dea F, Kent G, Stone E. A comparison of nonionic, low-osmolality radiocontrast agents with ionic, high-osmolality agents during cardiac catheterization. New Engl J Med 1992; 326:431–436.

Batavia AI. Of wheelchairs and managed care. Health Affairs 1999; 18(6): 177–82.

Bates DW. Drugs and adverse drug reactions: how worried should we be? JAMA 1998; 279: 1216–17.

Bates DW, Cullen DJ, Laird N, et al. Incidence of adverse drug events and potential adverse drug events. JAMA 1995; 274: 429–34.

Bates DW, Gawande AA. Error in medicine: what have we learned? Ann Intern Med 2000; 132: 763–767.

Bates DW, Leape LL, Cullen DJ, et al. Effect of computerized physician order entry and a team intervention on prevention of serious medication errors. JAMA 1998; 280: 1311–16.

Bates DW, Spell N, Cullen, DJ. The costs of adverse drug events in hospitalized patients. JAMA 1997; 277: 307–311.

Beauchamp TL, McCullough LB. Medical Ethics: The Moral Responsibilities of Physicians. Englewood Cliffs: Prentice-Hall, 1984.

Beckman HB, Markakis KM, Suchmen AL, Frankel RM. The doctor–patient relationship and malpractice: lessons from plaintiff depositions. Arch Intern Med 1994; 154; 1365–70.

Beebe SA, Britton JR, Britton HL, Fan P, Jepson B. Neonatal mortality and length of newborn hospital stay. Pediatrics 1996; 98: 231–235.

Beecher HK. Ethics and clinical research. New Engl J Med 1966; 274:1354–1360.

Bennett JC. Inclusion of women in clinical trials—policies for population subgroups. New Engl J Med 1993; 329: 288–292.

Bercu BB. The growing conundrum: growth hormone treatment of the non-growth hormone deficient child. JAMA 1996; 276: 567–68.

Berenson RA. Beyond competition. Health Affairs 1997; 16(2): 171–80.

Bergh J. Where next with stem-cell-supported high-dose therapy for breast cancer? Lancet 2000; 355: 944–45.

Bergthold LA. Medical necessity: do we need it? Health Affairs 1995; 14(4): 180–90.

Berkowitz RL. Should every pregnant woman undergo ultrasonography? New Engl J Med 1993; 329: 874–875.

Bernard GR, Sopko G, Cerra F, Demling R, et al. Pulmonary artery catheterization and clinical outcomes: NHLBI and FDA workshop report. JAMA 2000; 283: 2568–72.

Berwick DM. Quality of health care. Part 5: payment by capitation and the quality of care. New Engl J Med 1996; 335: 1227–1231.

Berwick DM. Harvesting knowledge from improvement. JAMA 1996(b); 275: 877–878.

Berwick DM. We can cut costs and improve care at the same time. Medical Economics 1996(c); 73(15): 180, 185–187.

Bindman AB. Can physician profiles be trusted? JAMA 1999; 281: 2142–2143.

Bischoff WE, Reynolds TM, Sessler CN, et al. Handwashing compliance by health care workers: the impact of introducing an accessible, alcohol-based hand antiseptic. Arch Intern Med 2000; 160: 1017–1021.

Blanchard TP. Medicare medical necessity determinations revisited: abuse of discretion and abuse of process in the war against Medicare fraud and abuse. St. Louis University Law Journal 1999; 43(1): 91–135.

Blendon RJ, Brodie M, Benson J. What should be done now that national health system reform is dead? JAMA 1995; 273: 243–44.

Blum JD. An analysis of legal liability in health care utilization review and case management. Houston Law Review 1989; 26: 191–228.

Blumberg LJ. Who pays for employer-sponsored health insurance? Health Affairs 1999; 18(6): 58–61.

Blumenthal D. Part 6: the role of physicians in the future of quality of management. New Engl J Med 1996; 335: 1328–1331.

Blumenthal D. Health care reform at the close of the 20th century. New Engl J Med 1999; 340: 1916–20.

Blumstein JF. Rationing medical resources: a constitutional, legal, and policy analysis. In: President's Commission for the Study of Ethical Problems in Medicine and Biomedical and Behavioral Research, Securing Access to Health Care, vol. 3, 349–394; Washington D.C.: U.S. Government Printing Office, 1983.

Blumstein JF, Sloan FA. Redefining government's role in health care: is a dose of competition what the doctor should order. Vanderbilt Law Review 1981; 34: 849–926.

Bodenheimer T. Disease management—promises and pitfalls. New Engl J Med 1999; 340: 1202–05.

Bodenheimer T. The American health care system: the movement for improved quality in health care. New Engl J Med 1999(b); 340: 488–492.

Bodenheimer T, Sullivan K. How large employers are shaping the health care marketplace (first of two parts). New Engl J Med 1998; 338: 1003–7.

Bodenheimer T, Sullivan K. How large employers are shaping the health care marketplace (second of two parts). New Engl J Med 1998(b); 338: 1084–87.

Bootman JL, Harrison DL, Cox E. The health care cost of drug-related morbidity and mortality in nursing facilities. Arch Intern Med 1997; 157: 2089–96.

Borenstein DB. Does managed care permit appropriate use of psychotherapy? Psychiatric Services 1996; 47: 971–74.

Bovbjerg R. The medical malpractice standard of care: HMOs and customary practice. Duke Law Journal 1975; 1975: 1375–1414.

Bovbjerg R. Legislation on medical malpractice: further developments and a preliminary report card. University of California, Davis Law Review 1989; 22: 499–556.

Bovbjerg RR, Schumm JM. Judicial policy and quantitative research: Indiana's statute of limitations for medical practitioners. Indiana Law Review 1998; 31: 1051–1106.

Bratzler DW, Raskob GE Murray CK, Bumpus LJ, Piatt DS. Underuse of venous thromboembolism prophylaxis for general surgery patients: physician practices in the community hospital setting. Arch Intern Med 1998; 158: 1909–1912.

Bree RL, Kazerooni EA, Katz SJ. Effect of mandatory radiology consultation on inpatient imaging use. JAMA 1996; 276: 1595–98.

Brennan TA. Practice guidelines and malpractice litigation: collision or cohesion? Journal of Health Politics, Policy and Law 1991; 16(1): 67–85.

Brennan TA, Colin MS, Burstin HR. Relation between negligent adverse events and the outcomes of medical-malpractice litigation. New Engl J Med 1996; 335: 1963–1967.

Brennan TA, Leape LL, Laird NM, et al. Incidence of adverse events and negligence in hospitalized patients: results of the Harvard Medical Practice Study I. New Engl J Med 1991; 324: 370–76.

Brewbaker WS. Medical malpractice and managed care organizations: the implied warranty of quality. Law and Contemporary Problems 1997; 60: 117–157.

Broadhead WE. Misdiagnosis of depression. Archives of Family Medicine 1994; 3: 319–320.

Brody B. Ethical Issues in Drug Testing, Approval, and Pricing. New York: Oxford University Press, 1995.

Brown JL. Note, statutory immunity for volunteer physicians: a vehicle for reaffirmation of the doctor's beneficent duties—absent the rights talk. Widener Law Symposium Journal 1996; 1: 425–64.

Bungard TJ, Ghali WA, Teo KK, et al. Why do patients with atrial fibrillation not receive warfarin? Arch Intern Med 2000; 160: 41–46.

Burnum JF. Medical practice a la mode. New Engl J Med 1987; 317: 1220–1222.

Burstin HR, Lipsitz SR, Brennan TA. Socioeconomic status and risk for substandard medical care. JAMA 1992; 268: 2383–87.

Burton EC, Troxclair DA, Newman WP. Autopsy diagnoses of malignant neoplasms: how often are clinical diagnoses incorrect? JAMA 1998; 280: 1245–48.

Burton TM. An HMO checks up on its doctors' care and is disturbed itself. Wall St J July 8, 1998; A-1, A-8.

Burton TM. UnitedHealth to end ruling on treatments. Wall St J, Nov 9, 1999; A-3, A-18.

Butler SM. A tax reform strategy to deal with the uninsured. JAMA 1991; 265: 2541–44.

Butler SM, Haislmaier EF, eds. Critical Issues: A National Health System for America. Washington: The Heritage Foundation, 1989.

Butler SM, Moffit RE. The FEHBP as a model for a new Medicare program. Health Affairs 1995; 14(4): 47–61.

Cabana MD, Rand CS, Powe NR et al. Why don't physicians follow clinical practice guidelines? JAMA 1999; 282: 1458–65.

Cain HP. Moving Medicare to the FEHBP model, or how to make an elephant fly. Health Affairs 1999; 18(4): 25–39.

Califf RM, O'Connor CM. β-blocker therapy for heart failure: the evidence is in, now the work begins. JAMA 2000; 283: 1335–37.

Cantor CA. Fiduciary liability in emerging health care. DePaul Business Law Journal 1997; 9: 189–220.

Caplan AL. When evil intrudes. Hastings Center Report 1992; 22(6): 29–32.

Cerminara KL. Protecting participants in and beneficiaries of ERISA-governed managed health care plans. Univ of Memphis Law Review 1999; 29: 317–361.

Chase-Lubitz JF. The corporate practice of medicine doctrine: an anachronism in the modern health care industry. Vanderbilt Law Review 1987; 40: 445–88.

Chassin MR. Standards of care in medicine. Inquiry 1988; 25: 437–53.

Chassin MR. Is health care ready for six sigma quality? Milbank Quarterly 1998; 76(4): 565–591.

Chassin MR, et al. Does inappropriate use explain geographic variations in the use of health care services? JAMA 1987; 258: 2533–37.

Chassin MR, Brook RH, Park RE, et al. Variations in the use of medical and surgical services by the medicare population. New Engl J Med 1986; 314: 285–290.

Chassin MR, Galvin RW, National Roundtable on Health Care Quality. The urgent need to improve health care quality. JAMA 1998; 280: 1000–1005.

Cheney K. What you can learn from an M.D. mutiny in a managed-care plan. Money, December 1995; 21.

Chin MH. Health outcomes and managed care: discussing the hidden issues. Am J Managed Care 1997; 3(5): 756–762.

Chittenden WA. Malpractice liability and managed health care: history and prognosis. Tort and Insurance Law Journal 1991; 26: 451–496.

Classen DC. Clinical decision support systems to improve clinical practice and quality of care. JAMA 1998; 280: 1360–1361.

Classen DC, Pestotnik SL, Evans RS, Lloyd JF, Burke JP. Adverse drug events in hospitalized patients: excess length of stay, extra costs, and attributable mortality. JAMA 1997; 277: 301–306.

Cleary PD, Greenfield S, Mulley AG, et al. Variations in length of stay and outcomes for six medical and surgical conditions in Massachusetts and California. JAMA 1991; 266: 73–79.

Clousson JP, Butz JT. A new look for the corporate practice of medicine doctrine: *Berlin* v. *Sarah Bush Lincoln Health Care Center*. Journal of Health and Hospital Law 1996; 29(3): 174–192.

Cohen JJ. White coats should not have union labels. New Engl J Med 2000; 342: 431–34.

Coleman JL. Moral theories of torts: their scope and limits. Law and Philosophy 1982; 371–390.

Conrad RJ, Seiter PD. Health plan liability in the age of managed care. Defense Counsel Journal (Apr)1995; 62: 191–200.

Cook D, Giacomini M. The trials and tribulations of clinical practice guidelines. JAMA 1999; 281: 1950–51.

Cooter R, Freedman BJ. The fiduciary relationship: its economic character and legal consequences. New York University Law Review 1991; 66: 1045–1075.

Council on Ethical and Judicial Affairs. Recent opinions of the Council on Ethical and Judicial Affairs. JAMA 1986; 256: 2241.

Coyle JT. Psychotropic drug use in very young children. JAMA 2000: 283: 1059–60.

Crane M. When doctors are caught between dueling clinical guidelines. Medical Economics 1994; 71(15): 30–36.

Crane M. When a medical mistake becomes a media event. Medical Economics 1997; 74(11): 158–171.

Crespi GS. Good faith and bad faith in contract law: reflections on *A Cautionary Tale* and *Border Wars*. Texas Law Review 1994; 72: 1277–1290.

Crothers LS. Professional standards review and the limitation of health services: an interpretation of the effect of statutory immunity on medical malpractice liability. Boston University Law Review 1974; 54: 931–944.

Culpepper L, Sisk J. The development of practice guidelines: a case study of otitis media with effusion. In: Boyle PH, ed. Getting Doctors to Listen: Ethics and Outcomes Data in Context. Washington DC: Georgetown University Press, 1998, 77–85.

Curran, WJ, Moseley, GB. The malpractice experience of health maintenance organizations. Northwestern University Law Review 1975; 70:69–89.

Cuttler L, Silvers JB, Singh J, et al. Short stature and growth hormone therapy: a national study of physician recommendation patterns. JAMA 1996; 276: 531–37.

Dalen JE. 'Conventional' and 'unconventional' medicine. Arch Intern Med 1998; 158: 2179–81.

Daly M. Attacking defensive medicine through the utilization of practice parameters. J Legal Medicine 1995; 16: 101–132.

Daniels N, Sabin JE. Limits to health care: fair procedures, democratic deliberation, and the legitimacy problem for insurers. Philosophy Public Aff 1997; 26:303–50.

Daniels N, Sabin JE. Last chance therapies and managed care: pluralism, fair procedures, and legitimacy. Hastings Center Report 1998; 28(2): 27–41.

Danzon PM. Medical malpractice: theory, evidence, and public policy. Cambridge, Mass.: Harvard University Press, 1985.

Davis DL, Love SM. Mammographic screening. JAMA 1994; 271: 152–153.

DeBusk RF, West JA, Miller NH, Taylor CB. Chronic disease management. Arch Intern Med 1999; 159: 2739–42.

Deedwania PC. Underutilization of evidence-based therapy in heart failure. an opportunity to deal a winning hand with ace up your sleeve. Arch Intern Med 1997; 157: 2409–2412.

Delbanco TL, Meyers KC, Segal EA. Paying the physician's fee: Blue Shield and the reasonable charge. New Engl J Med 1979; 301; 1314–20.

DeMott DA. Beyond metaphor: an analysis of fiduciary obligation. Duke Law Journal 1988; 819: 879–924.

Detsky AS. Regional variation in medical care. New Engl J Med 1995; 333: 589–590.

Deyo RA. Magnetic resonance imaging of the lumbar spine: terrific test or tar baby? New Engl J Med 1994; 331: 115–16.

Deyo RA, Psaty BM, Simon G, Wagner EH, Omenn GS. The messenger under attack—intimidation of researchers by special interest groups. New Engl J Med 1997; 336: 1176–1180.

Diamond TA. The tort of bad faith breach of contract: when, if at all, should it be extended beyond insurance transactions? Marquette Law Review 1981; 64: 425–454.

Donohoe MT. Comparing generalist and specialty care: discrepancies, deficiencies, and excesses. Arch Intern Med 1998; 158: 1596–1608.

Dowell MA. The corporate practice of medicine prohibition: a dinosaur awaiting extinction. J Health and Hosp Law 1994; 27(12): 369–384.

Dowell SF, Marcy SM, Phillips WR, Gerber MA, Schwartz B. Principles of judicious use of antimicrobial agents for pediatric upper respiratory tract infections. Pediatrics 1998; 101: 163–53.

Dowell SF, Marcy SM, Phillips WR, Gerber MA, Schwartz B. Otitis media—principles of judicious use of antimicrobial agents. Pediatrics 1998(b); 101: 1650–171.

Du X. Increase in the use of breast-conserving surgery (letter). JAMA 1999; 282: 326.

Durham ML. Partnerships for research among managed care organizations. Health Affairs 1998; 17(1): 111–122.

Durieux P, Nizard R, Ravaud P, et al. A clinical decision support system for prevention of venous thromboembolism. JAMA 2000; 283: 2816–21.

Durning S, Cation L. The educational value of autopsy in a residency training program. Arch Intern Med 2000; 160: 997–999.

ECRI. High-dose chemotherapy with autologous bone marrow transplantation and/or blood cell transplantation for the treatment of metastatic breast cancer. Health Technology Assessment Information Service: Executive Briefings, February 1995, at p. 10.

Eddy DM. Variations in physician practice: the role of uncertainty. Health Affairs 1984; 3(2): 74–89.

Eddy DM. Applying cost-effectiveness analysis: the inside story. JAMA 1992; 268: 2575–2582.

Eddy DM. Broadening the responsibilities of practitioners: the team approach. JAMA 1993(a); 269: 1849–1855.

Eddy DM. Three battles to watch in the 1990s. JAMA 1993(b); 270: 520–526.

Eddy DM. Principles for making difficult decisions in difficult times. JAMA 1994; 271: 1792–98.

Eddy DM. Benefit language: criteria that will improve quality while reducing costs. JAMA 1996; 275: 650–657.

Editorial. Consumer-first health care. Wall St J, July 21, 1994; A-12.

Edmonson MB, Stoddard JJ, Owens LM. Hospital readmission with feeding-related problems after early postpartum discharge of normal newborns. JAMA 1997; 278: 299–303.

Eichhorn JH. Prevention of intraoperative anesthesia accidents and related severe injury through safety monitoring. Anesthesiology 1989; 70: 572–77.

Eichhorn JH, Cooper JB, Cullen DJ, Maier WR, Philip JH, Seeman RG. Standards for patient monitoring during anesthesia at Harvard Medical School. JAMA 1986; 256: 1017–20.

Ellis JH, Cohan RH, Sonnad SS, Cohan NS. Selective use of radiographic low-osmolality contrast media in the 1990s. Radiology 1996; 200: 297–311.

Ellman IM, Hall M. Redefining the terms of health insurance to accommodate varying consumer risk preferences. Am J Law & Med 1994; 20: 187–201.

Elson RB, Connelly DP. Computerized patient records in primary care: their role in mediating guideline-driven physician behavior change. Arch Family Medicine 1995; 4: 698–705.

Elstein AS, Christensen C, Cottrerll JJ, Polson A, Ng M. Effects of prognosis, perceived benefit, and decision style on decision making and critical care on decision making in critical care. Crit Care Med 1999; 27: 58–65.

Enthoven AC, Kronick R. A consumer-choice health plan or the 1990s: universal health insurance in a system designed to promote quality and economy (first of two parts). New Engl J Med 1989; 320: 29–37.

Enthoven AC, Singer SJ. Managed competition and California's health care economy. Health Affairs 1995; 15(1): 39–57.

Enthoven AC, Singer SJ. The managed care backlash and the task force in California. Health Affairs 1998; 17(4): 95–110.

Enthoven AC, Vorhaus CB. A vision of quality in health care delivery. Health Affairs 1997; 16(3): 44–57.

Entman SS, Glass CA, Hickson GB, Githens PB, Whetten-Goldstein K, Sloan FA. The relationship between malpractice claims history and subsequent obstetric care. JAMA 1994; 272: 1588–91.

Epstein A. Performance reports on quality—prototypes, problems, and prospects. New Engl J Med 1995; 333: 57–61.

Epstein RA. Medical malpractice: the case for contract. American Bar Foundation Research Journal 1976; 1: 87–149.

Epstein RA. Medical malpractice, imperfect information, and the contractual foundation for medical services. Law and Contemporary Problems 1986; 49: 201–212.

Epstein RA. Market and regulatory approaches to medical malpractice: the Virginia obstetrical no-fault statute. Virginia Law Review 1988; 74:1451–1474.

Epstein RA. Mortal Peril: Our Inalienable Right to Health Care? New York: Addison-Wesley Publishing Company, Inc., 1997.

Epstein RS. From outcomes research to disease management: a guide for the perplexed. Ann Intern Med 1996; 124: 832–837.

Epstein RS, Sherwood LM. From outcomes research to disease management: a guide for the perplexed. Ann Intern Med 1996; 124: 832–37.

Etheredge L, Jones SB, Lewin L. What is driving health system change? Health Affairs 1996; 15(4): 93–104.

Evans RG. Manufacturing consensus, marketing truth: guidelines for economic evaluation. Ann Int Med 1995; 123: 59–60.

Evans RS, Pestotnik SL, Classen DC, et al. A computer-assisted management program for antibiotics and other antiinfective agents. New Engl J Med 1998; 338: 232–38.

Ewigman BG, Crane JP, Frigoletto FD, LeFevre ML, Bain RP, McNellis D, Radius Study Group. Effect of prenatal ultrasound screening on perinatal outcome. New Engl J Med 1993; 329: 821–827.

Farmer A. Medical practice guidelines: lessons from the United States. British Medical Journal 1993; 397: 313–317.

Farnsworth EA. Contracts, 2nd ed. Boston: Little, Brown and Company, 1990.

Farrell MG. ERISA preemption and regulation of managed health care: the case for managed federalism. Am J Law & Med 1997; 23: 251–89.

Feinman J, Feldman M. Pedagogy and politics. Georgetown Law Journal 1985; 73: 875–89.

Feinstein AR. Clinical judgment revisited: the distraction of quantitative methods. Ann Int Med 1994; 1230: 799–805.

Feinstein AR. System, supervision, standards, and the 'epidemic' of negligent medical errors. Arch Intern Med 1997; 157: 1285–89.

Feinstein AR, Horwitz RI. Problems in the 'evidence' of 'evidence-based medicine'. Am J Med 1997; 103: 529–35.

Feldman SR, Ward TM. Psychotherapeutic injury: reshaping the implied contract as an alternative to malpractice. North Carolina Law Review 1979; 58: 64–96.

Feldstein PJ, Wickizer TM, Wheeler JRC. Private cost containment: The effects of utilization review programs on health care use and expenditures. New Engl J Med 1988; 318: 1310–1314.

Felsenthal E. When HMOs say no to health coverage, more patients are taking them to court. Wall St J, May 17, 1996; B-1, B-6.

Ferguson JH, Dubinsky M, Kirsch PJ. Court-ordered reimbursement for unproven medical technology: circumventing technology assessment. JAMA 1993; 269: 2116–2121.

Field MJ, Gray BH. Should we regulate 'utilization-management?' Health Affairs 1989; 8(4): 103–112.

Finkelstein BS, Silvers JB, Marrero U, Neuhauser D, Cuttler L. Insurance coverage, physician recommendations, and access to emerging treatments: growth hormone therapy for childhood short stature. JAMA 1998; 279: 663–68.

Fisher ES, Welch HG. Avoiding the unintended consequences of growth in medical care: how might more be worse? JAMA 1999; 281: 446–453.

Fisher ES, Welch HG, Wennberg JE. Prioritizing Oregon's hospital resources: an example based on variations in discretionary medical utilization. JAMA 1992; 267: 1925–1931.

Fisher ES, Wennberg JE, Stukel TA, Sharp MA. Hospital readmission rates for cohort of medicare beneficiaries in Boston and New Haven. New Engl J Med 1994; 331: 989–95.

Fix AD, Strickland GT, Grant J. Tick bites and Lyme disease in an endemic setting. JAMA 1998; 279: 206–210.

Flint GL, Jr. ERISA: extracontractual damages mandated for benefit claims actions. Arizona Law Review 1994; 36: 611–666.

Fortess EE, Kapp MB. Medical uncertainty, diagnostic testing, and legal liability. Law, Medicine & Health Care 1985; 13: 213–218.

Fox DM, Schaffer DC. Health policy and ERISA: interest groups and semipreemption. Journal of Health Politics, Policy and Law 1989; 14: 239–60.

Fox PD, Snyder R, Dallek G, Rice T. Should Medicare HMO benefits be standardized? Health Affairs 1999; 18(4): 40–52.

Fox R. Training for uncertainty. In: Merton M, Reader G, Kendall P, eds. The Student-Physician. Cambridge, Mass.: Harvard University Press, 1957, 207–241.

Frader J, Caniano DA. Research and innovation in surgery. In: McCullough L, Jones JW, Brody BA. Surgical Ethics. New York: Oxford Univrsity Press, 1998, 216–241.

Frances DC, Go AS, Dauterman KW, et al. Outcome following acute myocardial infarction. Arch Intern Med 1999; 159: 1429–36.

Frank RG, McGuire TG, Newhouse JP. Risk contracts in managed mental health care. Health Affairs 1995; 14(3): 50–64.

Frankel J. Medical malpractice law and health care cost containment: lessons for reformers from the clash of cultures. Yale Law Journal 1994; 103: 1297–1331.

Fraser GL, Stogsdill P, Dickens JD, Wennberg DE, Smith, RP, Prato BS. Antibiotic optimization: an evaluation of patient safety and economic outcomes. Arch Intern Med 1997; 157: 1689–94.

Freeman TB, Vawter DE, Leaverton PE, et al. Use of placebo surgery in controlled trials of a cellular-based therapy for Parkinson's disease. New Engl J Med 1999; 341: 988–992.

Freeman VG, Rathore SS, Weinfurt KP, Schulman KA, Sulmasy DP. Lying for patients: physician deception of third-party payers. Arch Intern Med 1999; 159: 2263–2270.

Freudenheim M. Five Minnesota health insurers to standardize treatments. New York Times, March 13, 2001, C-1.

Friedberg M, Saffran B, Stinson TJ, Nelson W, Bennett CL. Evaluation of conflict of interest in economic analysis of new drugs used in oncology. JAMA 1999; 282: 1453–57.

Friedman E. Capitation, integration, and managed care: lessons from early experiments. JAMA 1996; 275: 957–62.

Friedman MA, Woodcock J, Lumpkin MM, Shuren JE, Hass AE, Thompson LJ. The safety of newly approved medicines: do recent market removals mean there is a problem? JAMA 1999; 281: 1728–34.

Friedmann D. The efficient breach fallacy. J. Legal Studies 1989; 18: 1–24.

Fuchs VR. The 'rationing' of medical care. New Engl J Med 1984; 311: 1572–1573.

Furberg CD. Should dihydropyridines be used as first-line drugs in the treatment of hypertension? the con side. Arch Intern Med 1995; 155: 2157–2161.

Furrow BR. The causes of "wrongful life" suits: ruminations on the diffusion of medical technologies. Law Med & Health Care 1982; 10: 11–14.

Furrow BR. Broadcasting clinical guidelines on the internet: will physicians tune in? Am J Law & Med 1994; 25: 403–21.

Furrow BR. Managed care orgnizations and patient injury: rethinking liability. Georgia Law Review 1997; 31(2): 419–509.

Furrow BR, Greaney TL, Johnson SH, Jost TS, Schwartz RL. Health Law: Cases, Materials and Problems, 3rd ed. St. Paul: West Publishing Co., 1997.

Furrow BR, Johnson SH, Jost TS, Schwartz RL. Liability and Quality Issues in Health Care. St. Paul: West Publishing Co., 1997.

Gabel J. Ten ways HMOs have changed during the 1990s. Health Affairs 1997; 16(3): 134–45.

Garber AM. No price too high? New Engl J Med 1992; 327: 1676–1678.

Garber AM. Can technology assessment control health spending? Health Affairs 1994; 13(3): 115–26.

Garibaldi R. Computers and the quality of care—a clinician's perspective. New Engl J Med 1998; 338: 259–60.

Garnick DW, Hendricks AM, Brennan TA. Can practice guidelines reduce the number and costs of malpractice claims? JAMA 1991; 266: 2856–2860.

Garrison G. House Bill 335—managed care in Missouri. UMKC Law Rev 1998; 66: 775–807.

Gawande A. When machines become doctors, will doctors become machines? Medical Economics 1998; 75(19): 144–155.

Gawande AA, Blendon RJ, Brodie M, Beson JM, Levitt L, Hugick L. Does dissatisfaction with health plans stem from having no choices? Health Affairs 1998; 17(5): 184–94.

Gazmarian JA, Koplan JP, Cogswell ME, et al. Maternity experiences in a managed care organization. Health Affairs 1997; 16(3): 198–208.

Gellins AC, Rosenberg N, Moskowitz AJ. Capturing the unexpected benefits of medical research. New Engl J Med 1998; 339: 693–97.

Gentry C. Aetna may adopt UnitedHealth's model to give doctors more say on treatment. Wall St. J. Nov 11, 1999; B-25.

Gerber PC, Bijlefeld M. Watch out for these malpractice hot spots. Physician's Management 1996; 36(5): 37–50.

Gerbert B, Maurer T, Berger T, et al. Primary care physicians as gatekeepers in managed care: primary care physicians' and dermatologists' skills at secondary prevention of skin cancer. Arch Dermatol 1996; 132: 1030–38.

Gergen M. A cautionary tale about contractual good faith in Texas. Texas Law Review 1994; 72: 1235–75.

Gifford DR, Holloway RG, Frankel MR, Albright CL, Meyerson R, Griggs RC, et al. Improving adherence to dementia guidelines through education and opinion leaders: a randomized, controlled trial. Ann Intern Med 1999; 131: 237–46.

Gifford F. Outcomes research and practice guidelines: upstream issues for downstream users. Hastings Center Report 1996; 26(2): 38–44.

Gilmore G. The Death of Contract. Columbus: Ohio State University Press, 1974.

Ginzberg E. A hard look at cost containment. New Engl J Med 1987; 316: 1151–1154.

Giordani LC. A cost containment malpractice defense: implications for the standard of care and for indigent patients. Houston Law Review 1989; 26: 1007–1032.

Glassman PA, Jacobson PD, Asch S. Medical necessity and defined coverage benefits in the Oregon health plan. American Journal of Public Health 1997; 87:1053–1058.

Glassman PA, Model KE, Kahan JP, Jacobson PD, Peabody JW. The role of medical necessity and cost-effectiveness in making medical decisions. Ann Intern Med 1997;126: 152–56.

Glazer WM. Psychiatry and medical necessity. Psychiatric Annals 1992; 22: 362–366.

Glazier AK. Genetic predispositions, prophylactic treatments and private health insurance: nothing is better than a good pair of genes. Am J Law & Med 1997; 23: 45–68.

Gleason SC. Health system deregulation: some aspects of health care system reform need not be held hostage. JAMA 1995; 274: 1483–86.

Gold HS, Moellering RC. Antimicrobial-drug resistance. New Engl J Med 1996; 335: 1445–53.

Gold MR, Hurley R, Lake T, Ensor T, Berenson R. A national survey of the arrangements managed-care plans make with physicians. New Engl J Med 1995; 333: 1678–83.

Goldfarb S. Physicians in control of the capitated dollar: do unto others. Ann Intern Med 1995; 123: 546–47.

Goldsmith JC. The illusive logic of integration. Healthcare Forum Journal 1994; 37(5): 26–31.

Goldsmith MF. Anesthesiology led in establishing standards of care, now plans practice parameter strategies. JAMA 1992; 267: 1575–1576.

Goldzweig CL, Mittman BS, Carter GM et al. Variations in cataract extraction rates in Medicare prepaid and fee-for-service settings. JAMA 1997; 277: 1765–68.

Gonzales R, Steiner JF, Lum A, Barrett PH. Decreasing antibiotic use in ambulatory practice. JAMA 1999; 281: 1512–19.

Gonzoles R, Steiner JF, Sande MA. Antibiotic prescribing for adults with colds, upper respiratory tract infections, and bronchitis by ambulatory care physicians. JAMA 1997; 278: 901–904.

Goodman JC, Musgrave GL. Patient Power. Washington, DC: Cato Institute, 1992.

Goodwin JS, Goodwin JM. The tomato effect: rejection of highly efficacious therapies. JAMA 1984; 251: 2387–2390.

Gorovitz S, Macintyre A. Toward a theory of medical fallibility. Hastings Center Report 1975; 5(6): 13–23.

Gosfield AG. Clinical practice guidelines and the law: applications and implications. In: CB Callaghan, ed. Health Law Handbook, 1994 ed. Deerfield Ill.: Thomson Legal Publishing, Inc., 59–95 (reprinted in, and with pagination of, NHLA's Legal Issues Related to Clinical Practice Guidelines).

Gosfield AG. The legal subtext of the managed care environment: a practitioner's perspective. Jour Law Med & Ethics 1995; 23: 230–35.

Gottlieb M. The managed care cure-all shows its flaws and potential. New York Times, October 1, 1995, A-1, A-16.

Gottsegen SW. A new approach for the interpretation of insurance contracts—*Great American Insurance Co.* v. *Tate Construction Co.* Wake Forest Law Review 1981; 17: 140–152.

Gotzsche PC, Olsen O. Is screening for breast cancer with mammography justifiable? Lancet 2000; 355: 129–34.

Gradishar WJ. High-dose chemotherapy and breast cancer. JAMA 1999; 282: 1378–80.

Grandinetti DA. What it takes for big groups to succeed. Medical Economics 1997; 74(7): 87–98.

Green JA. Minimizing malpractice risks by role clarification: the confusing transition from tort to contract. Ann Intern Med 1988; 109: 234–241.

Greenfield S, Nelson EC, Subkoff M, et al. Variations in resource utilization among medical specialties and systems of care: results from the medical outcomes study. JAMA 1992; 267: 1624–1630.

Grimes DA. Technology follies: the uncritical acceptance of medical innovation. JAMA 1993; 269: 3030–3033.

Grimshaw JM, Russell IT. Effect of clinical guidelines on medical practice: a systematic review of rigorous evaluations. Lancet 1993; 342: 1317–1322.

Gronfein WP, Kinney ED. Controlling large malpractice claims: the unexpected impact of damage caps. Journal of Health Politics, Policy and Law 1991; 16(3): 441–464.

Grumet GW. Health care rationing through inconvenience: the third party's secret weapon. New Engl J Med 1989; 321: 607–611.

Guadagnoli E, Hauptman PJ, Avanian JZ, Pashos CL, McNeil BJ, Cleary PD. Variation in the use of cardiac procedures after acute myocardial infarction. New Engl J Med 1995; 333: 573–578.

GUSTO Investigators. An international randomized trial comparing four thrombolytic strategies for acute myocardial infarction. New Engl J Med 1993(a); 329: 673–682.

GUSTO Investigators. The effects of tissue-plasminogen activator, streptokinase, or both on coronary-artery patency, ventricular function, and survival after acute myocardial infarction. New Engl J Med 1993(b); 329: 1615–1622.

Hadorn DC. Response to Callahan. In: Hadorn DC, ed. Basic Benefits and Clinical Guidelines. Boulder: Westview Press, 1992; 48–49.

Hadorn DC. Necessary-care guidelines. In: Hadorn DC, ed. Basic Benefits and Clinical Guidelines. Boulder: Westview Press, 1992(b); 13–29.

Hafferty FW, Light DW. Professional dynamics and the changing nature of medical work. Journal of Health and Social Behavior 1995 (extra issue): 132–153.

Hall JB. Use of the pulmonary artery catheter in critically ill patients: was invention the mother of necessity? JAMA 2000; 283: 2577–78.

Hall MA. Institutional control of physician behavior: legal barriers to health care cost containment. Univ of Pennsylvania Law Review 1988; 137: 431–536.

Hall MA. The malpractice standard under health care cost containment. Law Medicine & Health Care 1989; 17: 347–355.

Hall MA. The ethics of health care rationing. Public Affairs Quarterly 1994; 8(1): 33–50.

Hall MA. Rationing health care at the bedside. New York University Law Review 1994(b); 69(4–5): 693–780.

Hall MA. A theory of economic informed consent. Georgia Law Review 1997(a); 31(2): 511–586.

Hall MA. Making Medical Spending Decisions. New York: Oxford University Press, 1997(b).

Hall MA, Anderson GF. Health insurers' assessment of medical necessity. University of Pennsylvania Law Review 1992; 140: 1637–1712.

Hall MA, Smith TR, Naughton M, Ebbers A. Judicial protection of managed care consumers: an empirical study of insurance coverage disputes. Seton Hall Law Review 1996; 26: 1055–68.

Hamm CW, Reimers J, Ischinger T, Rupprecht HJ, Berger J, Bliefeld W. A randomized study of coronary angioplasty compared with bypass surgery in patients with symptomatic multivessel coronary disease. New Engl J Med 1994; 331: 1037–1043.

Hanson MJ, Callahan D. The Goals of Medicine: The Forgotten Issues in Health Care. Washington, D.C.: Georgetown University Press, 1998.

Hardison JE. To be complete. New Engl J Med 1979; 300: 193.

Hardwig J. Robin Hoods and good samaritans: the role of patients in health care distribution. Theoretical Medicine 1987; 8: 47–59.

Harper FV, James F. Accidents, fault and social insurance. In: Morris H, ed. Freedom and Responsibility. Stanford: Stanford Univ. Press, 1961, 267–73.

Harris JM, Jr. Disease management: new wine in new bottles? Ann Intern Med 1996; 124: 838–842.

Hartert TV, Windom HH, Peebles S, Jr., Freidhoff LR, Togias A. Inadequate outpatient medical therapy for patient with asthma admitted to two urban hospitals. Am J Med 1996; 100: 386–394.

Havighurst CC. Doctors and hospitals: an antitrust perspective on traditional relationships. Duke Law Journal 1984; 1984: 1071–1162.

Havighurst CC. Private reform of tort-law dogma: market opportunities and legal obstacles. Law and Contemporary Problems 1986; 49: 143–172.

Havighurst CC. Altering the applicable standard of care. Law and Contemporary Problems 1986(b); 49: 265–275.

Havighurst CC. Practice guidelines for medical care: the policy rationale. St. Louis University Law Journal 1990; 34: 777–819.

Havighurst CC. Practice guidelines as legal standards governing physician liability. Law & Contemporary Problems 1991; 54: 87–117.

Havighurst CC. Prospective self-denial: can consumers contract today to accept health care rationing tomorrow? University of Pennsylvania Law Review 1992; 140: 1755–180.

Havighurst CC. Legal and political considerations II. In: Hadorn DC, ed. Basic Benefits and Clinical Guidelines. Boulder: Westview Press, 1992(b); 119–127.

Havighurst CC. Health Care Choices: Private Contracts as Instruments of Health Reform. Washington, D.C.: The AEI Press, 1995.

Havighurst CC. Making health plans accountable for the quality of care. Georgia Law Review 1997; 31(2): 587–647.

Havighurst CC. Vicarious liability: relocating responsibility for the quality of medical care. Am J Law & Med 2000; 26: 7–29.

Havighurst CC, Blumstein JF, Brennan TA. Health Care Law and Policy, 2nd ed. New York: Foundation Press, 1998.

Havranek DP, Graham GW, Pan Z, Lowes B. Process and outcome of outpatient management of heart failure: a comparison of cardiologists and primary care providers. Am J Managed Care 1996; 2(Supp.): S6–S12.

Hayward LR. Revising Washington's corporate practice of medicine doctrine. Washington Law Rev 1996; 71: 403–30.

Hayward RSA, Wilson MC, Tunis SR, Bass EB, Guyatt G. Users' guides to the medical literature: VIII. how to use clinical practice guidelines: A. are the recommendations valid? JAMA 1995; 274: 570–74.

Helvestine WA. Legal implications of utilization review. In: Gray BH, Fields MJ, eds. Controlling Costs and Changing Patient Care? The Role of Utilization Review. Washington, DC: National Academy Press, 1989, 169–204.

Henderson JA, Siliciano JA. Universal health care and the continued reliance on custom in determining medical malpractice. Cornell Law Review 1994; 79: 1382–1404.

Henning JM. The role of clinical practice guidelines in disease management. American Journal of Managed Care 1998; 4(12): 1715–1722.

Hershey. Fourth-party audit organizations: practical and legal considerations, Law Med, & Health Care 1986; 14: 54–65.

Hibbard JH, Jewett JJ, Legnini MW, Tusler M. Choosing a health plan: do large empoyers use the data? Health Affairs 1997; 16(6): 172–80.

Hickson GB, Clayton EW, Entman SS, Miller CS, Githens PB, Whetten-Goldstein K, Sloan FA. Obstetricians' prior malpractice experience and patients' satisfaction with care. JAMA 1994; 272: 1583–87.

Hickson GB, Clayton EW, Githens PB, Sloan FA. Factors that prompted families to file medical malpractice claims following perinatal injuries. J Am Med Assn 1992; 267: 1359–1363.

Hillman AL. Managing the physician: rules versus incentives. Health Affairs 1991; 10(4): 138–146.

Hillman AL, Eisenberg JM, Pauly MV, Bloom BS, Glick H, Kinosian B, Schwartz JS. Avoiding bias in the conduct and reporting of cost-effectiveness research sponsored by pharmaceutical companies. New Engl J Med 1991; 324: 1362–65.

Hirshfeld EB. Should ethical and legal standards for physicians be changed to accommodate new models for rationing health care? University of Pennsylvania Law Review 1992; 140: 1809–1846.

Hirshfeld EB. The case for physician direction in health plans. Annals of Health Law 1994; 3: 81–102.

Hirshfeld EB. Physicians, unions, and antitrust. Journal of Health Law 1999; 32(1): 43–73.

Hirshfeld EB, Harris GH. Medical necessity determinations: the need for a new legal structure. Health Matrix 1996; 6(3): 3–52.

Hirshfeld JW. Low-osmolality contrast agents—who needs them? New Engl J Med 1992; 326:482–484.

Hlatky MA. Patient preferences and clinical guidelines. JAMA 1995; 273: 1219–20.

Hofer TP, Hayward RA, Greenfield S, et al. The unreliability of individual physician 'report cards' for assessing the costs and quality of care of a chronic disease. JAMA 1999; 281: 2098–2105.

Hoffman S. A proposal for federal legislation to address health insurance coverage for experimental and investigational treatments. Oregon Law Review 1999; 78(1): 203–274.

Holder AR. Medical Malpractice Law, 2d. ed. New York: John Wiley & Sons, 1978.

Holder AR. Medical insurance payments and patients involved in research. IRB 1994; 16 (1–2): 19–22.

Holoweiko M. When an insurer calls your treatment experimental. Medical Economics 1995; 72(17): 171–182.

Horn SD, Sharkey PD, Phillips-Harris C. Formulary limitations and the elderly: results from the managed care outcomes project. Am J Managed Care 1998; 4: 1105–13.

Horn SD, Sharkey PD, Tracy DM, Horn CE, James B, Goodwin F. Intended and unintended consequences of HMO cost-containment strategies: results from the managed care outcomes project. Am J Managed Care 1996; 2: 253–264.

Hornbein TF. The setting of standards of care. JAMA 1986; 256: 1040–1041.

Hornberger J. Wrone E. When to base clinical policies on observational versus randomized trial data. Ann Intern Med 1997; 127: 697–703.

Horton R. After Bezwoda. Lancet 2000; 355: 942–43.

Horwitz J, Brennan TA. No-fault compensation for medical injury: a case study. Health Affairs 1995; 14(4): 164–179.

Huber P. Liability: The Legal Revolution and Its Consequences. New York: Basic Books, 1988.

Hueston WJ. Antibiotics: neither cost effective nor "cough" effective. J Fam Pract 1997; 44: 261–65.

Hume D. A Treatise of Human Nature. Selby-Bigge, ed. Oxford: Clarendon Press, 1973.

Hunt DL, Haynes RB, Hanna SE, Smith K. Effects of computer-based clinical decision support systems on physician performance and patient outcomes: a systematic review. JAMA 1998; 280: 1339–1346.

Hunt DL, Jaeschke R, McKibbon KA, et al. Using electronic health information resources in evidence-based practice. JAMA 2000; 283: 1875–79.

Huycke LI, Huycke MM. Characteristics of potential plaintiffs in malpractice litigation. Ann Int Med 1994; 120: 792–98.

Hyams AL, Shapiro DW, Brennan TA. Medical practice guidelines in malpractice litigation: an early retrospective. Journal of Health Politics, Policy and Law 1996; 21(2): 289–313.

Iezzoni LI. Assessing quality using administrative data. Ann Intern Med 1997; 127: 666–674.

Iglehart JK. The American health care system: managed care. New Engl J Med 1992; 326: 742–747.

Iglehart JK. Medicaid and managed care. New Engl J Med 1995; 332: 1727–1731.

Institute of Medicine, Committee on Utilization Management by Third Parties, Gray BH, Field MJ, eds. Controlling Costs and Changing Patient Care? The Role of Utilization Management. Washington, D.C.: National Academy Press, 1989.

Institute of Medicine To Err Is Human. Washington, D.C.: National Academy Press, 1999.

Jacobson PD, Cahill MT. Applying fiduciary responsibilities in the managed care context. Am J Law & Med 2000; 26: 155–173.

Jacobson P, Kanna M. Cost-effectiveness analysis in the courts: recent trends and future prospects. Journal of Health Policy, Politics, & Law 2001; 26: 291–325.

Jacobson PD, Pomfret SD. Form, function, and managed care torts: achieving fairness and equity in ERISA jurisprudence. Houston Law Review 1998; 35: 985–1078.

Jacobson PD, Rosenquist CJ. The introduction of low-osmolar contrast agents in radiology. JAMA 1988; 260: 1586–1592.

James F. The experimental treatment exclusion clause: a tool for silent rationing? Journal of Legal Medicine 1991; 12: 359–418.

James FE. Blue Cross plans coverage limits on many tests. Wall St J, Apr. 1, 1987; 31, col.2.

Jeffrey N. Corrective or cosmetic? plastic surgery stirs a debate. Wall St J, June 25, 1998; B-1, B-15.

Jensen MC, Brant-Zawadzki MN, Obuchowski N, Modic MT, Malkasian D, Ross JS. Magnetic resonance imaging of the lumbar spine in people without back pain. New Engl J Med 1994; 331: 69–73.

Jerry RH. Remedying insurers' bad faith contract performance: a reassessment. University of Connecticut Law Review 1986; 18: 271–321.

Jerry RH. The wrong side of the mountain: a comment on bad faith's unnatural history. Texas Law Review 1994; 72: 1317–44.

Jerry RH. Understanding Insurance Law, 2nd ed. New York: Matthew Bender, 1996.

Johnson JK, Jr. An evaluation of changes in the medical standard of care. Vanderbilt Law Review 1970; 23: 729–53.

Johnson WG, Brennan TA, Newhouse JP, Leape LL, Lawthers AG, Hiatt HH, Weiler PC. The economic consequences of medical injuries: implications for a no-fault insurance plan. JAMA 1992; 267: 2486–2492.

Jonsen AR, Siegler M, Winslade WJ. Clinical Ethics, 3rd ed. New York: McGraw-Hill, 1992.

Joshi N, Milfred D. The use and misuse of new antibiotics. Arch Intern Med 1995; 155: 569–577.

Kahn CN. The AHCPR after the battles. Health Affairs 1998; 17(1): 109–10.

Kahn KL. Above all "do no harm": how shall we avoid errors in medicine? JAMA 1995; 274: 75–76.

Kalb PE. Controlling health care costs by controlling technology: a private contractual approach. Yale Law Journal 1990; 99: 1109–1126.

Kam K. Why doctors get sued. Hippocrates 1995; 9(10): 42–53.

Kapp M. Legal and ethical implications of health care reimbursement by diagnosis related groups. Law, Medicine & Health Care 1984; 12: 245–253.

Kapur K, Joyce GF, van Vorst KA, Escarce JJ. Expenditures for physician services under alternative models of managed care. Medical Care Research and Review 2000; 57: 161–181.

Kassirer J. The use and abuse of practice profiles. New Engl J Med 1994; 330: 634–636.

Kassirer J. Managed care and the morality of the marketplace. New Engl J Med 1995; 333: 50–52.

Kassirer JP, Angell M. The *Journal's* policy on cost-effectiveness analyses. New Engl J Med 1994; 331: 669–70.

Katz J. The Silent World of Doctor and Patient. New York: The Free Press, 1984.

Katzman GL, Dagher AP, Patronas NJ. Incidental findings on brain magnetic resonance imaging from 1000 asymptomatic volunteers. JAMA 1999; 282: 36–39.

Keeton RE, O'Connell J. Why shift loss? In: Feinberg J, Gross H, eds. Philosophy of Law. Encino, Calif.: Dickenson Publishing Company, 1975, 389–92.

Keeton W, Dobbs D, Keeton R, Owen D. Prosser and Keeton on Torts, 5th ed. St. Paul: West Publishing Co., 1984.

Keister LW. With health costs finally moderating, employers' focus turns to quality. Managed Care 1995; 4(10): 20–24.

Kenagy JW, Berwick DM, Shore MF. Service quality in health care. JAMA 1999; 281: 661–65.

Kerlikowske K, Grady D, Rubin SM, Sandrock C, Ernster VL. Efficacy of screening mammography. JAMA 1995; 273: 149–154.

Kerlikowske K, Salzmann P, Phillips KA, Cauley JA, Cummings SR. Continuing screening mammography in women aged 70 to 79 years: impact on life expectancy and cost-effectiveness. JAMA 1999; 282: 2156–63.

Kerr EA, Mittman BS, Hays RD, Siu AL, Leake, B, Brook RH. Managed care and capitation in California: how do physicians at financial risk control their own utilization? Ann Int Med 1995; 123: 500–504.

Kessler DA, Rose JL, Temple RJ, Schapiro R, Griffin JP. Therapeutic-class wars—drug promotion in a competitive marketplace. New Engl J Med 1994; 331: 1350–53.

Kessler DP, McClellan M. Do doctors practice defensive medicine? American Journal of Economics 1996; 111: 353–390.

King JH Jr. In search of a standard of care for the medical profession: the "accepted practice" formula. Vanderbilt Law Review 1975; 28: 1214–76.

King JH. The Law of Medical Malpractice, 2d ed. St. Paul: West Publishing Co., 1986.

King JY. No fault compensation for medical injuries. J Contemporary Health Law & Policy 1992; 8: 227–236.

King RT, Jr. In marketing of drugs, Genentech tests limits of what is acceptable. Wall St J, January 10, 1995; A-1, A-4.

King SB, Lembo NJ, Weintraub WS, et al. A randomized trial comparing coronary angioplasty with coronary bypass surgery. New Engl J Med 1994; 331: 1044–50.

Kinney ED, Gronfein WP. Indiana's malpractice system: no-fault by accident? Law and Contemporary Problems 1991; 54 (1): 169–193.

Kirsner RS, Federman DB. Lack of correlation between internists' ability in dermatology and their patterns of treating patients with skin disease. Arch Dermatol 1996; 132: 1043–46.

Kleinman LC, Boyd EA, Heritage JC. Adherence to prescribed explicit criteria during utilization review: an analysis of communications between attending and reviewing physicians. JAMA 1997; 278: 497–501.

Kleinman LC, Kosecoff J, Dubois RW, Brook RH. The medical appropriateness of tympanostomy tubes proposed for children younger than 16 years in the United States. JAMA 1994; 271: 1250–1255.

Kletke PR, Emmons DW, Gillis KD. Current trends in physicians' practice arrangements. JAMA 1996; 276: 555–560.

Knotterus W. California negotiated health care: implications for malpractice liability. San Diego Law Review 1984; 21: 455–76.

Kohn LT, Corrigan JM, Donaldson MS, eds. To Err Is Human: Building a Safer Health System. Washington, DC: National Academy Press, 1999.

Kolata G. Women rejecting trials for testing a cancer therapy. New York Times, Feb. 15, 1995, C8.

Kolata G, Eichenwald K. Hope for sale: business thrives on unproven care, leaving science behind. New York Times, October 3, 1999, A-1, column 2.

Kong SX, Wertheimer AI. Outcomes research: collaboration among academic researchers, managed care organizations, and pharmaceutical manufacturers. Am J Managed Care 1998; 4: 28–34.

Kornblum GO. The current state of bad faith and punitive damage litigation in the U.S. Tort and Insurance Law Journal 1988; 23: 812–841.

Korobkin R. The efficiency of managed care "patient protection" laws: incomplete contracts, bounded rationality, and market failure. Cornell Law Review 1999; 85: 1–88.

Koutoulogenis A. The invisible man: a call to empower individual participants and beneficiaries against fiduciary breaches in ERISA plans. John Marshall Law Review 1998; 31: 553–582.

Krimsky S. Conflict of interest and cost-effectiveness analysis. JAMA 1999; 282: 1474–75.

Krumholz HM, Murillo JE, Chen J, et al. Thrombolytic therapy for eligible elderly patients with acute myocardial infarction. JAMA 1997; 277: 1683–88.

Kuczewski MG, DeVita M. Managed care and end-of-life decisions. Arch Intern Med 1998; 158: 2424–2428.

Kuszler, PC. Telemedicine and integrated health care delivery: compounding medical liability. Am J Law & Med. 1999; 25: 297–326.

Kuttner R. The American health care system: employer-sponsored health coverage. New Engl J Med 1999; 340: 248–52.

Laffel G, Berwick DM. Quality in health care. JAMA 1992; 268: 407–409.

Landon BE, Wilson IB, Cleary PD. A conceptual model of the effects of health care organizations on the quality of medical care. JAMA 1998; 279: 1377–82.

Lane DA, Kauls LS, Ickovics JR, Naftolin F, Feinstein AR, Early postpartum discharges: impact on distress and outpatient problems. Arch Fam Med 1999; 8: 237–242.

Lange RA, Hillis LD. Use and overuse of angiography and revascularization for acute coronary syndromes. New Engl J Med 1998; 338: 1838–39.

Larson E. The soul of an HMO. Time 1996; 147(4): 44–52.

Lave JR, Peele PB, Black JE, Evans JH, Amersbach G. Changing the employer-sponsored health plan system: the views of employees in large firms. Health Affairs 1999; 18(4): 112–117.

Law SA. Health care in Hawai'i: an agenda for research and reform. Am J Law & Med 2000; 26: 205–233.

Lawthers AG, Localio AR, Laird NM, Lipsitz S, Hebert L, Brennan TA. Physicians' perceptions of the risk of being sued. J Health Politics, Policy and Law 1992; 17(3): 463–482.

Lazarou J, Pomeranz BH, Corey PN. Incidence of adverse drug reactions in hospitalized patients. JAMA 1998: 279: 1200–05.

Leahy RE. Rational health policy and the legal standard of care: a call for judicial deference to medical practice guidelines. California Law Review 1989; 77: 1483–1528.

Leape LL. Error in medicine. JAMA 1994; 272: 1851–57.

Leape LL. Translating medical science into medical practice: do we need a national medical standards board? JAMA 1995; 273: 1534–37.

Leape LL, Bates DW, Cullen DJ, et al. Systems analysis of adverse drug events. JAMA 1995; 274: 435–43.

Leape LL, Brennan, Laird NM, et al. The nature of adverse events in hospitalized patients: results of the Harvard Medical Practice Study II. New Engl J Med 1991; 324: 377–384.

Leape LL, Cullen DJ, Clapp MD, Burdick E, Demonaco HJ, Erickson JI, Bates DW. Pharmacist participation on physician rounds and adverse drug events in the intensive care unit. JAMA 1999; 282: 267–270.

Leape LL, Park RE, Solomon DH, Chassin MR, Kosecoff J, Brook RH. Relation between surgeons' practice volumes and geographic variation in the rate of carotid endarterectomy. New Engl J Med 1989; 321: 653–657.

Leape LL, Park RE, Solomon DH, Chassin MR, Kosecoff J, Brook RH. Does inappropriate use explain small-area variations in the use of health care services? JAMA 1990; 263: 669–672.

Leape LL, Woods DD, Hatlie MJ et al. Promoting patient safety by preventing medical error. JAMA 1998; 280: 1444–47.

Lederle FA, Applegate WA, Grimm RH, Jr. Reserpine and the medical marketplace. Arch Intern Med 1993; 153: 705–706.

Lee KL, Califf RM, Simes J, Van de Weft F, Topol EJ. Holding GUSTO up to the light. Ann Intern Med 1994; 120: 876–881.

Lee KL, Clapp-Channing NE, Sutherland W, Pilote L, Armstrong PW. Use of medical resources and quality of life after acute myocardial infarction in Canada and the United States. New Engl J Med 1994; 331: 1130–1135.

Legorreta AP, Christian-Herman J, O'Connor RD, et al. Compliance with national asthma management guidelines and specialty care. Arch Intern Med 1998; 158: 457–464.

Leibenluft RF. Attempts to "level the playing field"—developments in HMO merger, enforcement, antitrust exemptions, and physician unions. AHLA Health Law Digest Aug. 1999; 27(8): 3–15.

Leider HL. Influencing physicians: the three critical elements of a successful strategy. Am J Managed Care 1998; 4: 583–88.

Lesar TS, Briceland L, Stein DS. Factors related to errors in medication prescribing. JAMA 1997; 277: 312–17.

Lesar TS, Lomaestro BM, Pohl H. Medication-prescribing errors in a teaching hospital. Arch Intern Med 1997; 157: 1569–76.

Levinson W. Physician–patient communication: a key to malpractice prevention. JAMA 1994; 272: 1619–20.

Levinson W, Roter DL, Mullooly JP, Dull VT, Frankel RM. Physician–patient communication: the relationship with malpractice claims among primary care physicians and surgeons. JAMA 1997; 277: 553–59.

Leviton LC, Goldenberg RL, Baker C et al. Methods to encourage the use of antenatal corticosteroid therapy for fetal maturation. JAMA 1999; 281: 46–52.

Lewin JC, Sybinsky PA. Hawaii's employer mandate and its contribution to universal access. JAMA 1993; 269: 2538–2543.

Lewis LM, Lasater LC, Ruoff B. Failure of a chest pain clinical policy to modify physician evaluation and management. Ann Emerg Med 1995; 25: 9–14.

Light DW. Is competition bad? New Engl J Med 1983; 309: 1315–1319.

Light DW. The practice and ethics of risk-rated health insurance. JAMA 1992; 267: 2503–2508.

Light DW. Life, death and the insurance companies. New Engl J Med 1994; 330: 498–500.

Lindfors KK, Rosenquist J. The cost-effectiveness of mammographic screening strategies. JAMA 1995; 274: 881–884.

Liner RS. Physician deselection: the dynamics of a new threat to the physician–patient relationship. Am J Law & Med 1997; 23: 511–37.

Lippman ME. High-dose chemotherapy plus autologous bone marrow transplantation for metastatic breast cancer. New Engl J Med 2000; 342: 1119–1120.

Lipson DJ, De Sa JM. Impact of purchasing strategies on local health care systems. Health Affairs 1996; 15(2): 62–76.

Liu LL, Clemens CJ, Shay DK, Davis RL, Novack AH. The safety of newborn early discharge: the Washington state experience. JAMA 1997; 278: 293–298.

Lober CW. Dermatology: positioned for health care reform. Arch Dematol 1996; 132: 1065–1067.

Localio AR, Lawthers AG, Brennan TA, et al. Relation between malpractice claims and adverse events due to negligence: results of the Harvard Medical Practice Study III. New Engl J Med 1991; 325: 245–51.

Long SH, Marquis MS. Pooled purchasing: who are the players? Health Affairs 1999; 18(4): 105–111.

Louderback CM. Standards for limiting the tort of bad faith breach of contract. University of San Francisco Law Review. 1982; 16: 187–227.

Lowes R. Straightforward UR—or a "machine of denial"? Medical Economics 2000; 77(9): 180–206.

Lowes RL. These doctors pay their dues—to a union. Medical Economics 1998; 75(2): 157–158, 161–162.

Luft HS. Modifying managed competition to address cost and quality. Health Affairs 1995; 15(1): 23–38.

Lundberg GD. Low-tech autopsies in the era of high-tech medicine. JAMA 1998; 280: 1273–74.

Macklin R. The ethical problems with sham surgery in clinical research. New Engl J Med 1999; 341: 992–996.

Macneil IR. The New Social Contract: An Inquiry into Modern Contractual Relations. New Haven: Yale University Press, 1980.

Mangan D. Will doctor unions finally take hold? Medical Economics 1995; 72(14): 115–120.

Mangione S, Nieman LZ. Cardiac auscultatory skills of internal medicine and family practice trainees: a comparison of diagnostic proficiency. JAMA 1997; 278: 717–22.

Mann ME. Physicians and surgeons—standard of care—medical specialist may be found negligent as a matter of law despite compliance with the customary practice of the specialty. Vanderbilt Law Review 1975; 28: 441–51.

Marcus SA. Trade unionism for doctors: an ideal whose time has come. New Engl J Med 1984; 311: 1508–1511.

Mariner WK. Patients' rights after health care reform: who decides what is medically necessary? American Journal of Public Health 1994; 84: 1515–20.

Mariner WK. Business vs. medical ethics: conflicting standards for managed care. Journal of Law, Medicine & Ethics 1995; 23: 236–246.

Mark DB, Naylor CD, Phil D, Hlatky MA, Califf RM, Topol EJ, Granger CB, Knight D, Nelson CL, Marrie TH, Lau CY, Wheeler SL, et al. A controlled trial of a critical pathway for treatment of community-acquired pneumonia. JAMA 2000; 283: 749–55.

Mars S. The corporate practice of medicine: a call for action. Health Matrix 1997; 7: 241300.

Marsh FH. Health care cost containment and the duty to treat. The Journal of Legal Medicine 1985; 6: 157–189.

Martinez B. Care guidelines used by insurers face scrutiny. Wall St J, September 14, 2000; B-1, B-4.

May WE. Consensus or coercion. JAMA 1985; 254: 1077.

Mayer T, Cates RJ. Service excellence in health care. JAMA 1999; 282: 1281–83.

McCoid AH. The care required of medical practitioners. Vanderbilt Law Review 1959; 12: 549–632.

McDonald RK. My practice almost destroyed me. Medical Economics 1996; 73(5): 181–87.

McGarvey MR. Tough choices: the cost-effectiveness of sildenafil. Annals of Internal Medicine 2000; 132: 267–290.

McGivney WT. Proposal for assuring technology competency and leadership in medicine. Journal of the National Cancer Institute 1992; 84: 742–44.

McGlynn EA, Naylor D, Anderson GM, Leape LL, Park RE, Hilborne LH, Bernstein SJ, Goldman BS, Armstrong PW, Keesey JW, McDonald L, Pinfold SP, Damberg C, Sherwood MJ, Brook RH. Comparison of the appropriateness of coronary angiography and coronary artery bypass graft surgery between Canada and New York State. JAMA 1994; 272: 934–940.

Mehlman MJ. Rationing expensive lifesaving medical treatments. Wisconsin Law Review 1985; 1985: 239–302.

Mehlman MJ. Fiduciary contracting: limitations on bargaining between patients and health care providers. University of Pittsburgh Law Review 1990; 51:365–417.

Mehlman MJ. The patient–physician relationship in an era of scarce resources: is there a duty to treat? Connecticut Law Review 1993; 25: 349–391.

Menken M. What improved my patient communications? Getting sued. Medical Economics 1992; 68(7): 54–56.

Menzel PT. Strong Medicine: The Ethical Rationing of Health Care. New York: Oxford University Press, 1990.

Merkatz RB, Temple R, Sobel S, et al. Women in clinical trials of new drugs. New Engl J Med 1993; 329: 292–296.

Meyer M, Murr A. Not my health care. Newsweek, Jan. 10, 1994; 123(2): 36–38.

Miller MG, Miller LS, Fireman B, Black SB. Variation in practice for discretionary admissions. JAMA 1994; 271: 1493–1498.

Miller RH. Competition in the health system: good news and bad news. Health Affairs 1996; 15(2): 107–20.

Miller TE. Managed care regulation: in the laboratory of the states. JAMA 1997; 278: 1102–1109.

Miller TE, Sage WM. Disclosing physician financial incentives. JAMA 1999; 281: 1424–1430.

Milliman & Robertson, Practice Guidelines: Quality Care in a Cost Efficient Manner (1994).

Mirvis DM, Chang CF, Hall CJ, Zaar GT, Applegate WB. TennCare—health system reform for Tennessee. JAMA 1995; 274: 1235–1241.

Mold JW, Stein HF. The cascade effect in the clinical care of patients. New Engl J Med 1986; 314: 512–514.

Monane L, Kanter DS, Glynn RJ, Avorn J. Variability in length of hospitalization for stroke. Arch Neurol 1996; 53: 875–880.

Morain C. When managed care takes over, watch out! Medical Economics 1995; 72(20): 38–47.

Morhane M, Matthias DM, Nagle BA, Kelly MA. Improving prescribing patterns for the elderly through an online drug utilization review intervention. JAMA 1998; 280: 1249–52.

Morlock LL, Malitz FE. Do hospital risk management programs make a difference?: relationships between risk management program activities and hospital malpractice claims experience. Law and Contemporary Problems 1991; 54 (2): 1–22.

Morreim EH. Stratified scarcity and unfair liability. Case Western Reserve Law Review 1985–86; 36(4): 1033–57.

Morreim EH. Cost containment and the standard of medical care. California Law Review 1987; 75(5): 1719–63.

Morreim EH. Stratified scarcity: Redefining the standard of care. Law, Medicine and Health Care 1989; 17(4): 356–367.

Morreim EH. The law of nature and the law of the land: of horses, zebras, and unicorns. The Pharos 1990; 53(2): 2–6.

Morreim EH. Balancing Act. Dordrecht: Kluwer Academic Publishers, 1991(a) (reprinted in paperback, Washington, DC: Georgetown University Press, 1995).

Morreim EH. Gaming the system: dodging the rules, ruling the dodgers. Arch Intern Med 1991(b); 151(3): 443–447.

Morreim EH. Economic disclosure and economic advocacy: New duties in the medical standard of care. Journal of Legal Medicine 1991(c); 12(3): 275–329.

Morreim EH. Rationing and the law. In: Strosberg MA, Wiener JM, Baker R, Fein IA, eds. Rationing America's Medical Care: The Oregon Plan and Beyond. Washington, D.C.: Brookings Institution, 1992(a), 159–184.

Morreim EH. Whodunit? causal liability of utilization review for physicians' decisions, patients' outcomes. Medicine and Health Care 1992(b); 20(1): 40–56.

Morreim EH. Profoundly diminished life: the casualties of coercion. Hastings Center Report 1993; 24(1): 33–42.

Morreim EH. Redefining quality by reassigning responsibility. American Journal of Law and Medicine 1994(a); 20: 79–104.

Morreim EH. Moral justice and legal justice in managed care: the ascent of contributive justice. Journal of Law, Medicine, and Ethics 1995(a); 23(3): 247–265.

Morreim EH. Diverse and perverse incentives in managed care; bringing the patient into alignment. Widener Law Symposium Journal 1995(b); 1(1): 89–139.

Morreim EH. Futilitarianism, exoticare, and coerced altruism: the ADA meets its limits. Seton Hall Law Review 1995(c); 25: 101–149.

Morreim EH. At the intersection of medicine, law, economics, and ethics: the art of intellectual cross-dressing. In: Carson RA, Burns CR, eds: Perspectives on Philosophy in Medicine. Philosophy and Medicine Series, vol. 50; Dordrecht: Kluwer Academic Publishers, 1997(a); 299–325.

Morreim EH. Medicine meets resource limits: Restructuring the legal standard of care. University of Pittsburgh Law Review 1997(b); 59(1): 1–95.

Morreim EH. Managed care, ethics, and academic health centers: maximizing potential, minimizing drawbacks. Academic Medicine 1997(c); 72(5): pp. 332–340.

Morreim EH. To tell the truth: disclosing the incentives and limits of managed care. American Journal of Managed Care 1997(d); 3(1): 35–43.

Morreim EH. Revenue streams and clinical discretion. Journal of the American Geriatrics Society 1998; 46(3): 331–337.

Morreim EH. Benefits decisions in ERISA plans: diminishing deference to fiduciaries, and an emerging problem for PSOs. Tennessee Law Review 1998(b); 65(2): 511–553.

Morreim EH. Playing doctor: corporate medical practice and medical malpractice. Michigan Journal of Law Reform 1999; 32(4): 939–1040.

Morreim EH. Saving lives, spending money: shepherding the role of technology. In: Wear S, Bono JJ, Logue G, McEvoy A, ed.; Ethical Issues in Health Care on the Frontiers of the Twenty-First Century. Philosophy and Medicine Series; Dordrecht: Kluwer Academic Publishers, 2000, 99. 63–110.

Morreim EH. Quality of life: erosions and opportunities under managed care. Journal of Law Medicine & Ethics 2000(b); 28: 144–158.

Morreim EH. Confusion in the courts: managed care financial structures and their impact on medical care. Tort & Insurance Law Journal 2000(c); 35(3): 699–728.

Morris AH. Developing and implementing computerized protocols for standardization of clinical decisions. Ann Intern Med 2000; 132: 373–383.

Mort TC, Yeston NS. The relationship of pre mortem diagnoses and post mortem findings in a surgical intensive care unit. Crit Care Med 1999; 27: 299–303.

Moser M. Why are physicians not prescribing diuretics more frequently in the management of hypertension? JAMA 1998; 279: 1813–16.

Muir DM. ERISA remedies: chimera or congressional compromise? Iowa Law Review 1995; 81: 1–53.

Murata SK. Here come big changes in your patients' insurance. Medical Economics 1996; 73(7): 185–190.

Natsch S, Kullberg BJ, Meis JFGM, van der Meer JW. Earlier initiation of antibiotic treatment for severe infections after interventions to improve the organization and specific guidelines in the emergency department. Arch Intern Med 2000; 160: 1317–1320.

Naylor CD. Better care and better outcomes: the continuing challenge. JAMA 1998; 279: 1392–94.

Nease RF, Kneeland T, O'Connor GT, Sumner W, et al. Variation in patient utilities for outcomes of the management of chronic stable angina: implications for clinical practice guidelines. JAMA 1995; 273: 1185–90.

Nelson AF, Quiter ES, Solberg LI. The state of research within managed care plans: 1997 survey. Health Affairs 1998; 17(1): 128–138.

Neuhauser D, Lewicki AM. What do we gain from the sixth stool guaiac? New Engl J Med 1975; 293: 226–228.

Neumann PJ, Zinner DE, Paltiel AD. The FDA and regulation of cost-effectiveness claims. Health Affairs 1996; 15(3): 54–71.

Newcomer LN. Physician, measure thyself. Health Affairs 1998; 17(4): 32–35.

Newcomer LN. Medicare pharmacy coverage: ensuring safety before funding. Health Affairs 2000; 19(2): 59–62.

Note. Rethinking medical malpractice law in light of medicare cost-cutting. Harvard Law Review 1985; 98: 1004–22.

Novack DH, Detering BJ, Arnold R, et al. Physicians' attitudes toward using deception to resolve difficult ethical problems. JAMA 1989; 261: 2980–2985.

Novak J. How we wrote our own managed-care success story. Medical Economics 1998; 75(15): 116–27.

Nuland SB. The hazards of hospitalization. Wall St J, December 2, 1999; A-22.

Nutting PA, Beasley JW, Werner JJ. Practice-based research networks answer primary care questions. JAMA 1999; 281: 686–88.

Nyquist A, Gonzales R, Steiner JF, Sande MA. Antibiotic prescribing for children with colds, upper respiratory tract infections, and bronchitis. JAMA 1998; 279: 875–877.

Oberfield SE. Growth hormone use in normal, short children—a plea for reason. New Engl J Med 1999; 340: 557–59.

Oberman L. Risk management strategy: liability insurers stress practice guidelines. Amer Med News September 5, 1994; 1, 42, 43.

O'Brien CL. Direct contracting: potential legal and regulatory barriers. Minnesota Medicine 1996; 79: 21–25.

O'Connell J. The interlocking death and rebirth of contract and tort. Michigan Law Review 1977; 75: 659–85.

O'Connell J. Neo-no-fault remedies for medical injuries: coordinated statutory and contractual alternatives. Law & Contemporary Problems 1986: 49: 125–141.

O'Connor GT, Quinton HB, Traven ND, Ramuno LD, Dodds TA, Marciniak TA, Wennberg JE. Geographic variation in the treatment of acute myocardial infraction: the cooperative cardiovascular project. JAMA 1999; 281: 627–633.

Obstbaum SA. Should rates of cataract surgery vary by insurance status? JAMA 1997; 277: 1807–08.

Ogrod ES. Compensation and quality: a physician's view. Health Affairs 1997; 16(3): 82–86.

Orentlicher D. Paying physicians more to do less: financial incentives to limit care. University of Richmond Law Review 1996; 30(1): 155–197.

Orentlicher D. Medical malpractice: treating the causes instead of the symptoms. Medical Care 2000; 38: 247–49.

Orient J. Your Doctor Is Not In: Healthy Skepticism about National Health Care. New York: Crown Publishers Inc. 1994.

Orlowski JP, Wateska L. The effect of pharmaceutical firm enticements on physician prescribing patterns. Chest 1992; 102(1):270–3.

Ortolon K. Coming in first. Texas Medicine 1997; 93(7): 26–30.

Overbay A, Hall MA. Insurance regulation of providers that bear risk. Am J Law & Med1996; 22: 361–387.

Overhage JM, Tierney WM, McDonald CJ. Computer reminders to implement perventive care guidelines for hospitalized patients. Arch Intern Med 1996; 156: 1551–1556.

Ozar DT. Profession and professional ethics. In: Reich WT, ed. Encyclopedia of Bioethics, vol 4. New York: MacMillan Library Reference, 1995, 2103–2112.

Page L. Lawsuit puts spotlight on hospital discharge criteria. Amer Med News, March 27, 2000; 1, 29, 35.

Parker J. Corporate practice of medicine: last stand or final downfall? J Health and Hosp Law 1996; 29(3): 160–73.

Pashos CL, Normand SLT, Garfinkle JB, et al. Trends in the use of drug therapies in patients with acute myocardial infarction: 1988 to 1992. J Am Coll Cardiol 1994; 23: 1023–30.

Pauly MV, Goodman JC. Tax credits for health insurance and medical savings accounts. Health Affairs 1995; 14(1): 126–39.

Pearson RN. The role of custom in medical malpractice cases. Indiana Law Journal 1976; 51: 528–57.

Pearson SD, Goulart-Fisher D, Lee TH. Critical pathways as a strategy for improving care: problems and potential. Ann Int Med 1995; 123: 941–48.

Pearson SD, Sabin JE, Emanuel EJ. Ethical guidelines for physician compensation based on capitation. New Engl J Med 1998; 339: 689–693.

Pellegrino E. Altruism, self-interest, and medical ethics. JAMA 1987; 258: 1939–1940.

Pellegrino E, Thomasma D. A Philosophical Basis of Medical Practice. New York: Oxford University Press, 1981.

Peregrine MW, Schwartz RJ. The business judgment rule and other protections for the conduct of not-for-profit directors. Journal of Health Law 2000; 33: 455–484.

Perry K. Where salaried practice feels like private practice. Medical Economics 1994; 71(17): 65–75.

Perry S, Thamer M. Medical innovation and the critical role of health technology assessment. JAMA 1999; 282: 1869–1872.

Peters PG. The quiet demise of deference to custom: malpractice law at the millenium. Washington and Lee Law Review 2000; 57: 163–205.

Peters WP, Rogers MC. Variation in approval by insurance companies of coverage for autologous bone marrow transplantation for breast cancer. New Engl J Med 1994; 330: 473–477.

Petersen SK. No-fault and enterprise liability: the view from Utah. Ann Intern Med 1995; 122: 462–463.

Philp T. When juries play doctor, verdicts can be bitter pills. Sacramento Bee, Nov. 9, 1998.

Pilote L, Califf RM, Sapp S, Miller DP, Mark DB, Weaver D, Gore JM, Armstrong PW, Ohman M, Topol EJ, for the GUSTO-1 Investigators. Regional variation across the United States in the management of acute myocardial infarction. New Engl J Med 1995; 333: 565–572.

Pincus CR. Where health care is headed now. Medical Economics 1995; 72(19): 33–41.

Pitsenberger WH. "An apparently irrational distinction": a suggestion for using equal protection arguments to overcome conflicts in ERISA preemption. Journal of Health Law 1999; 32: 307–338.

Pomfret SD. Emerging theories of liability for utilization review under ERISA health plans. Tort & Insurance Law Journal 1998; 34: 131–166.

Poses RM, Cebul RD, Witgon RS, et al. Controlled trial using computerized feedback to improve physicians' diagnostic judgments. Acad Med 1992; 67: 345–347.

Posner J. Trends in medical malpractice insurance, 1970–1985. Law and Contemporary Problems 1986; 49(2): 37–56.

Powe NR. Low- versus high-osmolality contrast media for intravenous use: a health care luxury or necessity? Radiology 1992; 183:21–22.

Power EJ. Identifying health technologies that work. JAMA 1995; 274: 205.

Pretzer M. Hate those Medicare denials? try moving. Medical Economics 1995; 72(7): 92–101.

Quinn JL. Physician collective bargaining: all eyes are on Texas. Journal of Health Law 2000; 33: 141–155.

Rai AK. Reflective choice in health care: using information technology to present allocation options. Am J Law & Med 1999; 25: 387–402.

Ransohoff DF, Harris RP. Lessons from the mammography screening controversy: can we improve the debate? Ann Intern Med 1997; 127: 1029–1034.

Rapoport J, Teres D, Steingrub J, Higgins T, McGee W, Lemeshow S. Patient characteristics and ICU organizational factors that influence frequency of pulmonary artery catheterization. JAMA 2000; 283: 2559–67.

Raschke RA, Gollihare B, Wunderlich TA et al. A computer alert system to prevent injury from adverse drug events. JAMA 1998; 280: 1317–20.

Ray WA. Policy and program analysis using administrative data banks. Ann Intern Med 1997; 127: 712–18.

Reinhardt UE. American values: are they blocking health-system reform? Medical Economics 1992(a); 69(21): 126–148.

Reinhardt UE. You pay when business bankrolls health care. Wall St J, Dec 2, 1992(b); A-14.

Reinhardt UE. Employer-based health insurance: a balance sheet. Health Affairs 1999; 18(6): 124–132.

Reiser SJ. Criteria for standard versus experimental therapy. Health Affairs 1994; 13(3): 127–136.

Rennie D. Thyroid storm. JAMA 1997; 277: 1238–43.

Report to the Board of Trustees, AMA. Direct contracting with employers: a strategy to increase physician involvement in the current health care market. Board of Trustees Report 27–A-95, 1995.

Retchin SM, Brown RS, Yeh SCJ, Chu D, Moreno L. Outcomes of stroke patients in Medicare fee for service and managed care. JAMA 1997; 278: 119–124.

Retchin SM, Penberthy L, Desch C, Brown R, Jerome-D'Emilia B, Clement D. Perioperative management of colon cancer under Medicare risk programs. Arch Intern Med 1997; 157: 1878–84.

Reuben DB. Learning diagnostic restraint. New Engl J Med 1984; 310: 591–593.

Reynolds RA, Rizzo JA, Gonzalez ML. The cost of medical professional liability. JAMA 1987; 257: 2776–2781.

Rice B. Where doctors get sued the most. Medical Economics 1995; 72(4): 98–100, 103–104, 107–110.

Rice B. Look who's on the malpractice hot seat now. Medical Economics 1996; 73(15): 193–205.

Riley GF, Potosky AL, Klabunde CN, Warren JL, Ballard-Barbash R. Stage at diagnosis and treatment patterns among older women with breast cancer: an HMO and fee-for-service comparison. JAMA 1999; 281: 720–26.

Robinson GO. Rethinking the allocation of medical malpractice risks between patients and providers. Law & Contemporary Problems 1986(a): 49: 173–199.

Robinson GO. The medical malpractice crisis of the 1970s: a retrospective. Law and Contemporary Problems 1986; 49(2): 5–35.

Robinson JC. Health care purchasing and market changes in California. Health Affairs 1995; 14(4):117–130.

Robinson JC. Blended payment methods in physician organizations under managed care. JAMA 1999; 282: 1258–63.

Robinson JC, Casalino LP. The growth of medical groups paid through capitation in California. New Engl J Med 1995; 333: 1684–87.

Robinson JC, Casalino LP. Vertical integration and organizational networks in health care. Health Affairs 1996; 15(1): 7–22.

Rodwin MA. Patient accountability and quality of care: lessons from medical consumerism and the patients' rights, women's health and disability rights movements. Am J Law & Med 1994; 20: 147–167.

Rodwin MA. Strains in the fiduciary metaphor: divided physician loyalties and obligations in a changing health care system. Am J Law & Med 1995; 21: 241–257.

Rodwin MA. Managed care and consumer protection: what are the issues? Seton Hall Law Review 1996; 26: 1007–54.

Roe BB. The UCR boondoggle: a death knell for private practice? New Engl J Med 1981; 305: 41–45.

Roemer J. Fighting back: how labor unions are helping physicians regain some of their lost power. Hippocrates 1998; 12(4): 50–52, 54–55, 59.

Rose S. Are we overtreating children with growth hormone? Endocrinologist 1995; 5: 113–17.

Rosenbaum S, Frankford DM, Moore B, Borzi P. Who should determine when health care is medically necessary? New Engl J Med 1999; 340: 229–32.

Rosenberg S, Allen DR, Handte JS, Jackson TC, Leto L, Rodstein BM, Stratton SC, Westfall G, Yasser R. Effect of utilization review in a fee-for-service health insurance plan. New Engl J Med 1995; 333: 1326–30.

Rosoff AJ. The business of medicine: problems with the corporate practice doctrine. Cumberland Law Review 1987; 17: 485–503.

Rosoff AJ. The role of clinical practice guidelines in health care reform. Health Matrix 1995; 5: 369–96.

Ross JW. Practice guidelines: texts in search of authority. In: Boyle PH, ed. Getting Doctors to Listen: Ethics and Outcomes Data in Context. Washington, DC: Georgetown University Press, 1998, pp. 41–70.

Rossbacher HH, Cahill JS, Griffis LL. ERISA's dark side: retiree health benefits, false employer promises and the protective judiciary. DePaul Business Law Journal 1997; 9: 305–348.

Rost K, Smith R, Matthews DB, Guise B. The deliberate misdiagnosis of major depression in primary care. Archives of Family Medicine 1994; 333–337.

Rouco R. Available remedies under ERISA section 502(a). Alabama Law Review 1994; 45: 631–673.

Rowlings PA, Williams SP, Antman KH, et al. Factors correlated with progression-free survival after high-dose chemotherapy and hematopoietic stem cell transplantation for metastatic breast cancer. JAMA 1999; 282: 1335–43.

Russell PS, Kaplan LJ. The American Academy of Dermatology's response to managed care and capitation. Arch Dermatol 1996; 132: 1125–1127.

Sabin JE, Daniels N. Determining 'medical necessity' in mental health practice. Hastings Center Report 1994; 24(6): 5–13.

Sage WM. "Health Law 2000": the legal system and the changing health care market. Health Affairs 1996; 15(3): 9–27.

Sage WM. Enterprise liability and the emerging managed health care system. Law and Contemporary Problems 1997; 60 (1&2): 159–210.

Sage WM. Regulating through information: disclosure laws and American health care. Columbia Law Review 1999; 99: 1701–1829.

Sage WM, Hastings KE, Berenson RA. Enterprise liability for medical malpractice and health care quality improvement. Am J Law & Medicine 1994; 20: 1–28.

Sage WM, Jorling JM. A world that won't stand still: enterprise liability by private contract. DePaul Law Review 1994; 43: 1007–1043.

Salem-Schatz S, Moore G, Rucker M, Pearson SD. The case for case-mix adjustment in practice profiling: when good apples look bad. JAMA 1994; 272: 871–874.

Salzmann P, Kerlikowske K, Phillips K. Cost-effectiveness of extending screening mammography guidelines to include women 40 to 49 years of age. Ann Intern Med 1997; 127: 955–965.

Samsa GP, Matchar DB, Goldstein LB et al. Quality of anticoagulation management among patients with atrial fibrillation. Arch Intern Med 2000; 160: 967–973.

Schaber GD, Rohwer CD. Contracts, 2nd ed. St. Paul: West Publishing Co., 1984.

Schauffler HH, Brown C, Milstein A. Raising the bar: the use of performance guarantees by the Pacific Business Group on Health. Health Affairs 1999; 18(2): 134–142.

Schauffler HH, Rodriguez T. Exercising purchasing power for preventive care. Health Affairs 1996; 15(1): 73–85.

Scheetz A. Access to hospice care. J Am Geriatrics Society 1995; 43: 1174.

Schreter RK. Ten trends in managed care and their impact on the biopsychosocial model. Hospital and Community Psychiatry 1993; 44: 325–27.

Schroeder SA. The legacy of SUPPORT. Ann Intern Med 1999; 131: 780–81.

Schroeder SA, Cantor JC. On squeezing balloons: cost control fails again. New Engl J Med 1991; 325: 1099–1100.

Schuck PH. Malpractice liability and the rationing of care. In: President's Commission for the Study of Ethical Problems in Medicine and Biomedical and Behavioral Research, Securing Access to Health Care, vol. 3, pp. 413–418; Washington D.C.: U.S. Government Printing Office, 1983.

Schuster MA, McGlynn EA, Brook RH. How good is the quality of health care in the United States? Milbank Quarterly 1998; 74: 517–63.

Schwartz B, Mainous AG, Marcy SM. Why do physicians prescribe antibiotics for children with upper respiratory tract infections? JAMA 1998; 279: 881–82.

Schwartz JS. The role of professional medical societies in reducing practice variations. Health Affairs 1984; 3(2): 90–101.

Schwartz RK, Soumerai SB, Avorn J. Physician motivations for nonscientific drug prescribing. Soc Sci Med 1989; 28(6): 577–582.

Schwartz WB, Komesar NK. Doctors, damages and deterrence. New Engl J Med 1978; 298: 1282–1289.

Shah SR. Loosening ERISA's preemptive grip on HMO medical malpractice claims: a response to *PacifiCare of Oklahoma* v. *Burrage*. Minnesota Law Review 1996; 80: 1545–1577.

Shaneyfelt TM, Mayo-Smith MF, Rothwangl J. Are guidelines following guidelines? the methodological quality of clinical practice guidelines in the peer-reviewed medical literature. JAMA 1999; 281: 1900–05.

Shapiro MF, Wenger NS. Rethinking utilization review. New Engl J Med 1995; 333: 1353–54.

Shapiro RS, Simpson DE, Lawrence SL, Talsky AM, Sobocinski KA, Schiedermayer DL. A survey of sued and nonsued physicians and suing patients. Arch Intern Med 1989; 149: 2190–2196.

Shekelle PG, Kahan JP, Bernstein SJ, et al. The reproducibility of a method to identify the overuse and underuse of medical procedures. New Engl J Med 1998; 338: 1888–95.

Shewry S, Hunt S, Ramey J, Bertko J. Risk adjustment: the missing piece of market competition. Health Affairs 1996; 15(1): 171–181.

Shuman E. Expertise in law, medicine, and health care. Journal of Health Policy, Politics, & Law 2001; 26: 267–290.

Siliciano JA. Wealth, equity and the unitary medical malpractice standard. Virginia Law Review 1991; 77:439–487.

Slomski AJ. How business is flattening health costs. Medical Economics 1994; 71(13): 87–100.

Slomski AJ. How doctors cope in the land of 10,000 mergers. Medical Economics 1995; 72(13): 194–210.

Slomski AJ. Here they come: price-conscious patients. Medical Economics 1996; 73(8): 40–46.

Smith KJ, Roberts MS. The cost-effectiveness of sildenafil. Annals of Internal Medicine 2000; 132: 933–937.

Sommers PA. Malpractice risk and patient relations. J Family Practice 1985; 20(3): 299–301.

Soumerai SB, Avorn J. Principles of educational outreach (academic detailing) to improve clinical decision making. JAMA 1990; 263: 549–556.

Soumerai SB, McLaughlin TJ, Gurwitz JH, et al. Effect of local medical opinion leaders on quality of care for acute myocardial infarction: a randomized controlled trial. JAMA 1998; 279: 1358–63.

Soumerai SB, McLaughlin TJ, Ross-Degnan D, Caswteris CS, Bollini P. Effects of limiting Medicaid drug-reimbursement benefits on the use of psychotropic agents and acute mental health services by patients with schizophrenia. New Engl J Med 1994; 331: 650–55.

Soumerai SB, Ross-Degnan D, Avorn J, McLaughlin TJ, ChoodnovskiyI. Effects of Medicaid drug-payment limits on admission to hospitals and nursing homes. New Engl J Med 1991; 325: 1072–77.

Soumerai SB, Ross-Degnan D, Fortess EE, Abelson J. A critical analysis of studies of state drug reimbursement policies: research in need of discipline. Milbank Quarterly 1993; 7(2): 217–52.

Sox HC, Woolf SH. Evidence-based practice guidelines from the US Preventive Services Task Force. JAMA 1993; 269: 2678.

Stadtmauer EA, O'Neill A, Goldstein LJ, et al. Conventional-dose chemotherapy compared with high-dose chemotherapy plus autologous hematopoietic stem-cell transplantation for metastatic breast cancer. New Engl J Med 2000; 342: 1069–1076.

Starr P. The Social Transformation of American Medicine. New York: Basic Books Inc, 1982.

Steinberg EP, Moore RD, Powe NR, et al. Safety and cost effectiveness of high-osmolality as compared with low-osmolality contrast material in patients undergoing cardiac angiography. New Engl J Med 1992; 326:425–430.

Steinberg EP, Tunis S, Shapiro D. Insurance coverage for experimental technologies. Health Affairs 1995; 14(4): 143–58.

Stelfox HT, Chua G, O'Rourke K, Detsky AS. Conflict of interest in the debate over calcium-channel antagonists. New Engl J Med 1998; 338: 101–6.

Stern JB. Bad faith suits: are they applicable to health maintenance organizations? West Virginia Law Review 1983; 85: 911–928.

Stern RS. Managed care and the treatment of skin diseases. Arch Dermatol 1996; 132: 1039–1042.

Stevens C. Guidelines spread, but how much impact will they have? Medical Economics 1993; 70(13): 66–89.

Stone AA. Law's influence on medicine and medical ethics. New Engl J Med 1985; 312: 309–312.

Streja DA, Hui RL, Streja E, McCombs JS. Selective contracting and patient outcomes: a case study of formulary restrictions for selective serotonin reuptake inhibitor antidepressants. Am J Managed Care 1999; 5: 1133–42.

Stross JK. Guidelines have their limits. Ann Intern Med 1999; 131: 304–306.

Studdert DM, Brennan TA. The problems with punitive damages in lawsuits against managed-care organizations. New Engl J Med 2000; 342: 280–84.

Studdert DM, Sage WM, Gresenz CR, Hensler DR. Expanded managed care liability: what impact on employer coverage? Health Affairs 1999; 18(6): 7–27.

Studdert DM, Thomas EJ, Burstin HR, Zbar Bi, Orav EJ, Brennan TA. Negligent care and malpractice claiming behavior in Utah and Colorado. Medical Care 2000; 38: 250–260.

Suchman Al, Eiser A, Goold SD, Stewart KJ. Rationale, principles, and educational approaches of organizational transformation. Journal of General Internal Medicine 1999; 14(S-1): S51–57.

Sugarman PR, Yarasbus VA. Admissibility of managed care financial incentives in medical malpractice cases. Tort & Insurance Law Journal 1999; 34(3): 735–760.

SUPPORT Principal Investigators. A controlled trial to improve care for seriously ill hospitalized patients: the Study to Understand Prognoses and Preferences for Outcomes and Risks of Treatments (SUPPORT). JAMA 1995; 274: 1591–1598.

Swisher PN. A realistic consensus approach to the insurance law doctrine of reasonable expectations. Tort & Insurance Law Journal 2000; 35: 729–779.

Tancredi L. Designing a no-fault alternative. Law & Contemporary Problems 1986: 49: 277–286.

Tannock IF. Treating the patient, not just the cancer. New Engl J Med 1987; 317: 1534–35.

Task Force on Principles for Economic Analysis of Health Care Technology. Economic analysis of health care technology: a report on principles. Ann Intern Med 1995; 122: 61–70.

Taubes G. The breast-screening brawl: controversy over regular mammogram screening for women in their forties. Science 1997; 275: 1056.

Terry K. Is this the best way to divide HMO income? Medical Economics 1994; 71(19): 26B-26F.

Terry K. Look who's guarding the gate to specialty care. Medical Economics 1994(b); 71(16): 124–32.

Terry K. Teaming up with employers against HMOs. Medical Economics 1995; 72(19): 54, 59–63, 68–72.

Terry K. Can functional-status surveys improve your care? Medical Economics 1996; 73(14): 126–44.

Terry K. Surprise! Capitation can be a boon. Medical Economics 1996(b); 73(7): 126–138.

Terry K. Look who's rating doctors on clinical quality—patients. Medical Economics 1998; 75(7): 50–51.

Terry NP. Cyber-malpractice: legal exposure for cybermedicine. Am J Law & Med 1999; 25: 327–66.

Theodos TF. The patients' bill of rights: women's rights under managed care and ERISA preemption. Am J Law & Med 2000; 26: 89–108.

Thurow LC. Learning to say "No". New Engl J Med 1984; 311: 1569–1572.

Thurow LC. Medicine versus economics. New Engl J Med 1985; 313: 611–614.

Tiano LV. The legal implications of HMO cost containment measures. Seton Hall Legislative Journal 1990; 14: 79–102.

Trauner JB, Chesnutt JS. Medical groups in California: managing care under capitation. Health Affairs 1996; 15(1): 159–70.

Trueman DL. Managed care liability today: laws, cases, theories, and current issues. Journal of Health Law 2000; 33: 191–262.

Truog RD, Brett AS, Frader J. The problem with futility. New Engl J Med 1992; 326: 1560–1564.

Tu JV, Naylor CD, Kumar D, DeBuono BA, McNeil BJ, Hannan EL, and the Steering Committee of the Cardiac Care Network of Ontario. Coronary artery bypass graft surgery in Ontario and New York state: which rate is right? Ann Intern Med 1997; 126: 13–19.

United States General Accounting Office, Medicare Part B: Inconsistent Denial Rates for Medical Necessity Across Six Carriers, GAO/T-PEMD-94-17, Mar. 1, 1994.

United States General Accounting Office, Medicare Part B: Regional Variation in Denial Rates for Medical Necessity, GAO/PEMD-95-10, Dec. 19, 1994.

Van de Werf F. Variations in patient management and outcomes for acute myocardial infarction in the United States and other countries. JAMA 1995; 273: 1586–1591.

Veatch RM. A Theory of Medical Ethics. New York: Basic Books, 1981.

Veatch RM. Why physicians cannot determine if care is futile. J Am Geriatr Soc 1994; 42: 871–874.

Veatch RM, Spicer CM. Medically futile care: the rule of the physician in setting limits. Am J Law & Med 1992; 18: 15–36.

Wadlington W. Legal responses to patient injury: a future agenda for research and reform. Law and Contemporary Problems 1991; 54 (2): 199–223.

Wadlington W, Waltz J, Dworkin R. Cases and Materials on Law and Medicine. Mineola, N.Y.: The Foundation Press, 1980.

Wang TJ, Stafford RS. National patterns and predictors of β-blocker use in patients with coronary artery disease. Arch Intern Med 1998; 158: 1901–1906.

Wasserstrom RA. Strict liability in the criminal law. In: Morris H, ed. Freedom and Responsibility. Stanford: Stanford University Press, 1961.

Weaver J. The best care other people's money can buy. Wall St J, Nov 19,1992; A-14.

Webster JR, Feinglass J. Stroke patients, "managed care," and distributive justice. JAMA 1997; 278: 161–62.

Weiler PC, Newhouse JP, Hiatt HH. Proposal for medical liability reform. JAMA 1992; 267: 2355–2358.

Weiner JP, deLissovoy G. Razing a tower of babel: a taxonomy for managed care and health insurance plans. Journal of Health Politics, Policy and Law 1993; 18(1): 75–103.

Weiner JP, Parente ST, Garnick DW, Fowles J, Lawthers AG, Palmer H. Variation in office-based quality: a claims-based profile of care provided to medicare patients with diabetes. JAMA 1995; 273: 1503–1508.

Weingarten SR. Using practice guideline compendiums to provide better preventive care. Ann Int Med 1999; 130: 454–58.

Weingarten SR, Riedinger MS, Hobson P et al. Evaluation of a pneumonia practice guideline in an interventional trial. Am J Respir Crit Care Med 1996; 153: 1110–1115.

Weiss RB, Rifkin RM, Stewart FM, et al. High-dose chemotherapy for high-risk primary breast cancer: an on-site review of the Bezwoda study. Lancet 2000; 355: 999–1003.

Welch HG, Miller ME, Welch WP. An analysis of inpatient practice patterns in Florida and Oregon. New Engl J Med 1994; 330: 607–612.

Welch WP, Miller ME, Welch HG, Fisher ES, Wennberg JE. Geographic variation in expenditures for physicians' services in the United States. New Engl J Med 1993; 328: 621–627.

Wells KB, Sherbourne C, Schoenbaum M, et al. Impact of disseminating quality improvement programs for depression in managed primary care. JAMA 2000; 283: 212–220.

Wells KB, Sturm R. Care for depression in a changing environment. Health Affairs 1995; 14(3): 78–89.

Wennberg JA. AHCPR and the strategy for health care reform. Health Affairs 1992(a); 11(4): 67–71.

Wennberg JE. Which rate is right? New Engl J Med 1986; 314: 310–311.

Wennberg JE. The paradox of appropriate care. JAMA 1987; 258: 2568–2569.

Wennberg JE. Outcomes research, cost containment, and the fear of rationing. New Engl J Med 1990; 323: 1202–1204.

Wennberg JE. Unwanted variations in the rule of practice. JAMA 1991; 265: 1306–1307.

Wennberg JE., ed. The Dartmouth Atlas of Health Care in the United States. Chicago: American Hospital Publishing: 1996.

Wennberg JE. Why treatment varies so greatly. Medical Economics 1997; 74(3): 40–56.

Wennberg JE. Understanding geographic variations in health care delivery. New Engl J Med 1999; 340: 52–53.

Wennberg JE, Freeman JL, Culp WJ. Are hospital services rationed in New Haven or overutilized in Boston? Lancet 1987; 1: 1185–1188.

Wennberg JE, Freeman JL, Shelton RM, Bubolz TA. Hospital use and mortality among Medicare beneficiaries in Boston and New Haven. New Engl J Med 1989; 321: 1168–1173.

Wennberg DE, Kellett MA, Dickens JD, Malenka DJ, Keilson LM, Keller RB. The association between local diagnostic testing intensity and invasive cardiac procedures. JAMA 1996; 275: 1161–1164.

Wethly FC. New York Conference of Blue Cross & Blue Shield Plans v. Travelers Insurance Co.: vicarious liability malpractice claims against managed care organizations escaping ERISA'S grasp. Boston College Law Review 1996; 37: 813–860.

Wetzell S. Consumer clout. Minnesota Medicine 1996; 79(2): 15–19.

White G. Tort Law in America. New York: Oxford University Press, 1980.

White LJ. Clinical uncertainty, medical futility and practice guidelines. J Am Geriatr Soc 1994; 42: 899–901.

White PH. Innovative no-fault tort reform for an endangered specialty. Virginia Law Review 1988; 74: 1487–1526.

Whyte HE, Fitzhardinge PM, Shennen AT, et al. Extreme immaturity: outcome of 568 pregnancies of 23–26 weeks' gestation. Obstetrics and Gyenecology 1993; 82: 1–7.

Wiehl JG, et al. Legal issues related to systems integration. In: Integrated Health Care Delivery Systems, Fine A, ed. New York: Thompson Publishing Group, 1993, pp. 9–38.

Williams PC. Abandoning medical malpractice. Journal of Legal Medicine 1984; 5: 549–94.

Wing KR. American health policy in the 1980's. Case Western Reserve Law Review 1986; 36: 608–685.

Winslow R. Studies show doctors underprescribe beta blockers for heart attack patients. Wall St J, August 19, 1998; B-5.

Wong ET, Lincoln TL. Ready! Fire! . . . Aim! JAMA 1983; 250: 2510–2513.

Wooley SC. Managed care and mental health: the silencing of a profession. International Journal of Eating Disorders 1993; 14: 387–401.

Woolf SH. Practice guidelines: a new reality in medicine: II. methods of developing guidelines. Arch Intern Med 1992; 152: 946–952.

Woolf SH. Practice guidelines: a new reality in medicine. III. impact on patient care. Arch Intern Med 1993(a); 153: 2646–2655.

Woolf SH, Lawrence RS. Preserving scientific debate and patient choice: lessons from the consensus panel on mammography screening. JAMA 1997; 278: 2105–2108.

Woolhandler S, Himmelstein DU. Extreme risk—the new corporate proposition for physicians. New Engl J Med 1995; 333: 1706–1708.

Woosley RL. Centers for education and research in therapeutics. Clin Pharmacol Ther 1994; 55: 249–55.

Wynia MK, Cummins DS, VanGeest JB, Wilson IB. Physician manipulation of reimbursement rules for patients: between a rock and a hard place. JAMA 2000; 283: 1858–1865.

Yacht AC. Collective bargaining is the right step. New Engl J Med 2000; 342: 429–31.

Younger PA, Conner C, Cartwright KK. Managed Care Law Manual. Gaithersburg, Md.: Aspen Publishers, 1994.

Zalta E. Utilization review works—most of the time. Medical Economics 1991; 68(13): 23–27.

Zito JM, Safer DJ, dosReis S, Gardner JF, Boles M, Lynch F. Trends in the prescribing of psychotropic medications to preschoolers. JAMA 2000; 283: 1025–30.

Zoloth-Dorfman L. Standing at the gate: managed care and daily ethical choices. Managed Care Medicine 1994; 1(6): 26–38.

Zoloth-Dorfman L, Rubin S. The patient as commodity: managed care and the question of ethics. Journal of Clinical Ethics 1995; 6: 339–57.

Zuckerman S. Medical malpractice: claims, legal costs, and the practice of defensive medicine. Health Affairs 1984; 3: 128–33.

TABLE OF CASES

INDEX